D1569719

CHRONIC OBSTRUCTIVE PULMONARY DISEASE
Current Concepts

JOHN E. HODGKIN, M.D.
Clinical Professor of Medicine, University of California, Davis
Medical Director, Center for Health Promotion and Rehabilitation
Medical Director, Respiratory Care and Pulmonary Rehabilitation
St. Helena Hospital, St. Helena, California

THOMAS L. PETTY, M.D.
Professor of Medicine and Director, Webb-Waring Lung Institute
University of Colorado Health Sciences Center, Denver, Colorado

1987
W. B. SAUNDERS COMPANY
Philadelphia / London / Toronto / Sydney / Tokyo / Hong Kong

W. B. Saunders Company: West Washington Square
Philadelphia, PA 19105

Library of Congress Cataloging in Publication Data

Hodgkin, John E. (John Elliott), 1939–

Chronic obstructive pulmonary disease.

1. Lungs—Diseases, Obstructive.   2. Chronic diseases.
  I. Petty, Thomas L., 1932–   .   II. Title. [DNLM: 1. Lung
Diseases, Obstructive. WF 600 H689c]

RC776.O3H63 1987   616.2′4   86–20425
ISBN 0–7216–1897–9

Editor: Dean Manke
Developmental Editor: David Kilmer
Designer: Bill Donnelly
Production Manager: Bill Preston
Manuscript Editor: David Prout
Illustration Coordinator: Walt Verbitski
Indexer: Ann Cassar

Chronic Obstructive Pulmonary Disease: Current Concepts   ISBN   0–7216–1897–9

Last digit is the print number: 9   8   7   6   5   4   3   2   1

Contributors

WILLIAM M. ANDERSON, M.D.
Assistant Professor of Medicine, Louisiana State University School of Medicine, and Director, Medical Intensive Care Unit, Veteran's Administration Hospital, Shreveport, Louisiana.

BEN V. BRANSCOMB, M.D., F.A.C.P., F.C.C.P.
Alabama Professor of Medicine in Emphysema and Respiratory Disease, Division of Pulmonary and Critical Care Medicine, University of Alabama School of Medicine, Birmingham, Alabama.

BENJAMIN BURROWS, M.D.
Professor of Internal Medicine and Director, Division of Respiratory Sciences, University of Arizona College of Medicine, Tucson, Arizona.

IAN A. CAMPBELL, B.Sc., M.D. (Lond.), F.R.C.P. (Edin.)
Consultant in Thoracic Medicine, Llandough and Sully Hospitals, Cardiff, United Kingdom.

REUBEN M. CHERNIACK, M.D.
Professor of Medicine, University of Colorado Health Sciences Center, and Director, Pulmonary Physiology Unit, National Jewish Center for Immunology and Respiratory Medicine, Denver, Colorado.

ALLEN B. COHEN, M.D., Ph.D.
Professor of Medicine and Executive Associate Director, University of Texas Health Center at Tyler, Tyler, Texas.

GERARD J. CRINER, M.D.
Assistant Professor of Medicine, University of Maryland Hospital, Baltimore, Maryland; Research Pulmonary Fellow, Pulmonary Center, Boston University School of Medicine, Boston, Massachusetts.

DONALD L. DUDLEY, M.D.
Clinical Professor, Neurological Surgery, University of Washington, and Medical Director, Washington Institute of Neurosciences, Seattle, Washington.

iii

CHARLES F. GEORGE, M.D., F.R.C.P.C.
Attending Physician, Department of Respiratory Medicine, St. Boniface General Hospital, Winnipeg, Manitoba.

RONALD B. GEORGE, M.D.
Professor of Medicine, Louisiana State University School of Medicine, Shreveport, Louisiana.

EDWARD M. GLASER, Ph.D.
President, Human Interaction Research Institute, Los Angeles, California; and Visiting Professor, Claremont Graduate School, Claremont, California.

JOHN E. HODGKIN, M.D.
Clinical Professor of Medicine, University of California, Davis; Medical Director, Center for Health Promotion and Rehabilitation, and Medical Director, Respiratory Care and Pulmonary Rehabilitation, St. Helena Hospital, St. Helena, California.

LEONARD D. HUDSON, M.D.
Professor of Medicine, and Head, Respiratory Disease Division, Department of Medicine, University of Washington, Seattle, Washington.

STEVEN IDELL, M.D., Ph.D.
Assistant Professor of Medicine, Director, Medical Intensive Care Unit, University of Texas Health Center at Tyler, Tyler, Texas.

HELENA B. JONES, M.D.
Senior Fellow, Respiratory Disease Division, Department of Medicine, University of Washington, Seattle, Washington.

RICHARD E. KANNER, M.D.
Associate Professor of Medicine; Division of Respiratory, Critical Care and Occupational Medicine; University of Utah School of Medicine; Salt Lake City, Utah.

MEIR H. KRYGER, M.D., F.R.C.P.C.
Associate Professor, University of Manitoba, and Medical Director, Sleep Laboratory, St. Boniface General Hospital, Winnipeg, Manitoba

BARRY J. MAKE, M.D.
Associate Professor of Medicine, Pulmonary Center, Boston University School of Medicine, and Director, Respiratory Care Center, The University Hospital at the Boston University School of Medicine, Boston, Massachusetts.

WILLIAM F. MILLER, M.D.
Professor of Internal Medicine, The University of Texas Health Science Center at Dallas, Southwestern Medical School, Dallas, Texas.

THOMAS L. PETTY, M.D.
Professor of Medicine, and Director, Webb-Waring Lung Institute, University of Colorado Health Sciences Center, Denver, Colorado.

MITCHELL L. RHODES, M.D.
Associate Dean of Graduate Medical Education and Professor of Medicine, University of Health Sciences, The Chicago Medical School, North Chicago, Illinois.

PAUL A. SELECKY, M.D.
Clinical Associate Professor of Medicine, UCLA School of Medicine, Los Angeles, California; and Medical Director, Pulmonary Department, Hoag Memorial Hospital Presbyterian, Newport Beach, California.

DOROTHY L. SEXTON, Ed.D., R.N.
Associate Professor and Chairperson, Medical-Surgical Nursing Program, Yale University School of Nursing, New Haven, Connecticut.

IRWIN ZIMENT, M.D.
Professor of Medicine, UCLA School of Medicine, Los Angeles, California; and Chief of Medicine, Olive View Medical Center, Sylmar, California.

Foreword

The roots of this book can be traced to the 1950s. At that time, a relatively small number of chest physicians in the United States recognized that patients suffering from chronic obstructive pulmonary disease (COPD) could be treated most effectively for their emphysema, chronic bronchitis, or bronchial asthma through a systematized, comprehensive pulmonary rehabilitation program, rather than focusing only on providing relief for their airways obstruction problems.

In 1967, a research grant from the Social and Rehabilitation Service (SRS) of the Department of Health, Education, and Welfare enabled the Human Interaction Research Institute (HIRI), located in Los Angeles, to undertake a national survey of current practices with regard to the diagnosis, treatment, and rehabilitation of COPD patients. When the survey results became available, HIRI followed through under an SRS research grant (No. RD-2571-G-67) by arranging a multidisciplinary conference of persons engaged in the study and treatment of patients with COPD. The conferees included chest physicians, internists, pulmonary physiologists, an allergy-immunology specialist, respiratory nurse specialists, physiatrists, physical therapists, a psychiatrist, a psychologist, and vocational rehabilitation counselors. The proceedings from that conference were published in 1968 under the title *A Pilot Study to Determine the Feasibility of Promoting the Use of a Systematized Care Program for Patients with Chronic Obstructive Pulmonary Disease*. The lively discussion and conclusions/recommendations from this conference constituted a kind of state-of-the-art document.

The above study was carried forward from 1973 to 1978 under a National Science Foundation (NSF) grant (No. DAR73-07767-A06) entitled "Strategies for Facilitating Knowledge Utilization in the Biomedical Field." NSF's interest was not in COPD per se, but rather in learning more about how to most effectively facilitate the dissemination and utilization of a very promising development in medical technology. Under that grant, the 11-person project team (Oscar Balchum, Ben Branscomb, Donald Dudley, Edward Glaser, Albert Haas, John Hodgkin, Irving Kass, Philip Kimbel, William Miller, Thomas Petty, and Barry Shaw) coauthored a state-of-the-art paper in *JAMA* (1975), which was subsequently expanded into a monograph, *Chronic Obstructive Pulmonary Disease: Current Concepts in Diagnosis and Comprehensive Care*, edited by Dr. Hodgkin and published in 1979 by the American

College of Chest Physicians (ACCP). This, in turn, was followed by three papers in *Chest* (1980) entitled "Psychological Concomitants to Rehabilitation in Chronic Obstructive Pulmonary Disease, Part I: Psychosocial and Psychological Considerations," "Part II: Psychosocial Treatment," and "Part III: Dealing with Psychiatric Disease," by D. Dudley, E. Glaser, B. Jorgenson, and D. Logan. The final product from this study was a paper Glaser published in the *Journal of Applied Behavioral Science* (1980) describing in detail the procedure for developing these state-of-the-art documents, entitled "Using Behavioral Science Strategies for Defining the State-of-the-Art." Two members of the project research team that developed the *JAMA* article and ACCP documents have gone on to further update the state-of-the-art: Dr. Hodgkin as primary editor of *Pulmonary Rehabilitation: Guidelines to Success* (Butterworth, 1984), and Dr. Petty as editor of *Chronic Obstructive Pulmonary Disease,* 2nd edition (Marcel Dekker, 1985).

Departing now from the above historical "root tracings", it seems that adaptation here of the following portion from the preface of the ACCP monograph would still be timely, accurate, and relevant:

> This document is written primarily for the physicians who are most likely to see the majority of pulmonary disease patients: those in family practice, internal medicine, allergy-immunology, and chest medicine. Since different individuals have differing degrees of familiarity with the subject matter, some may find certain material to be well known, while others may feel that the information in certain sections may be beyond their resources to carry out in a busy private practice situation. We have tried to keep the nonresearch setting in mind; that is, to synthesize a consensus of available knowledge and "best practice" with regard to diagnosis and treatment of COPD in almost any medical setting. In addition, we hope that portions of the monograph will also be useful to respiratory nurses, respiratory therapists, physical therapists, occupational therapists, social workers, psychologists, vocational counselors, and dietitians.
>
> The two principal objectives of a comprehensive respiratory care program are to: (1) control and alleviate as much as possible the symptoms of respiratory impairment, and (2) teach the patient how to achieve optimal capability for carrying out his/her activities of daily living. There is evidence that patients treated by a systematized care program of the type summarized herein are likely to remain functional for longer periods of time and become better able to cope with the demands of their daily living.
>
> The focus of this state-of-the-art communication on diagnosis and systematized care of patients suffering from emphysema, chronic bronchitis, and asthma is on the individual and his particular situation, not just on the manifestations of the disease. It includes concern for the patient's life or living situation and personality. Thus, systematized care involves not only selection of the most appropriate medications for treating airway obstruction, but also bronchial hygiene, chest physical therapy, rehabilitation medicine, consideration of metabolic and nutritional factors, and patient and family education.

It would be fitting now to continue with a quotation from Dr. Petty's Foreword to Dr. Hodgkin's *Pulmonary Rehabilitation: Guidelines to Success:*

> Those who understand pulmonary rehabilitation recognize that we do not treat emphysema, rather we treat patients with emphysema. Thus the fully

integrated approach presented in this text is ideally designed to explain and inform, and, in fact, to inspire those who wish to serve the dyspneic patient better than ever before.

Much of what we do in medicine aims to prevent premature morbidity and mortality. Rehabilitative techniques accomplish this and, in fact, it would be best if this preventive approach would begin even before disabling symptoms occur. This could be accomplished today in the office of every primary care physician by careful patient assessment and by simple measurements of lung function.

Finally, from the Preface to Dr. Hodgkin's 1984 book:

There is no better area than pulmonary rehabilitation to demonstrate the value of team care. Patients with respiratory disorders can benefit from the talents of many health care disciplines in both the assessment of the individual and the development of a treatment plan.

It was this recognition of the importance of multiple disciplines in evaluating and caring for patients with pulmonary disease that led us to develop this book.

In this book, *Chronic Obstructive Pulmonary Disease: Current Concepts,* Dr. Hodgkin and Dr. Petty along with a distinguished group of contributing authors have updated the approach to diagnosis and treatment of COPD. This state-of-the-art book should be of immense practical value to health care professionals who treat these individuals with chronic respiratory impairment.

EDWARD M. GLASER, PH.D.
President
Human Interaction Research Institute
Los Angeles, California

Preface

The number of individuals with Chronic Obstructive Pulmonary Disease (COPD) has increased markedly over the last decade. Fortunately, there has been a corresponding increase in knowledge regarding the treatment of obstructive airways disease during this same period.

The Human Interaction Research Institute under the direction of Edward M. Glaser, Ph.D., has been interested in expanding the knowledge base of physicians and allied health professionals as to the best way to diagnose and treat COPD patients since the late 1960s. In the Foreword of this book, Dr. Glaser describes the process by which *Chronic Obstructive Pulmonary Disease: Current Concepts in Diagnosis and Comprehensive Care*, edited by John E. Hodgkin and published by the American College of Chest Physicians in 1979, was developed. This current book reflects our desire to provide a state-of-the-art discussion regarding the diagnosis and treatment of COPD, incorporating new information that has become available since the ACCP book was published.

In addition to covering the usual approach to diagnosis and treatment of COPD, there are special chapters dealing with such things as smoking cessation, relaxation techniques and biofeedback, exercise training, sleep disturbances, sexuality, preoperative evaluation, and home care. A chapter on pulmonary rehabilitation emphasizes the important role of allied health professionals in assessing patients with COPD and aiding the physician in the development of an appropriate treatment program. Recognizing the important ethical and moral questions raised when dealing with those patients who are severely impaired, a chapter dealing with the final stages of disease has been included. The final chapter in the book discusses issues deserving further investigation.

We wish to thank our authors for their willingness to contribute to our book. Their expertise has allowed us to present this update on current concepts relating to the evaluation and care of patients with COPD. We also want to express our thanks to Carol Lewis and Jeanne Cleary, who assisted with the clerical challenges of typing chapters and corrresponding with the multiple authors, and to Dean Manke and David Prout of Saunders, who assisted with the development of the book.

Finally, we would like to acknowledge the many contributions made to the field of pulmonary medicine by our colleague Irving Kass, M.D., who was an integral member of the team that developed the book on COPD published by ACCP in 1979. Dr. Kass, who died on August 28, 1984, helped to pioneer the important role of pulmonary rehabilitation programs in enhancing the quality of life of individuals with chronic obstructive pulmonary disease.

JOHN E. HODGKIN, M.D.
THOMAS L. PETTY, M.D.

Contents

xiii

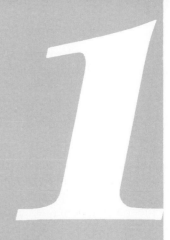

DEFINITIONS AND EPIDEMIOLOGY OF COPD

THOMAS L. PETTY
JOHN E. HODGKIN

This chapter presents our view of the contemporary definition of chronic obstructive pulmonary disease (COPD) along with a brief summary of the epidemiology.

DEFINITIONS

More than 20 years ago, an attempt to define the clinical condition of chronic airflow obstruction caused by loss of or damage to alveolar walls and inflammation of the conducting airways resulted in an official statement by the American Thoracic Society.[1] *Chronic bronchitis* was defined in clinical terms of chronic cough and expectoration when other specific causes of cough, e.g., tuberculosis or tumor, could be excluded. *Emphysema* was defined in pathologic terms of enlargement or destruction of alveolar units. Neither definition considered progressive airflow obstruction (or limitation) as a fundamental feature of this clinical or pathologic state. A restatement of these original definitions was made at the 1965 Aspen Emphysema Conference.[2]

The problem with these early definitions is that many patients with cough and expectoration have normal airflow, as emphasized by Bates and colleagues.[3] While this symptom complex is a major nuisance, those patients with normal airflow do not have premature morbidity and mortality as do individuals with the same symptom complex *plus* airflow obstruction as judged by simple measures, such as the forced expiratory volume in one second (FEV₁). Also, lungs from patients with extensive emphysema at postmortem examination often revealed no morphologic basis for airflow obstruction, i.e., no compromise of the internal diameters of the conducting airways.[4, 5] Most importantly, a pathologic definition for an important clinical state was not of much use to clinicians, and the accuracy of death certificates in identifying emphysema proved to be poor.[5]

More recent longitudinal studies strongly suggest that two parallel processes are responsible for cough, expectoration, and dyspnea on exertion.[6] One—mucosal inflammation—causes cough and excessive mucus formation, and the other—alveolar damage—is related to reduced airflow. Both inflammatory narrowing of airways (bronchitis and bronchiolitis) and reduced recoil could limit airflow.[7, 8] This concept, however, was first suggested by Laennec in his famous 1835 treatise on diseases of the chest. Over 150 years ago, he wrote:

> In emphysema, the air makes its escape from the air cells much slower than in a healthy state of the organ. This seems to indicate either more difficult communication between air contained in the air cells and that of the bronchi or else diminished elasticity of the air cells themselves. *Perhaps both these causes conspire to produce the effect in question* [italics added].

What a marvelous insight! Today, we recognize the origins of airflow from fully inflated lungs. Figure 1–1 presents these basic concepts that define the mechanisms of airflow and the reasons for airflow limitation or obstruction. A reduced elastic recoil (from damage to the alveolar tissue) or compromise of the conducting air passages may limit airflow.

As careful clinical studies with serial physiologic measurements demonstrate, measurements of airflow are extremely important as disease indicators and for estimates of prognosis.[9] Structure-function correlations of lungs derived from postmortem examination added to our knowledge of the basic disease state.[10]

The site of airflow obstruction is believed to begin in the small airways, based on studies that identified the anatomic location of airflow abnormalities.[11] This work supported the earlier notion that bronchiolitis was an essential step in the pathogenesis of the disease states termed chronic bronchitis and emphysema.[12]

The revelation that many patients with mild, and thus presumably early, abnormalities of airflow also demonstrated bronchial hyperreactivity added another complicating factor.[13] Responsiveness to bronchodilators and to bronchoconstrictive pharmacologic agents such as methylcholine was previously conceptually reserved for another group of airway disorders loosely referred to as bronchial asthma. Newer concepts concerning the basic nature of bronchial hyperreactivity and the various factors in bronchoprovocation (other than allergic agents) have expanded our views concerning asthma. Clearly, patients with intermittent acute episodes of wheezing and dyspnea and reversible airflow obstruction could be classified as asthmatic, but those with dyspnea on exertion, chronic cough, wheezing, expectoration, and irreversible airflow abnormalities could not be so easily segregated.

Although everyone who reads this book may not agree, the following pragmatic definitions and concepts, which were first presented in another monograph,[14] are of potential use to the clinician.

COPD* is an all-inclusive and nonspecific term referring to the condition in patients who have chronic cough and expectoration and various degrees of exertional dyspnea as well as a significant and progressive reduction in expiratory airflow, as measured by the forced expiratory volume in one second (FEV_1). This airflow abnormality *does not* show major reversibility in response to pharmacologic agents. Hyperinflation and a reduced diffusing capacity may be present. Both inflammatory damage to airways (bronchitis) and alveoli (emphysema) are present at postmortem examination. Terms such as chronic obstructive airways disease (COAD), chronic obstructive lung disease (COLD), chronic airflow (or airways) obstruction (CAO), and chronic airflow limitation (CAL) all mean the same thing.

Chronic Obstructive Bronchitis refers to patients with cough and expectoration along with a reduced FEV_1 that does not improve significantly following bronchodilator inhalation. Simple chronic cough and expectoration

---

*The first use of this term was apparently in Briscoe WA, Nash ES: The slow space in chronic obstructive pulmonary disease. *Annals of the New York Academy of Sciences* 1965;121: 706–722.

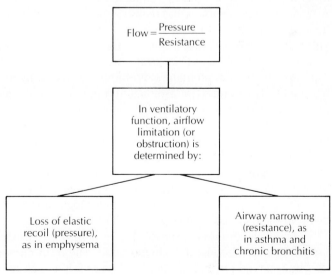

Figure 1–1. Mechanisms of airflow and causes of airflow limitation.

with normal airflow is *not included* in this definition. Simple chronic bronchitis with no airflow obstruction has a good prognosis, meaning there is not the same social and economic impact to patients, their families, or society. Chronic obstructive bronchitis is distinguished from asthmatic bronchitis (see below) only by the degree of reversibility in response to pharmacologic agents. Patients with chronic obstructive bronchitis do not have physiologic or roentgenographic evidence of hyperinflation. Diffusion tests are normal or near-normal.

Emphysema. This term refers to patients who have various degrees of dyspnea on exertion and irreversible airflow abnormalities as measured by FEV_1. In addition, these patients *also* demonstrate abnormalities at the air/blood interface as judged by carbon monoxide uptake tests (diffusion tests) and hyperinflation (judged clinically by physical examination, size of lungs on x-ray films, and measurements of total lung capacity).

Participants at a 1984 National Heart, Lung, and Blood Institute, Division of Lung Diseases Workshop, retained the American Thoracic Society's definition of emphysema,[1] but with the qualification that obvious fibrosis should be absent.

> Emphysema is defined as a condition of the lung characterized by abnormal, permanent enlargement of airspaces distal to the terminal bronchiole, accompanied by the destruction of their walls, and without obvious fibrosis.[15]

Chronic bronchitis and emphysema, of course, often coexist. Most clinicians will thus continue to use the COPD designation for this reason.

Asthmatic Bronchitis. Many patients with a productive cough and exertional dyspnea also have a significant reversibility in response to inhaled beta agonists, methylxanthines, and corticosteroids (either used alone or in combination). Population studies conducted by Ben Burrows of the University of Arizona have also shown that many of these patients have increased levels of IgE, which suggests that an immune reaction is sometimes involved in the pathogenesis of bronchial asthma. Progressive airflow obstruction, as judged by accelerated losses in FEV_1 over time, occur in longitudinal studies, and it is almost certain that premature morbidity and mortality results from asthmatic bronchitis. The concept of asthmatic bronchitis as a clinical entity may be of profound importance in early stages of the disease when airflow abnormalities are just beginning to occur. This may be the start of airways inflammation from smoking and other causes, which results in bronchial hyperreactivity and may be reversible by avoiding the irritating factors and by using bronchodilators. Regular use of bronchodilators in asthmatic bronchitis may forestall or prevent irreversible changes to both airways and alveoli. This must be the final common pathway resulting in physiologic impairment, disability, and death from so-called "endstage" COPD.

In later stages of the disease, chronic obstructive bronchitis and asthmatic bronchitis may become indistinguishable. The term chronic bronchitis might best be reserved for those patients with chronic cough and expectoration but no airflow obstruction, i.e., simple chronic bronchitis.

Thus, airflow limitation, which is chronic and not completely reversible, is a key indicator of these disease states and fundamental to identification and in establishing prognosis and guiding therapy.

Gordon Snider from Boston was the summarizer of the 1983 Aspen Lung Conference on COPD and commented in his final remarks:

> I suggest that COPD may be defined as a pulmonary process characterized by non-specific changes in the lung parenchyma and bronchi, which may give rise to one or more of chronic productive cough, wheezing and dyspnea, and which may lead to emphysema and airflow obstruction; airflow obstruction need not be present at all times during the process (a stage in the evaluation). Note that this definition includes emphysema and chronic bronchitis without airflow obstruction; as accepted in scientific terminology, the term "obstructive" is given a special meaning. The term chronic airflow limitation is appropriate for patients who have demonstrable airflow obstruction. Of course, further characterization of patient populations by roentgenographic, physiologic or clinical criteria is always appropriate, and in many circumstances, is essential.[16]

Thus, we are closer to a consensus on definitions than ever before—the bottom line becomes the degree of airflow obstruction (or limitation) as measured by FEV_1, the age of the patient when the abnormality is found, the degree of reversibility, and the rate of change of the FEV_1 over time (at least in our judgment).

EPIDEMIOLOGY

The epidemiology of COPD is now well documented.[17] Data from the National Health Interview Survey estimate that at least 7.5 million Americans have chronic bronchitis, more than 2 million have emphysema, and at least 6.5 million more have some form of asthma.[18] Data from the Tecumseh Community Health Survey of over 9000 men and women in all age groups revealed approximately 14% of adult males and 8% of adult females with chronic bronchitis, obstructive airways disease, or both. In addition, days of disability (as defined by restricted activity) are considerable and averaged 12 days per year for patients with chronic bronchitis, 68 days per year in patients with emphysema, and roughly 17 days per year for asthmatics.[17] In 1981, there were at least 60,000 deaths from chronic obstructive pulmonary disease and related conditions, making this the fifth leading cause of death. However, it is certain that the reporting of deaths from COPD is grossly underestimated each year, and probably 150,000 deaths for 1981 would be a more realistic figure.[17] All estimates point to the fact that deaths are increasing from chronic obstructive pulmonary disease.[17, 18] The estimated economic cost for COPD in 1979 was 6.5 billion dollars, and health care costs are rising for this spectrum of disease. Therefore, there is no question of the importance of this disease spectrum as a major health problem for our country, and it represents a major challenge to physicians who care for these patients in their clinics and offices.

SUMMARY AND COMMENTARY

COPD is a common and vexing disorder. It affects the lives of many families and both challenges and frustrates primary care physicians and specialists alike. The pathogenesis is much better understood than before. COPD is probably a result of a basic tissue defect or a deficit of defense mechanisms in lung tissue or both. COPD is precipitated and aggravated by external factors such as smoking and perhaps infection and other inhaled irritants. The course of the disease is probably 30 years or more in most cases. Survival is much shorter in individuals with $alpha_1$-antitrypsin deficiency. Unfortunately, COPD is usually first diagnosed in advanced stages. Proper management offers hope and substantial benefit to sufferers of this disorder, as subsequent chapters of this book testify. The future demands a better understanding of the pathogenesis of COPD as well as new therapeutic approaches directed at its prevention and earlier detection.

References

1. American Thoracic Society: Definitions and classification of chronic bronchitis, asthma and pulmonary emphysema. *Am Rev Respir Dis* 1962;85:762–768.
2. Petty TL (ed): Management of chronic obstructive lung diseases—conclusion of the eighth Aspen emphysema conference. U.S. Public Health Service Publication No. 1457, May 1966.
3. Bates DV, Bell G, Burnham C, Hazwober M, et al: Problems in studies of human exposure to air pollutants. *Can Med Assoc J* 1970;103:833–837.
4. Mitchell RS, Silvers GW, Dart GA, Petty TL, et al: Clinical and morphological correlations in chronic airway obstruction. *Am Rev Respir Dis* 1968;98:54–62.
5. Mitchell RS, Walker SH, Maisel JC: The causes of death in chronic airway obstruction. 1. The unreliability of death certificates and routine autopsies. *Am Rev Respir Dis* 1968;98:601–610.
6. Fletcher C, Peto R: The natural history of chronic airflow obstruction. *Brit Med J* 1977;1:1645–1648.
7. Macklem PT: Airway obstruction and collateral ventilation. *Physiol Rev* 1971;51: 308–436.
8. Thurlbeck WM: Smoking, airflow limitation and the pulmonary circulation, *Am Rev Respir Dis* 1980;122:183–186.
9. Burrows B: An overview of obstructive lung diseases. *Med Clin North Amer* 1981;65:455–471.
10. Thurlbeck WM: *Chronic Airflow Obstruction in Lung Disease.* Philadelphia, WB Saunders Co, 1976.
11. Hogg JL, Macklem PT, Thurlbeck W: Site and nature of airway obstruction in chronic obstructive lung disease. *N Engl J Med* 1968;278:1355–1360.
12. McLean KH: The pathogenesis of pulmonary emphysema. *Am J Med* 1958;25: 62–74.
13. Fanta CH, Ingram RH: Airway responsiveness and chronic airway obstruction. *Med Clin North Amer* 1981;65:473–487.
14. Petty TL: Definition, Clinical Assessment and Risk Factors, in *Chronic Obstructive Pulmonary Disease*, ed 2. New York, Marcel Dekker, 1985.
15. The definition of emphysema. Report of a National Heart, Lung, and Blood Institute, Division of Lung Diseases Workshop. *Am Rev Respir Dis* 1985;132:182–185.
16. Snider GL: Conference Summary; 26th Aspen Lung Conference Silver Anniversary, in Petty TL (ed): The First Aspen Lung Conference Revisited (The Past 25 Years and the Next). *Chest* 1984;85(Suppl): 84S–89S.
17. Higgins M: Epidemiology of COPD. State of the art. *Chest* 1984;85(suppl):3S–8S.
18. National Center for Health Statistics: *Ten-Year Review and Five-Year Plan*, vol 3. Bethesda, Md, National Heart, Lung and Blood Institute, 1983.

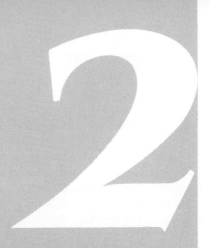

THE PATHOGENESIS
OF EMPHYSEMA

S. IDELL
A. B. COHEN

Emphysema is a pathologic process characterized by the destruction of alveolar septae and dilatation of the alveolar air spaces. This common medical problem is a major cause of disability and death. The discovery of the association between homozygous alpha-1-antiprotease (AAP) deficiency and emphysema was made over 20 years ago. The protease-antiprotease hypothesis has since been proposed to explain how pulmonary emphysema occurs by attributing its cause to the action of proteolytic enzymes on lung elastin, one of the major structural proteins of the lung. These proteolytic enzymes, called elastases, may exceed the control exerted by their natural inhibitors. Alternatively, there is evidence that oxidant-related lung injury may play a role in the development of emphysema. The following discussion is designed to inform practicing physicians about the progress that has been made in understanding the pathogenesis of emphysema.

ALPHA-1-ANTIPROTEASE IN MAN

The protease-antiprotease hypothesis was first proposed because it was determined that individuals with low blood concentrations of AAP tend to develop emphysema at an early age.[1] An understanding of this experiment of nature gives valuable clues to the pathogenesis of human emphysema.

Biology of AAP

This section reviews the biology of AAP in order to explain how proteolytic enzymes may be involved in the pathogenesis of emphysema. AAP is a serum protein capable of inhibiting many proteolytic enzymes. Enzymes inhibited by AAP can be divided into those with potential access to the lungs and those with no known access to the lungs. The first group consists of proteases that have been observed in the plasma, in the formed elements of the blood, or in the lungs, such as neutrophil elastase, alveolar macrophage cathepsin, plasmin, thrombin, Factors IX and XI, and pancreatic elastase. Enzymes that have not been demonstrated in either the circulation or in the lungs include the pancreatic enzymes, trypsin, and chymotrypsin.

AAP is produced in the liver. Patients with AAP deficiency have large amounts of AAP in their hepatocytes, within sacs of rough endoplasmic reticulum. The defect in the structure of AAP thus seems to impair the ability of the liver to transfer the AAP from the liver to the blood. Once in the blood, the AAP undergoes clearance at a normal rate.[2]

AAP deficiency has been detected in several other disease states, but its role in the pathogenesis of these diseases is unclear. Although AAP deficiency has been found in neonatal respiratory distress syndrome, levels of AAP rise to within the normal range after recovery. A relationship between variant types of AAP deficiency and the severity of asthma has also been suggested. In studies of bronchoalveolar lavage fluid obtained from patients with adult respiratory distress syndrome, AAP activity was greatly attenuated. Oxidation or proteolytic cleavage of AAP was shown to be the mechanism of this inactivation. The importance of these results in the evolution of lung injury awaits further study.

AAP has been demonstrated to occur at the sites of lung destruction in emphysema, and it is distributed into almost every body compartment in which albumin is found. Human alveolar macrophages contain AAP in a form that does not inhibit enzymes.[3] Functional AAP has also been found in alveolar lining material.[4]

Studies of the structure of AAP have provided valuable clues about the disease associated with its deficiency. When AAP is electrophoresed in acid-starch gels[5] or is fractionated by isoelectric focusing, multiple bands appear, even though AAP is composed of a single polypeptide chain. This heterogeneity is determined by the subject's genotype and provides evidence that AAP is a codominant allele and that both genes are expressed. Individuals who are homozygotes for the genotype (PiZZ) have low concentrations of AAP in their blood. The M and Z forms of AAP differ by only a single amino acid, and they arise from a point mutation in the structural gene for AAP.[6, 7] Therefore, as one gene usually codes for each protein, the AAP abnormality is almost certain to be the central defect in these patients.

Clinical Aspects of AAP Deficiency

AAP deficiency is a genetic disease. Patients who develop emphysema are homozygotes for the AAP deficiency gene (protease inhibitor phenotype of Pi type ZZ).

The AAP phenotype PiMM is the normal one, and the phenotype PiZZ is associated with a marked deficiency of AAP in the plasma. Investigators still disagree whether a heterozygous state for a "deficiency" allele for AAP (Pi type MZ) leads to obstructive airways disease. About 2% to 3% of the white U.S. population has the PiMZ phenotype. Several studies have been conducted to determine the prevalence of phenotypes in patients with emphysema. The results of these different studies are not in accord, although there seems to be a greater prevalence of MZ phenotypes in patients with emphysema. In pulmonary function studies of MZ heterozygotes based on population surveys, there is no consensus about an association between obstructive airway disease and the MZ phenotype. These large-scale studies found no correlation between either serum trypsin inhibitory capacity or AAP phenotype and pulmonary function abnormalities consistent with emphysema. However, two smaller studies did find that a decrease in airflow and abnormalities in lung scans were more common in individuals with intermediate trypsin inhibitory values than in normal individuals.

The symptoms of emphysema associated with AAP deficiency begin before the age of 40 in 60% of the cases and before the age of 50 in 90%.[8] This early occurrence contrasts with the peak incidence of 50 to 60 years of age in the more common type of emphysema. The earliest abnormalities in pulmonary function are detected by radiosotope ventilation-perfusion scans, which often detect abnormalities by the second decade of life. Spirometric tests, diffusing capacity, and elastic recoil are usually abnormal by the fifth decade.

Not all individuals who are AAP-deficient go on to develop emphysema. Therefore, other factors may contribute to the development of emphysematous changes. Smoking appears to be a significant factor. The mean age of onset of dyspnea was 44 years in nonsmokers and 35 years in smokers. Pulmonary function abnormalities and radiographic changes suggestive of emphysema are more pronounced and occur earlier in smokers as compared with nonsmokers. Infection may also play a role in the development of emphysema in some AAP-deficient individuals. In some patients, symptoms either occur for the first time or are substantially exacerbated after lobar pneumonia; however, this is uncommon.

In addition to the lung disease resulting from AAP deficiency, infants with the ZZ phenotype may develop hepatic cirrhosis and neonatal cholestasis, and adults with ZZ phenotype may develop cirrhosis and liver cancer. The prevalence of these associations are not yet known. In both infants and adults with the homozygous AAP deficiency (and, to a lesser degree, in individuals who have a heterozygous deficiency), subclinical morphologic liver changes have also been reported.

The diagnosis of AAP deficiency may be suspected in any individual who develops emphysema before age 50. Serum protein electrophoresis of individuals affected with the ZZ phenotype will demonstrate a plateau in the alpha globulin region. Serum AAP may be measured by radial immunodiffusion or as the serum trypsin inhibitory capacity. In individuals who have abnormalities in these studies, phenotyping may be obtained. Phenotyping is of potential value for genetic counseling of patients with emphysema or for family members of patients, and may be of greater value in the future if therapeutic trials become possible.

EXPERIMENTAL EVIDENCE FOR THE PROTEASE-ANTIPROTEASE HYPOTHESIS

Several pieces of evidence support the enzyme-inhibitor hypothesis. The human disease associated with AAP deficiency is one of the strongest arguments in its favor, and experimental support has also been developed.[9]

After the original description of the association of emphysema with low blood concentrations of AAP, Gross and colleagues performed a key experiment that led to the development of the protease-inhibitor hypothesis for the pathogenesis of emphysema.[10] After rats were injected intratracheally with papain, an initial hemorrhagic phase was followed by enlargement of air spaces associated with alveolar septal destruction. Figure 2–1 shows the lung destruction that occurred in similar experiments by Kimbel and Weinbaum (unpublished data). The development of these lesions was associated with functional changes characteristic of pulmonary emphysema, such as limitation of expiratory air flow and a decreased diffusing capacity. In this model, the destruction of lung parenchyma is directly related to the ability of the enzyme to attack elastin.[11] Similar lesions may be produced by introducing the enzymes into the bloodstream or into the trachea; however, much higher concentrations of elastase are required by the bloodstream than by the airway. It has therefore been suggested that emphysema may be caused by the unrestrained action of elastase on pulmonary tissues. The common variety of emphysema could be caused by excess elastase orginating from neutrophils, macrophages, platelets, microbes, or other sources.

Identification of the source of destructive enzymes in the lungs is the key to the development of specific therapy. Neutrophils have been implicated as the most likely source of the elastase that may cause emphysema. Recent investigations about the physiology of neutrophils in normal lungs have shown that low numbers of neutrophils enter the airspace. This small pool turns over rapidly enough to leave a residue of neutrophil elastase in the airspaces, which is probably sufficient to cause lung destruction and emphysema over

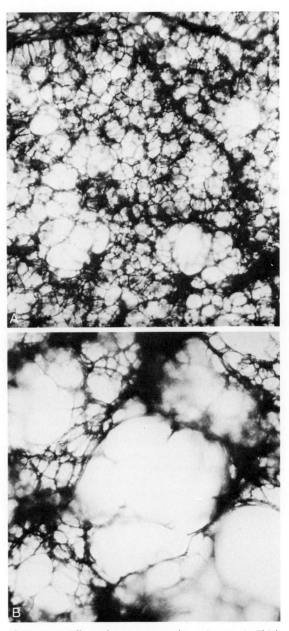

Figure 2–1. Effect of proteases on lung tissues. *A,* Thick section of normal lung. *B,* Thick section of a lung from a dog treated with papain three weeks before being killed. (Courtesy of Drs. P. Kimbel and G. Weinbaum.)

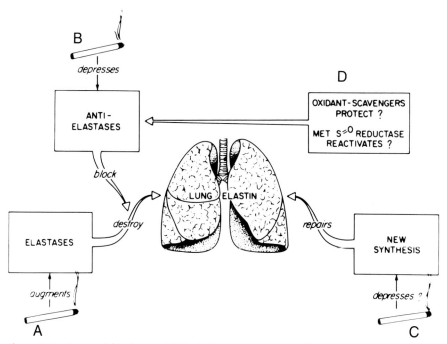

Figure 2–2. Proposed biochemical links between cigarette smoking and the pathogenesis of emphysema. *A,* Smoking recruits monocytes, macrophages, and (through macrophage chemotactic factors) polymorphonuclear neutrophils to the lung, elevating the connective tissue "burden" of elastolytic serine and metalloproteases. *B,* At the same time, oxidants in smoke plus those produced by smoke-stimulated lung phagocytes (as well as oxidizing products of chemical interactions between these two) inactivate bronchial mucus proteinase inhibitor and alpha$_1$-antiprotease, the latter representing the major antielastase "shield" of the respiratory units. *C,* Other unidentified, water-soluble, gas-phase components of cigarette smoke (cyanide? copper chelators?) inhibit lysyl oxidase-catalyzed oxidative deamination of epsilon-amino groups in tropoelastin and block formation of desmosine and presumably other cross-links during elastin synthesis, thus decreasing connective tissue repair. *D,* Antioxidants (ceruloplasmin? methionin-sulfoxide-reductase [met S=^{O} reductase]?) may protect or reactivate elastase inhibitors, and other unidentified factors may modulate the chemical lesions induced in the lung by smoking to influence the risk of developing COPD. (From Janoff A, Carp H, Laurent P, Raju L: The role of oxidative processes in emphysema. *American Review of Respiratory Disease* 127(2):S31, 1983, by permission.)

a long period of time if the elastase is not inhibited. The neutrophils may enter the lungs in response to one or both of the neutrophil chemotactic factors secreted by human alveolar macrophages and may release some of their elastase in response to another macrophage product.

Exposure of the lung to neutrophils and their products may be increased by smoking (Fig. 2–2). Bronchoalveolar lavage fluid from normal nonsmoking subjects contains only a few neutrophils, but bronchoalveolar lavage from cigarette smokers contains a higher percentage of neutrophils. Alveolar macrophages from cigarette smokers produce more chemotactic factors for neutrophils than those of nonsmokers, and more macrophages are found in lung washes of smokers than of nonsmokers (Fig. 2–3).[12, 13] Smokers have also been shown to have higher concentrations of leukocytes in their blood than nonsmokers.

Various other cells may be a source of emphysema-producing enzymes. For example, it has been found that alveolar macrophages from mice secrete elastase and increase this secretion in response to exposure to cigarette smoke. Macrophage elastase from human alveolar macrophages had not always been detected in culture supernatants. However, human alveolar macrophages take up neutrophil elastase selectively and may secrete it later. In addition, instillation of dog neutrophils, dog alveolar macrophages, rabbit neutrophils, and dog monocytes into dog lungs results in emphysema-like lesions.[14, 15] These experiments suggest that enzyme from one or more of these cell types may cause emphysema when excess ezyme is produced or when an inhibitor of the enzyme(s) is lacking. Margination of leukocytes in lung capillaries has also been shown to exert destructive effects on the lungs of rhesus monkeys. In these experiments, repeated injections of endotoxin caused leukocytes to sequester in the lungs, and this sequestration was accompanied by disruption of alveolar walls.

Morphologic observations likewise support the role of neutrophils and macrophages in the pathogenesis of emphysema. Increased numbers of phagocytes in the lungs are associated with smoking, the principal cause of emphysema in humans. Cigarette smoking causes neutrophils to accumulate within the alveolar septa in humans and experimental animals. Morphometric studies have also shown the presence of inflammatory cells in the small

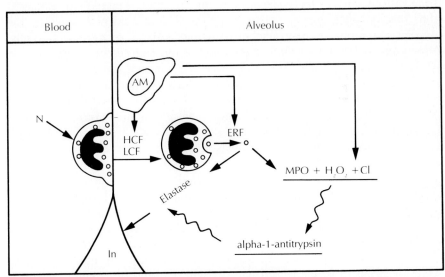

Figure 2–3. Putative events that occur in alveoli relating to macrophages, neutrophils, and lung tissues. Alveolar macrophage (AM), enzyme-releasing factor (ERF), high-molecular-weight chemotactic factor (HCF), low-molecular-weight chemotactic factor (LCF), and myeloperoxidase (MPO). (From Cohen AB, Rossi M: Neutrophils in normal lungs. *American Review of Respiratory Disease* 127:S2, 1983, by permission.)

airways of smokers.[16] Respiratory bronchiolitis associated with clusters of pigmented alveolar macrophages is a characteristic early lesion seen in the lungs of young smokers.[17] This lesion may antedate the development of centrilobular emphysema. Prolonged cigarette smoking is associated with progressive injury to the small airways, which may contribute to the development of airflow obstruction.

Certain microbes also secrete elastases, which may contribute to the development of emphysema, although this point is conjectural. Elastases are produced by *Pseudomonas aeruginosa* isolated from human infections. These elastases are not serine proteases and are therefore not inhibited by AAP. It is likely that other bacteria will be shown to secrete elastases as well. In addition, some bacteria produce enzymes that are inhibited by AAP, whereas others produce enzymes that destroy AAP.

ENZYME-INHIBITOR INTERACTIONS IN MAN

Recent investigations have focused on the behavior of proteolytic enzymes and their inhibitors in the microenvironment of the lung. Inhibitors of proteolytic enzymes have been found in the respiratory tract of man. In the airways, the major defenses against proteolytic enzymes are probably several low-molecular-weight peptides that occur in human bronchial mucus. These peptides have activity against neutrophil elastase and trypsin-like enzymes. AAP occurs in human alveolar macrophages[3] and in alveolar fluid.[4] The AAP isolated from alveolar fluid is able to inhibit enzymes, whereas that extracted from macrophages appears to be inactive. Recent evidence suggests that alveolar macrophages may synthesize active AAP in very small amounts. Alpha$_2$-macroglobulin is another inhibitor of most proteases, which is also synthesized in small amounts by alveolar macrophages, but probably enters the alveoli from plasma only in response to lung inflammation or injury.

The enzyme-inhibitor balance has been examined in purulent and nonpurulent sputum from patients with chronic bronchitis and in bronchoalveolar lavage fluid from normal individuals and those with a deficiency of AAP. When bronchoalveolar lavage fluid was obtained from these subjects using a technique involving the wedging of a bronchoscope into peripheral airways, the major inhibitor seen was AAP. Increased levels of AAP and bronchial mucus inhibitor have also been found in bronchoalveolar lavage of patients with adult respiratory distress syndrome. In these patients, active neutrophil elastase may be inhibited by AAP. As one would expect, individuals with low blood concentrations of AAP also had immeasurable amounts of AAP in their alveolar lavage. AAP, alpha$_2$-macroglobulin, and bronchial mucus inhibitors were all found in sputum from patients with chronic bronchitis. However, either the inhibitory capacity of the inhibitors in the mucus was saturated or they were destroyed and free elastase was demonstrated. While it has been suggested that the protease activity of purulent sputum can be ablated with

AAP, it has not been convincingly demonstrated that this occurs with all elastase activity in these sputa.

DAMAGE TO AAP BY OXIDANTS AND THEIR POTENTIAL ROLE IN HUMAN EMPHYSEMA

Oxidants apparently play a critical role in the development of human emphysema. The oxidant of one or more methionyl residues in AAP causes the molecule to lose its ability to inhibit elastases.[18] In addition, oxidants in cigarette smoke[19] and ozone suppress the elastase inhibitory capacity (EIC) of plasma in vitro. AAP in bronchoalveolar lavage from both human cigarette smokers[20] and rats exposed to cigarette smoke has been shown to lose its ability to inhibit elastase, but others have not been able to reproduce the human data. Oxidant levels in smoke are closely correlated with levels of tar and nicotine. These key observations provide a chemical link between the emphysema found in smokers and AAP-deficient patients. Furthermore, these observations suggest the possibility that elastase inhibitors might prevent the progression of emphysema in both groups of patients. Additionally, it has been noted that endogenously derived oxidants can result in impaired inhibition of elastase by AAP.[21] Investigations have shown that superoxides generated from neutrophils and macrophages can impair the EIC of AAP. Since the earlier pathologic lesion seen in smokers is the collection of macrophages in the respiratory bronchioles, the local destruction of AAP in this area may foster the development of centrilobular emphysema. Lung destruction does not follow the influx of neutrophils in infections of the lung because of the concomitant influx of inhibitors from the serum.

OTHER EXPERIMENTAL MODELS OF EMPHYSEMA

Other experimental models of emphysema exist.[22] It has been produced in animals by gaseous NO_2, NO_2 absorbed on activated carbon dust, phosgene, cigarette smoke, injection of chlorpromazine in horses and 3-methylindole into cattle and goats, intratracheal ingestion of phytohemagglutinin in rats, and induced vitamin A deficiency in weanling rats. In most cases, mechanisms or common denominators remain speculative. These different models have different points of primary attack, e.g., chlorpromazine causes bronchial artery obliteration, whereas phosgene causes a terminal bronchitis. These experiments therefore raise the possibility that the characteristic pathologic and physiologic derangements of emphysema may be a uniform consequence of different kinds of insults to the lung. Recently, the oxidant chloramine-T was used to develop a dog model of AAP deficiency. The chloramine-T inactivated the EIC of plasma AAP, and within 12 weeks of treatment, these dogs developed the pathologic derangements associated with emphysema. Two avenues for further investigation are raised by these experiments: (1) the testing of oxidants to determine if they produce emphysema by mechanisms other than their effect on the EIC of AAP, and (2) the use of the model to test the effects of therapeutic agents.

Oxidants in smoke also reduce elastin synthesis by interfering with the enzyme lysyl oxidase, which forms the cross-links that make elastin uniquely tough. Interruption of elastin synthesis causes greater lung destruction in animal models of emphysema.

These experiments suggest the possibility that the current emphasis on the protease-inhibitor hypothesis may be analogous to a man who enters a dark room with a flashlight and sees only one aspect of it. The protease-inhibitor hypothesis must ultimately be proved by preventing the progress of emphysema by restoring the protease-inhibitor balance in the lungs.

Since small airway disease is prevalent in smokers, one can ask whether it is causally related to the mechanism of production of emphysema. The data described above can be formulated into a logical connection between smaller airways disease and centrilobular emphysema.

Cigarette smoke causes chronic bronchitis and colonization of the large airway with bacteria. These bacteria are aspirated into small airways and alveoli, especially at night. The macrophages secrete leukotriene B_4 (LTB_4) which attracts neutrophils. The neutrophils degranulate dumping enzymes such as elastin and myeloperoxidase into small airways. The degranulation of neutrophils occurs in response to a peptide secreted by the alveolar macrophages. The myeloperoxidase and hydrogen peroxide along with oxidants in smoke inactivate AAP in the small airways, and the elastase degrades the elastin in the reinforcing rings at the entrances to respiratory bronchioles. The elastin peptides attract more monocytes into small airways to magnify the cycle. Eventually, emphysema emanates from these lung parenchymal areas surrounding small airways. This scenario uses available facts to construct a feasible hypothesis for why smokers develop centrilobular emphysema.

THE PROTEASE-INHIBITOR HYPOTHESIS AND THERAPY FOR EMPHYSEMA

One can logically deduce from the foregoing review that if AAP or a low-molecular-weight elastase inhibitor were given to patients who have either the global deficiency of AAP as in subjects with PiZZ phenotype or a local deficiency of AAP as occurs in the lungs of smokers, then the progressive lung destruction of emphysema might be arrested. About six years ago, the Lung Division of the National Heart, Lung, and Blood Institute (NHLBI) initiated a program designed to determine whether such therapy could be tried. Several working groups met to identify the most formidable obstacles to inhibitor therapy and to solve the problems.

Analysis of a large amount of data led to the consensus that degradation of lung elastin by elastases was probably important in the production of emphysema in patients with the ZZ phenotype for AAP and in the larger groups of patients with obstructive airways disease, which is commonly seen in cigarette smokers. Based on this assessment, the following was postulated:

1. AAP replacement in patients with pulmonary emphysema has a strong likelihood of preventing the progression of emphysema in patients with the PiZZ phenotype.

2. If such replacement therapy appears to be successful, then therapeutic trials of low-molecular-weight elastase inhibitors could be undertaken.

3. If safe elastase inhibitors become available, they could be tried in common forms of emphysema regardless of the results in patients with ZZ phenotypes for AAP.

The committee convened by the NHLBI recognized that a series of formidable problems had to be solved before clinical trials of the specific agents could be tried and identified five problem areas for replacement therapy:

1. Isolation of AAP on a clinical scale and proven safety for licensing.

2. Determination of the pharmacokinetics of AAP in humans.

3. Development and testing of the safety of elastase inhibitors.

4. Development of chemical markers of lung destruction.

5. Determination of the natural history of emphysema in patients with PiZ to determine if a study of replacement therapy is feasible.

The following progress has been made in the resolution of these problems:

1. Isolation of AAP from Blood Products. Although enough blood is currently fractionated in the United States to provide enought AAP to treat all patients deficient in this protein, relatively simple and inexpensive methods of fractionation for AAP have only recently been developed. In addition, the AAP gene has been cloned; therefore, newer technology may provide AAP for treating AAP-deficient patients.

2. Pharmacokinetics of AAP. A knowledge of the rate of disappearance, volumes of distribution, and proteolytic enzyme inhibitory capacity of the administered protein are essential to the development of replacement therapy of AAP in patients with this deficiency. Studies in humans have shown that PiM protein administered to MM subjects has a half-life in serum of between five and seven days. Isolated AAP has also proved effective in replacing the deficient protein in blood and bronchoalveolar lavage when given to these patients.

3. Development of Safe Elastase Inhibitors. In recent years, a number of elastase inhibitors have been synthesized. Classes of such compounds include alkylating agents (chlormethylketones), acylating agents (aza-peptides), and simple peptides. Some of these inhibitors exhibit a high reactivity and specificity for human leukocytic elastase while others are capable of inhibiting a broad range of serine proteases.

Studies of elastase inhibitors in animals have been encouraging. Prior intraperitoneal or oral administration of a peptide chlormethylketone has provided nearly complete protection from lung damage caused by an intratra-cheal injection of porcine pancreatic elastase. Data are also available showing that the application of a chlormethylketone shortly after the intratracheal administration of elastase reduces the severity of the elastase-induced lung damage in hamsters. Information on the toxicity and carcinogenicity of such elastase inhibitors is incomplete. At this time, none are sufficiently soluble, specific, or safe to make them candidates for therapeutic use.

4. Development of Chemical Markers of Lung Destruction. Present tests of lung function fail to discriminate between patients with irreversible disease and those in whom disease can be arrested. In order to assess accurately the efficacy of AAP replacement or the administration of protease inhibitors, sensitive assays of lung parenchymal destruction are needed. Immunologic measurements of plasma and/or urinary excretion of elastin degradation fragments have been undertaken in patients with emphysema and in animal models of the disease. Immunoassays for desmosine and elastin peptides have been developed. Preliminary work has shown that elastin peptides are elevated in some smokers, patients with emphysema, and elastase-treated animals.[23]

5. The Natural History of Emphysema in PiZZ Subjects and Replacement Therapy. It is necessary to know the natural history of emphysema in these individuals to determine the size of treated and control groups required for a clinical study and its duration. Recently, the natural history was examined by a retrospective study of longitudinal data of American and Swedish patients with AAP deficiency, and a workshop on the natural history of PiZ emphysema was sponsored by the Lung Division of the National Heart, Lung, and Blood Institute of the National Institutes of Health. Retrospective data on 298 PiZ individuals collected at several institutions in the United States and Sweden were reviewed.[24] Baseline FEV_1 values were compared with follow-up meas-urements obtained after more than 12 months had elasped, and linear regression analysis was carried out separately for each individual to determine the annual rate of change of the FEV_1. From these analyses, group mean rates of decline were calculated and the standard deviations of these rates deter-mined. The proportion of nonsmoking PiZ patients evaluated was 19.7%. This subpopulation is smaller than might be expected and may reflect a bias in case ascertainment, which selectively looked at a large proportion of pulmonary patients whose clinical disease may have been potentiated by smoking. PiZ subjects, particularly nonsmokers, and those who have escaped clinical disease sufficient to declare itself are therefore underrepresented. The resulting analysis is therefore skewed toward a description of the progression of disease in more severely affected PiZ individuals (Fig. 2–4).

Although cases collected in this manner pose problems in interpretation of the data, the rates of decline in FEV_1 observed in clinically significant but not end-stage PiZ disease are nearly twice the average rates of decline reported in "ordinary COPD." Therefore, PiZ subjects who develop significant airflow obstruction enter a phase of relatively rapid functional decline. In a study of pediatric patients with Pi phenotypes ZZ and SZ associated with severe and moderately severe AAP deficiency, no gross impairment in overall pulmonary

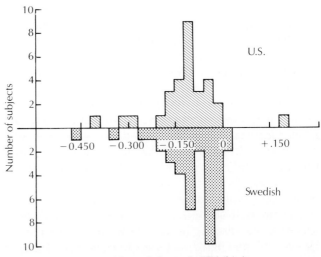

Figure 2–4. Annual change in one-second forced expiratory volume (FEV₁) for 30 U.S. and 41 Swedish subjects with homozygous alpha₁-antitrypsin deficiency, PiZ phenotype. All subjects were under age 65 and had a FEV₁ between 30% and 65% of that predicted. (From Buist AS, Burrows B, Eriksson S, Mittman C, Wu M: The natural history of air-flow obstruction in PiZ emphysema. *American Review of Respiratory Disease* 127:S43–45, 1983, by permission. Adapted from Morris JF, Koski A, Johnson LC: Spirometric standards for healthy nonsmoking adults. *American Review of Respiratory Disease* 103:57–67, 1971.)

function was found in a comparison with matched controls. This suggests that either functional decline may proceed slowly or that subclinical disease may escape detection early in the course of PiZ disease.

Replacement Therapy in Severe AAP

A recent trial of replacement therapy of AAP has been undertaken in five patients with severe AAP deficiency (PiZ phenotype and emphysema).[25, 26] Serum AAP levels were increased from mean pretreatment values of 37 mg/dl (± 4 mg/dl) to 108 mg/dl (± 12 mg/dl) two days after the intravenous infusion of 4 g of AAP. This regimen also resulted in a restoration of the antiprotease balance in the lungs. Analysis of bronchoalveolar lavage specimens revealed that lower respiratory tract AAP increased to about 60% of normal, associated with an equivalent restoration of functional antielastase activity. There were no significant untoward reactions to the infusion of the AAP concentrate, and none of the patients developed clinical or biochemical evidence of hepatitis. The application of replacement therapy of AAP to the long-term therapy of emphysema is the next step. Difficulties regarding the proper selection of patients and determination of clinical endpoints require resolution before undertaking such a study.

Since some individuals with PiZZ phenotype reach old age without developing disease, it appears impractical to attempt prevention in young, healthy PiZZ subjects. Also, since emphysema may be self-perpetuating in its later stages, it might be difficult to observe beneficial effects of antiproteolytic therapy at this stage. Ideal subjects for replacement therapy would be those with mild disease.

Techniques to obtain AAP from blood have recently been developed. The techniques are inexpensive, simple, and safe. These procedures result in a high yield of a product composed of less than 10% of contaminating proteins and withstands hepatitis sterilization procedures. Should future clinical trials document the value of replacement therapy of AAP for the treatment of emphysema, the methodologies necessary to implement this therapy on a broad scale appear to be available.

Synthetic Elastase Inhibitors. Reversible and irreversible elastase inhibitors have successfully been used to prevent emphysema in animal models. Peptide chlormethylketones were the first class of selective inhibitors of human leukocyte elastase. Acylating agents, sulfonyl fluorides, AAP analogues, heterocyclic elastase inhibitors, and a variety of other compounds serve as inhibitors of human leukocyte elastase. Although inhibitors to date have had chemical problems that preclude their use in patients, the overall prospects for the development of synthetic elastase inhibitors suitable for use in humans in the near future appear good. If the major cause of emphysema in smokers is the inactivation of AAP, one would hope that these agents could be used in this larger group of patients.

Danazol. Since diethylstilbestrol, an anabolic steroid, can increase the release of AAP from the liver, Gadek and colleagues attempted to achieve increased plasma concentrations of AAP with an anabolic steroid called danazol, which has fewer side effects.[25, 26] They achieved a mean increase of 37% in patients with PiZ phenotype. The concentrations of AAP were still far below those thought to be safe (those seen in individuals with PiMZ phenotype.) It is unclear whether these elevations will affect morbidity or mortality in patients with PiZ phenotype. However, one can be cautiously optimistic that other agents might be found to achieve greater release of AAP from the livers of patients with PiZ phenotype.

SUMMARY AND CONCLUSIONS

Many current investigations have suggested that pulmonary emphysema may result from an imbalance between proteases and inhibitors in the lungs of cigarette smokers and of patients who have a genetically determined deficiency of AAP. Significant advances have been made in the isolation of AAP in therapeutic quantities and in the design of elastase inhibitors. Advances have also been made in the understanding of the natural history of emphysema and in the development of chemical markers for lung destruction in patients who are developing emphysema. These advances provide the basis for future trials to prevent the progression of emphysema with specific therapeutic agents.

References

1. Eriksson S: Studies of alpha-1-antitrypsin deficiency. *Acta Med Scand* (suppl) 1965; 177:175.
2. Makino S, Reed CE: Distribution and elimination of exogenous alpha-1-antitrypsin. *J Lab Clin Med* 1970;75:741–746.
3. Cohen AB: Interrelationships between the human alveolar macrophage and alpha-1-antitrypsin. *J Clin Invest* 1973;52:2793–2799.
4. Tuttle WC, Jones RF: Fluorescent antibody studies of alpha-1-antitrypsin in adult human lung. *Am J Clin Path* 1975;64: 477–482.
5. Fagerhol MK, Gedda-Dahl T: Genetics of the Pi serum types. Family studies of the inherited variants of serum alpha-1-antitrypsin. *Hum Hered* 1969;19:354–359.
6. Jeppsson J: Amino acid subsitution Glu Lys in alpha-1-antitrypsin. *FEBS Lett* 1976; 65:195–197.
7. Yoshida L, Lieberman L, Gaidulis L, Ewing C: Molecular abnormality of human alpha-1-antitrypsin variant (PiZ) associated with plasma activity deficiency. *Proc Nat Acad Sci USA* 1976;73:1324–1328.
8. Larsson, C: Natural history and life expectancy in severe alpha-1-antitrypsin deficiency. PiZ. *Acta Med Scand* 1978; 204–345.
9. Janoff A: Elastases and emphysema. *Am Rev Respir Dis* 1985;132:417–433.
10. Gross P, Pfitzer EA, Toker E, Babyak M, et al: Experimental emphysema: its production with papain in normal and silicotic rats. *Arch Environ Health* 1965;11: 50–58.
11. Snider FL, Hayes JA, Franzblau C, Kagan HM, et al: Relationship between elastolytic activity and experimental emphysema-inducing properties of papain preparations. *Am Rev Respir Dis* 1974;110: 254–262.
12. Hunninghake GW, Gadek JE, Fales HM, Crystal RC: Human alveolar-derived chemotactic factor for neutrophils. Stimuli and partial characterization. *J Clin Invest* 1980;66:473–483.
13. Merrill WW, Naegel GP, Matthay RA, Reynolds HY: Alveolar macrophage derived chemotactic factor. *J Clin Invest* 1980;65:268–276.
14. Mass B, Ikeda T, Maranze D, Weinbaum G, et al: Induction of experimental emphysema, cellular and species specificity. *Am Rev Respir Dis* 1972;106:384–391.
15. Weinbaum G, Marco V, Ikeda T, Mass B, et al: Enzymatic production of experimental emphysema in the dog. Route of exposure. *Am Rev Respir Dis* 1974;109: 351–357.
16. Cosio MG, Hale K, Niewoehner DE: Morphologic and morphometric effects of prolonged cigarette smoking on the small airways. *Am Rev Respir Dis* 1980;22: 265–271.
17. Niewoehner DE, Kleinerman J, Rice DB: Pathologic changes in the peripheral airways of young cigarette smokers. *N Engl J Med* 1974;291:755–758.
18. Johnson D, Travis J: The oxidative inactivation of human alpha-1-antiproteinase inhibitor. Further evidence for methionine at the reactive center. *J Biol Chem* 1979; 254:4022–4026.
19. Carp H, Janoff A: Possible mechanisms of emphysema in smokers. In vitro suppression of serum elastase-inhibitor capacity by fresh cigarette smoke and its prevention by antioxidants. *Am Rev Respir Dis* 1978; 118:617–621.
20. Gadek JE, Fells FA, Crystal RG: Cigarette smoking induces functional antiprotease deficiency in the lower respiratory tract of humans. *Science* 1979;206:1314–1315.
21. Matheson NR, Wong PS, Travis J: Enzymatic inactivation of human alpha-1-proteinase inhibitor by neutrophil myeloperoxidase. *Biochem Biophys Res Commun* 1979;88:402–409.
22. Karlinsky JB, Snider GC: Animal models of emphysema. *Am Rev Respir Dis* 1978; 117:1109–1134.
23. Kucich U, Christner P, Weinbaum G, Rosenbloom J: Immunologic identification of elastin-derived peptides in the sera of dogs with experimental emphysema. *Am Rev Respir Dis* 1980;122:461–465.
24. Buist AS, Burrows B, Eriksson S, Mittman C, Wu M: The natural history of airflow obstruction in PiZ emphysema. *Am Rev Respir Dis* 1983;127:S43–S45.
25. Gadek, JE, Fells GA, Zimmerman RL, Rennard SI, Crystal RG: Antielastases of the human alveolar structures. Implications for the protease-antiprotease theory of emphysema. *J Clin Invest* 1981;68:889–898.
26. Gadek JE, Klein HG, Holland PV, Crystal RG: Replacement therapy of alpha-1-antitrypsin deficiency. *J Clin Invest* 1981; 68:1158.

HISTORY AND PHYSICAL EXAMINATION

HELENA B. JONES
LEONARD D. HUDSON

Obtaining a useful history and doing a thorough physical examination require attention and an understanding of disease pathogenesis and clinical correlations. If done carefully, this process is time-effective and rewarding, especially in the initial assessment of chronic obstructive pulmonary disease (COPD), in making therapeutic decisions, and in following the efficacy of treatment. In fact, history and physical examination are critical in evaluation of the patient with COPD. Although spirometry and arterial blood gases are obviously important adjuncts to evaluation, much of the initial assessment regarding diagnosis is based on history and physical examination. Most decisions regarding therapy, including whether or not to treat and whether changes in therapy should be made, are based on findings from the history.

The major categories of disease under the general heading of COPD are chronic bronchitis and emphysema, but bronchiectasis and elements of reversible airflow obstruction may also be included. These are primarily clinically defined disease entities, with the exception of emphysema which is defined pathologically. Therefore, their correct diagnosis depends on the physician's ability to elicit pertinent history and to recognize physical findings that will direct the examiner toward a specific diagnosis and appropriate therapeutic plan.

It is important to gain an understanding of the person being evaluated as well as of his disease to understand the greater context of the patient's life and the role played by the disease in his overall existence. For the most part, treatment of COPD is directed toward symptomatic improvement in the patient's respiratory disability rather than toward reversal of the disease process. Ensuring ongoing compliance with the therapeutic regimen becomes paramount in the treatment of the patient with COPD. Occupational, financial, sexual, and interpersonal issues are central to a patient's life and will directly affect his medical compliance as well as the ultimate outcome of his disability. These issues should therefore be explored by the physician as part of the initial and ongoing assessment of the patient.

Assessment of the efficacy of treatment of COPD is based, for the most part, on the patient's subjective sense of improvement and well-being. Careful attention to the patient's complaints and concerns becomes invaluable in following the course of the disease.

The ultimate goal of doing a comprehensive history and physical exam- ination is to correlate signs and symptoms with pulmonary abnormalities and limitations. This is not always objectively possible and requires the patience and skill of the physician.

HISTORY

There are six major symptoms of respiratory disease: cough, sputum production, dyspnea, wheezing, hemoptysis, and chest pain. These categories provide a practical framework for eliciting a comprehensive and useful pulmonary history. All are important in evaluating the patient with COPD although the first four predominate.

Cough is the most obvious symptom of pulmonary disease, readily apparent both to the patient and to others. Cough, caused by irritating stimuli in the airways, plays a major role in the defense against aspiration of foreign objects, infection, and exposure to environmental irritants. Cough is also caused by infiltrative processes such as neoplasms. The site of the stimulus can affect the type of cough produced. The cough caused by pharyngitis or by nasal and sinus secretions trickling down the posterior pharynx is usually dry, persistent, and painless and is occasionally worse at night, while the cough of acute laryngitis, although nonproductive, can be painful.

A persistent cough is abnormal, and carefully characterizing it can help lead to a diagnosis of the nature of the patient's pulmonary disease. A new, unexplained cough should always raise the specter of neoplasm in the physician's mind and requires a full evaluation. The following questions about a patient's cough can help characterize his disease. Does the cough occur during the day or at night? Is there a time of day when it is worse? Does it go on indefinitely or present with a paroxysm that, once completed, does not return immediately? Is it effective at raising sputum or is it an "unfinished cough," ineffective at clearing secretions? Do changes in the patient's position, temperature, or exposure to irritants bring on cough? Is it associated with laughter, exertion, or anything that increases the depth of respiration? Has the patient ever fainted during a paroxysm of coughing? Has the sound of the cough changed? Has its expulsive abilities decreased in association with a change in sound? Is the cough associated with wheezing?

The onset of cough in the patient with chronic bronchitis is usually insidious. The patient often denies coughing, even on direct questioning, assuming that it is a normal finding to have some morning cough ("I just have a cigarette cough"). Most typically, it is the patient with chronic bronchitis who will give a history of prolonged paroxysms of cough, culminating in production of sputum. Frequently, he will complain of an ineffective cough, resulting in ineffective clearing of sputum. His cough is usually worse in the morning, upon rising, and at night. He is seldom awakened from sleep by coughing. His is the cough that is stimulated by anything that increases the depth of respiration. The patient with chronic obstructive airways disease may give a very disturbing history of fainting while having a paroxysm of cough. The patient with bronchiectasis complains of a persistently loose cough, productive of copious amounts of sputum. Postural changes can bring on cough, presumably by causing drainage of sputum into the airways and causing irritation leading to cough. Patients with unilateral bronchiectasis frequently sleep on the affected side to prevent cough caused by dislodged sputum. A cough that has lost its expulsive ability might be caused by a vocal cord palsy and incomplete closure of the glottis and should alert the physician to the possibility of neoplasm.

Occasionally, chronic and persistent cough may signal that a patient has asthma and may respond to bronchodilators. In fact, cough can be the first symptom of asthma. Nocturnal cough may be caused by recurrent aspiration, either separate from or as a part of the general picture of COPD. Nocturnal cough may also be present in asthma. Chronic cough may also be psychogenic in origin. Chronic bronchitis is defined by the presence of a productive cough. Specifically, the presence of a cough productive of sputum on most mornings for three months of the year for two successive years has been accepted as the definition of chronic bronchitis. The patient with this definition of chronic bronchitis may have so-called simple bronchitis, so this finding does not necessarily denote the presence of airflow obstruction.

Noticeable sputum production is always abnormal. The normal person produces about 10 ml of sputum in 24 hours, most of which is swallowed, unnoticed.

It is useful to question patients about the amount, character, viscosity, taste, and odor of their sputum as well as the chronicity. The patient generally estimates the amount produced: A cupful would be very large, and a teaspoon would clearly be scant. One would expect a patient with bronchiectasis to complain of producing large amounts of sputum. Characterizing it is important in arriving at a diagnosis. Is the sputum serous, mucoid, purulent, or mucopurulent? What color is it? In chronic bronchitis the sputum is mucoid and generally gray, white, or clear. A change in its color or character is important to note. Mucopurulent or purulent sputum that has changed color to yellow or green implies the presence of an infection but can also be seen with allergies due to increased numbers of sputum eosinophils. Very viscid sputum is difficult to clear and may lead to consideration of therapies directed toward facilitating clearing of secretions. A foul taste or odor to the sputum also implies infection, such as a lung abscess or in bronchiectasis.

The physician must never overlook inquiring about the presence of hemoptysis. Since hemoptysis can be caused by cardiovascular as well as pulmonary diseases, obtaining a good history is of primary importance. Occasionally, the complaint of hemoptysis may actually be caused by bleeding from the upper airway (nasopharynx, oropharynx, or larynx). Again, a careful history is helpful in differentiating among the possible diagnoses. The most obvious cardiovascular reason for hemoptysis is mitral stenosis. Pulmonary causes include endobronchial lesions (malignant and benign), pulmonary infarction, tuberculosis, and other pulmonary infections, all of which can and do coexist with COPD. Bronchiectasis can produce frank bleeding, whereas chronic bronchitis is usually associated with blood-streaked sputum and is usually associated with an acute infection or increase in the severity of cough. A malignant lesion can cause any degree of bleeding. Other causes of hemoptysis include thoracic trauma and coagulopathy.

Dyspnea is the most subjective pulmonary symptom, difficult to quantify or to relate to objective findings. Ventilatory control and its pathophysiology has very complex neurological, chemical, and physical factors, and it is difficult to sort out the contribution of each of these factors to the patient's symptoms. However, individuals with brisk ventilatory drives generally sense dyspnea at a lower threshold of impairment than people with normal or blunted ventilatory drives.

A comprehensive history of dyspnea should include the pattern of onset, duration, associated symptoms (e.g., cough, chest pain, wheeze, or palpitations), precipitating factors (e.g., exercise, cough, or emotions), and whether it occurs at night. Paroxysmal dyspnea is associated with the sudden onset or worsening of airways obstruction. Nocturnal dyspnea that awakens the patient can be either cardiac in origin or caused by bronchospasm. When caused by bronchospasm, nocturnal dyspnea (often associated with a cough) is felt by some clinicians to imply a degree of reversibility. Any sudden onset of dyspnea, especially if associated with pleuritic chest pain, should evoke the possibility of a pulmonary embolus or of a pneumothorax, both of which have a higher incidence in patients with COPD. Documenting the degree of exercise needed to induce dyspnea is important in establishing a baseline from which the physician can follow the patient and can help sort out the organic versus the functional basis for a patient's dyspnea. Dyspnea at rest is most likely to be functional unless severe impairment is present.

The pattern of onset of dyspnea in the course of a patient's disease can be helpful in characterizing the disease. Dyspnea may be a prominent symptom, even early in the course of emphysema, and is insidious in onset, progresses slowly, occurs with decreasing amounts of exertion, and is not necessarily associated with cough or affected by the patient's position. Dyspnea can sometimes be decreased by assuming the posture commonly associated with COPD patients, who sit bending forward while bracing their hands or elbows against a table, bed, or their knees, which presumably optimizes respiratory mechanics. An important point to remember in patients' initial assessment and in following their progress or decline is that there is not necessarily a correlation between dyspnea and hypoxemia. In fact, a patient can be severely hypoxemic and not feel short of breath and vice versa. Dyspnea developing slowly over a workweek might point to an industrial irritant as a contributing factor.

Nonpulmonary diseases associated with dyspnea include metabolic acidosis of any etiology, anemia, hyperthyroidism, cardiovascular disease, neurologic disease, primary muscle diseases, and collagen vascular disorders associated with decreased chest wall compliance or with a restrictive pulmonary process. Obtaining a history of dyspnea should therefore be directed at sorting out all possible etiologies, whether primarily pulmonary or extrapulmonary disease.

When obtaining a history of wheezing, a hallmark of airway obstruction, it is of foremost importance to establish what is the patient's definition of wheezing. Once the physician is satisfied that the patient is indeed describing wheezing, further evaluation can proceed. In directing a history, it is important to remember that bronchospasm is not the sole cause of wheezing. It can also be caused by a tumor, aspiration of a foreign body, edema of the bronchial mucosa, inspissated mucus, infection, or other conditions. Thus, if a patient describes the sudden onset of wheezing, the physician should consider aspiration as a possible etiology. Positional wheezing raises the possibility of an endotracheal lesion. Absence of wheezing in a patient with COPD may imply primarily irreversible airflow obstruction and lack of response to bronchodilators. However, a trial of bronchodilators is still warranted.

Chest pain can have cardiovascular, esophageal, neuromuscular, infectious, and traumatic as well as various pulmonary causes. The presence of chest pain in the COPD patient implies another, concurrent, disease process. The following information, elicited in the history, can help differentiate among possible etiologies. The character of the pain, whether sharp or dull, its location, whether onset was sudden or gradual, association with fever, sputum production, hemoptysis, dyspnea, diaphoresis, and the effect of positional changes are all salient parts of a complete history. Thus, the gradual onset of a severe, aching, constant chest pain without cough, fever, or sputum production would lead the physician to suspect the possibility of an infiltrative process involving the chest wall or pleura, while the sudden onset of a sharp, pleuritic chest pain associated with dyspnea and diaphoresis might evoke the possibility of a pulmonary embolus. Pneumothorax may present with the sudden onset of a sharp pleuritic chest pain, followed by chest tightness, lateralizing to the involved side, associated with dyspnea. Pneumonia may be heralded by the onset of chest pain in association with fever, chills, and purulent sputum.

Details of the patient's past medical history can provide valuable insights into the patient's present disease. Inquiry about childhood asthma or cystic fibrosis should be included. Severe measles or whooping cough in childhood are associated with increased incidence of bronchiectasis, as is a history of tuberculosis. Recurrent pneumonias in the same area of the lung raise the possibility of localized disease including the spector of an obstructing lesion, although an obstructing neoplasm is more often associated with persistent rather than recurrent pneumonia. Recurrent sinusitis can be implicated in the pathogenesis of recurrent pulmonary infections and wheezing. A history of collagen vascular disease suggests the possibility of restrictive lung disease. Cardiovascular diseases, especially congestive heart failure of any etiology, can cause dyspnea, cough, and wheezing.

Family, social, and occupational histories are key elements in a full evaluation of a patient's health and are vital to the physician's ability to diagnose, treat, and counsel patients. The patient's smoking history is obviously important to establish. Genetic disorders such as $alpha_1$-antitrypsin deficiency, immotile cilia syndrome, and IgA deficiency can be associated with pulmonary disease, and their occurrence in a patient's family medical history should be noted. A thorough occupational history stressing exposure to known respiratory irritants or carcinogens is extremely important. Occupational exposures to animals, including pets as well as farm animals, can cause various diseases and can exacerbate existing COPD.

Close attention should be paid to the review of systems. Does the patient note bone pain, weakness, CNS symptoms, or hemoptysis that might be the harbingers of a pulmonary malignancy? Nightime symptoms, such as thrashing about, nightmares, morning headaches, or personality changes are seen in patients who suffer nocturnal hypoxemia or hypercapnia and may signal a deterioration in the patient's condition. Peripheral edema may mark progression to cor pulmonale in the patient with COPD.

PHYSICAL EXAMINATION

A comprehensive physical examination complements the detailed history and is obviously an integral part of patient evaluation. Physical findings can be quite sensitive and specific for the presence of disease and can aid in determining the direction of a diagnostic workup and the choice of therapy. In addition, the physician can frequently follow progression or change of the patient's disease by noting the evolution of physical findings. This is especially useful in the patient with COPD.

General Inspection

The initial impression that a patient gives can be eloquent and is worth careful attention and note. General appearance, hygiene, state of nutrition, affect, and posture should be acknowledged in the evaluation. The presence at rest of cough, wheezing, stridor, and general respiratory discomfort are important markers of the degree of disease. The degree of respiratory distress caused by minimal exertion as the patient undresses or moves over to the examining table can help objectively quantify respiratory limitations. The pattern and noise of breathing are worth noting; the patient with chronic bronchitis or asthma frequently makes noticeable noise while breathing, while the patient with emphysema breathes quietly. There is some correlation between degree of noise generated by breathing and FEV_1, since both are affected by high velocity and turbulence of flow in abnormally narrowed large airways. Patients with emphysema usually have quiet breathing because the caliber of large airways is normal during inspiration.

Respiratory rate and depth, the use of accessory respiratory muscles and whether they are hypertrophied, and the presence of pursed-lip breathing are clues to the degree of respiratory dysfunction. The normal pattern of breathing is synchronous motion of the abdomen and chest, outward with inspiration and inward during expiration. Those patients in whom an asynchronous breathing pattern is observed during an exacerbation of their disease have been found to have a poorer prognosis than those with a normal breathing pattern. They more frequently require intubation during the course of their acute illness and are more difficult to wean from the ventilator.[1] The presence of asynchronous motion of the chest and abdomen has been proposed as an indication for early intubation and mechanical ventilation during an acute exacerbation of disease. This finding implies inspiratory muscle fatigue including diaphragmatic ineffectiveness and poor ventilatory mechanics.[2] Overall prognosis seems to be worse in this group of patients; a significantly higher mortality has been noted compared to patients with COPD and a normal pattern of breathing.

A patient's posture while sitting is an indirect indication of ventilatory mechanics. Patients who sit leaning forward, grasping the edge of the bed or chair are dependent on their accessory respiratory muscles for adequate ventilation. By assuming this posture, they are fixing their shoulder girdle in order to be able to recruit the latissimus dorsi muscles for ventilation, to approximate their ribs during expiration.

Observation of jugular venous pressure and movement over the suprasternal and supraclavicular fossae during breathing can prove valuable in judging the degree of airflow obstruction. Excessive increases in intrathoracic pressure during expiration, as seen in patients with severe obstructive disease, result in visible jugular venous filling. These patients may also manifest excessive inward motion of tissues over the suprasternal and supraclavicular fossae and of the intercostal spaces during inspiration because of a large decrease in intrathoracic pressure. Hyperinflation of the lungs can result in pushing the liver down in the abdomen, but the overall breadth of the liver, as determined by percussion, should be normal.

Hypercapnia is suggested on physical examination by finding venous engorgement on funduscopic examination. Hypercarbia can also result in papilledema.[3] Peripheral venous engorgement occurs as well, more frequently involving the upper rather than the lower extremities. Finding engorged forearm veins in a patient who complains of frequent headaches should alert the examiner to the possibility of hypercapnia as the etiology. It is important to emphasize that other causes of papilledema and headache, such as CNS metastases, should be ruled out before these findings are entirely attributed to elevations in $Paco_2$. The presence of Horner's syndrome (ptosis, miosis, enophthalmos, and impaired sweating on one side) should bring to mind the possibility of a superior sulcus tumor.

Hypoxemia may be evident on physical examination by the presence of central cyanosis involving the soft palate, mouth, tongue, and lips. Peripheral cyanosis is seen in patients with long-standing hypoxemia that has resulted in a secondary erythrocytosis as well as in patients with cardiac diseases.

Both initial and follow-up evaluations of patients with COPD should include careful examination of the hands. The presence or absence of clubbing should be noted. Clubbing is defined as the loss of the angle between the nail and nail bed, sponginess to palpation of the nail bed, swelling of the terminal tuft of the finger, and increased curvature of the nail in late clubbing. It usually occurs to a greater degree in the fingers than the toes. Clubbing can occur as a familial trait or can occur in a variety of pulmonary and extrapulmonary diseases. It is important to remember that the presence of COPD alone does not explain the presence of clubbing. New onset clubbing should lead the physician to pursue the cause aggressively. Intrathoracic neoplasm, bronchiectasis, abscesses, cystic fibrosis, diffuse interstitial fibrosis as well as cyanotic congenital cardiac diseases, certain gastrointestinal and hepatic disorders, and thyroid diseases can cause clubbing. Unilateral wasting of the muscles of the hand associated with Horner's syndrome is seen in superior sulcus tumors with T1 lesions.

The head and neck examination should include dental and gingival evaluation, because poor oral health and hygiene predisposes the patient to recurrent aspiration and to pulmonary infections caused by oral flora. In the absence of oral pathology, fetid breath may indicate that the patient has an anaerobic infection. Palpable nodes, especially supraclavicular and scalene adenopathy, are abnormal and imply infection (e.g., tuberculosis), neoplasm, or inflammatory disease such as sarcoidosis.

Cardiovascular Examination

Cardiac examination can be elusive in the patient with COPD. Palpation of the heart is made difficult by the hyperinflated lung and respiratory noises, which can obscure heart sounds. In patients with mild COPD without a significant degree of hypoxemia, the cardiac findings do not differ from those found in normal people. However, in more advanced disease with chronic hypoxemia, signs of right ventricular failure, or cor pulmonale, can occur. These findings can be subtle and, because of the difficulties outlined above, can be overlooked. Given the therapeutic and prognostic implications that the diagnosis of cor pulmonale carries, careful attention must be given to the signs of right ventricular failure and pulmonary hypertension.

Central cyanosis and peripheral edema are the most obvious signs of cor pulmonale. In an ambulatory patient, edema is most typically found in the lower legs, feet, and ankles, whereas it may be found only over the sacrum or posterior aspect of the thighs in a bedridden patient. Edema distributed over the face, eyelids, conjunctiva (chemosis), and upper extremities should alert the examiner to a possible superior vena cava syndrome that is due to compression by a tumor. Increased jugular venous pressure, the large a wave of right ventricular hypertrophy, and v wave of tricuspid incompetence can be observed over the jugular veins of a patient with cor pulmonale. The heave of a hypertrophied right ventricle can be palpated in the left parasternal area. On auscultation, the right ventricular S4 can be heard in the same area. The pulsation of a hypertensive pulmonary artery is best palpated over the second left intercostal space where a loud P2 can also be heard. An S3, heard in inspiration over the right ventricle, is a sign of right ventricular failure. Hepatomegaly, secondary to passive congestion, is another hallmark of right ventricular failure.

Inspection of the Trachea and Chest Wall

Deviation of the trachea from the midline is usually associated with a disease process other than COPD. This could be due to either progressive scarring and collapse with volume loss, such as with tuberculosis, or associated with a mass lesion pushing the trachea to one side. In the patient with severe COPD, a downward movement on inspiration can be seen or palpated—the so-called tracheal tug. With progressive hyperinflation, the length of the trachea palpable between the cricoid cartilage and the upper border of the sternum is decreased.

On inspection of the chest, it is important to note the use of the accessory muscles to respiration. The use of the sternocleidomastoids and scalene muscles is an attempt to compensate for the overinflation by placing the chest cage at better mechanical advantage for inspiration. As noted above, excavation or recession of the supraclavicular fossae on inspiration reflects excessive negative swings in intrathoracic pressure seen in severe airflow obstruction. Another finding associated with hyperinflation is paradoxical movement of the lateral costal margin on inspiration or the so-called Hoover's sign. Usually, the costal margin of the rib cage moves outward on inspiration. However, when hyperinflation is present and the diaphragm is in a flattened position, the costal margins move inward. The barrel-chested appearance seen in the patient with with severe COPD is also a sign of marked hyperinflation. Kyphosis and scoliosis should be looked for since kyphosco-liosis can lead to restrictive ventilatory impairment and, if severe enough, cause significant ventilation/perfusion inhomogeneity.

During palpation of the chest, the degree of chest expansion should be checked. The excursion of the chest is symmetrically reduced in severe COPD due to hyperinflation with reduction in the vital capacity. Vocal fremitus can be reduced with hyperinflation.

Percussion should be performed with the finger placed firmly in the intercostal space and both sides of the chest compared. The percussion note is increased over areas of hyperinflated lung and decreased over a pleural effusion, areas of marked pleural thickening, or consolidation of the lung. The level of the diaphragm and the excursion of the diaphragm from full inspiration to complete expiration should be checked by percussion. If hyperinflation is present, the diaphragm is lower than usual, and the excursion of the diaphragm is decreased.

Auscultation of the Chest

On auscultation, first the intensity and quality of the breath sounds should be evaluated. The intensity of the breath sounds can be estimated by asking the patient to take a few deep breaths with the mouth open and then to perform a brief maximum voluntary ventilation maneuver, breathing rapidly in and out through the open mouth for a few seconds. The intensity of the breath sounds can be subjectively rated and roughly correlates with airflow obstruction and hyperinflation. Mild degrees of airflow obstruction are not reliably picked up by this method. However, normal breath-sound intensity essentially rules out severe degrees of airflow obstruction, and if breath-sound intensity is reduced, severe airflow obstruction is much more likely.[4] The breath sounds are also reduced over areas of pleural effusion, bullae, or pleural thickening.[5] Bronchial breath sounds, distinguished by expiration being heard equally as well as inspiration and by change in the quality of the breath sounds, are present over areas of consolidation. The presence of bronchial breath sounds is an important finding when consolidation is present on the chest x-ray film because, in order for bronchial breathing to be heard, the airway into the consolidated area of the lung must be open. Therefore, the presence or absence of bronchial breath sounds can be helpful in determining whether total obstruction of the airway with a postobstructive pneumonia or atelectasis might be present. If there is any suspicion of pneumonia, egophony and "E to A" change should be listened for over the suspected areas of involvement, looking for evidence of consolidation.

The presence of airflow obstruction can be determined on physical examination either by the presence of diffuse wheezing or the prolongation of airflow. Prolongation of airflow can be roughly judged by comparing the inspiratory-to-expiratory time period ratio. It is perhaps best judged by measuring the forced expiratory time (FET), defined as the time of hearing airflow while listening with the stethoscope over the trachea while the patient is doing a forced vital capacity maneuver.[6, 7] After instructing the patient to take as deep a breath as possible and then to blow it out as fast and as completely as possible, the period of time that airflow is heard is timed in seconds. In one study in which the results of the FET were compared to spirometry, none of the subjects had airflow obstruction if the FET was three seconds or less ($FEV_1/FVC > 65\%$).[6] If the FET was six seconds or longer, all subjects had airflow obstruction ($FEV_1/FVC < 65\%$), and the degree of airflow obstruction roughly correlated with longer FETs. If the FET was between three and six seconds, some subjects were normal while others were abnormal, and no definite determination of airflow obstruction could be made. The FET can be used both to screen for airflow obstruction and to follow patients with a reversible component of airflow obstruction in order to judge the effect of therapy. Obviously, when used as a screening technique, the results should be substantiated by spirometry.

Considerable confusion exists over the terminology used to describe adventitious or extra sounds on auscultation of the chest. Laënnec's original treatise on chest auscultation used the term "rales" as a generic description of any extra lung sound and then qualified each type of rale with an adjective.[8] Later, because of the lay use of the term to describe "death rattles" in an agonal patient, Laënnec substituted the word "rhonchi" as a generic term in place of rales. When his works were translated into English, a common usage developed in the United States in which rales and rhonchi were used to describe different types of adventitious sounds, with rhonchi being reserved for coarser sounds thought to originate from secretions in the larger airways. However, other diagnosticians continued to use Laënnec's original classification, with rales referring to several types of extra sounds modified by an adjective. However, the classification system that became prevalent in the United States described three basic types of adventitious sounds, all of which could be further modified. These consisted of: (1) rales (crepitations or crackles), used to describe discontinous, fine sounds thought to originate from the smaller airways, (2) rhonchi, used to describe coarser, discontinous, gurgling sounds caused by air passing secretions in the larger airways, and (3) wheezes, used to describe continuous musical sounds associated with narrowing of airways. Recently, a joint committee of the American Thoracic Society and American College of Chest Physicians endorsed a slate of standard definitions of pulmonary terminology and proposed just two terms to describe adventitious sounds: crackles and wheezes.[9] These make eminent sense, first, because of the descriptive nature of the word "crackles," which is very appropriate for the type of sounds previously referred to as crepitations or rales, and second, because of the virtually universal acceptance of the term "wheezes" and its clear description of high-pitched musical sounds. This, however, begs the question of what to call sounds emanating from the large airways associated with secretions. Although gurgles would make descriptive sense, this term has not been widely accepted, and until some other term is endorsed for more universal acceptance, the word "rhonchi" appears to remain with us to describe these types of sounds. Therefore, in this chapter, we will use the somewhat incongruous terms "crackles," "rhonchi" (or "gurgles"), and "wheezes."

Wheezing is an important sign of airflow obstruction. If it is heard diffusely over the chest, asthma or COPD is the usual cause. These diseases must be distinguished from wheezing originating high in the airway and transmitted throughout the lung fields, but if one is careful in the evaluation with this difference clearly in mind, the distinction can usually be made. Localized wheezing can occur from local airway obstruction from a number of other causes, including foreign bodies and neoplasms. Wheezing related to a laryngeal source may also be associated with stridor on inspiration as well as wheezing on expiration.

One study evaluated 100 patients referred to a pulmonary function laboratory for spirometry and correlated the presence or absence of wheezing with pulmonary function in order to determine the sensitivity and specificity of wheezing, both to predict the presence of obstruction and its reversibility.[10] Wheezes heard during unforced breathing are relatively specific for airflow obstruction (as defined by an $FEV_1/FVC < 70\%$) but are not sensitive. That is, of 83 patients with airflow obstruction by spirometry, 48 (58%) had wheezing on unforced breathing while 35 (42%) did not. On the other hand, of the 17 patients who did not have airflow obstruction by spirometry, only two (12%) had any wheezing on unforced breathing. Wheezing also correlated with reversibility of the airflow obstruction. Twenty-nine of 48 patients with wheezing (60%) showed at least a 15% improvement in FEV_1 after inhaled isoproterenol, compared with only 3 of 35 nonwheezing obstructed patients (8%) ($p < 0.001$). When wheezing during forced expiration was examined, 80 of the 83 patients (96%) with obstruction were found by spirometry to have wheezing, but so were 11 of 17 (65%) patients without airflow obstruction. It is possible, since these patients were being referred for spirometry, that they had either mild or small airway obstruction, and wheezing was sensitive in picking up obstruction, which did not meet the criteria of an FEV_1/FVC of $< 70\%$, but this possibility was not critically examined in the study. Therefore, wheezing on forced exhalation is relatively nonspecific, although quite sensitive. One of the implications of these data is that in a patient with COPD and airflow obstruction proved by spirometry, the absence of wheezing implies lack of reversibility as indicated by lack of response to an inhaled bronchodilator.

Rhonchi or gurgles (sounds originating from large areas related to secretions) are commonly heard in COPD patients and indicate probable chronic bronchitis. On the other hand, patients with severe emphysema without significant chronic bronchitis by history may have difficulty in clearing even a normal amount of secretions and may have audible rhonchi. Listening for rhonchi in addition to a history of sputum production is important in determining how aggressive to be with bronchial hygiene measures.

Crackles are also frequently heard in patients with COPD. Thus, the presence of crackles on chest auscultation does not reliably distinguish COPD from congestive heart failure as a cause of dyspnea.[11] However, there are some differences in the crackles between these two groups of patients, primarily in their timing during inspiration. Crackles in congestive heart failure and, in fact, in restrictive disease of any etiology tend to occur late in inspiration whereas crackles associated with severe airflow obstruction tend to be primarily heard in early inspiration.[12] The character of the crackles is less easy to distinguish in these two groups of patients.[11]

The descriptive words "wet" or "moist" as opposed to "dry" have no basis in the acoustic quality of crackles, and these adjectives have not allowed separation of the crackles of patients with congestive heart failure as opposed to COPD or pneumonia when listeners were "blinded" as to the diagnosis. It is probable that when the diagnostician thinks a patient has congestive heart failure, he or she calls these crackles wet. If the same crackles are heard in a patient considered to have some other diseases, they would be called dry.

The crackles heard in idiopathic pulmonary fibrosis appear to have a different quality and are often very loud. The current theory regards crackles as probably originating from the opening of small airways, regardless of the specific disease etiology. The differences in timing are probably due to differences in critical opening volumes of the abnormal airways.[13] Thus, the most important aspect in describing crackles is the timing of their occurrence during inspiration. Crackles in COPD occur in the first half of inspiration, and those in restrictive airways disease and congestive heart failure primarily occur during the second half of inspiration.

The other type of sound that may be heard on auscultation is a pleural friction rub. Pleural rubs have a leathery quality, much like the sound of two pieces of leather being rubbed together, and give the impression of being "closer to the ear" than other sounds originating from the chest. There is often both an inspiratory and expiratory component. Pleural rubs can be heard in any process that involves the pleural surface resulting in irritation and inflammation. Thus, they can be heard with pulmonary infarcts or with pneumonias that extend to the pleural surface. When an effusion develops, the pleural rub often disappears but may reappear as the effusion resolves and the inflamed pleural surfaces touch each other again.

SUMMARY

Obtaining an accurate history and performing a thorough physical examination are extremely important in evaluating the patient with COPD. A meticulous history in conjunction with a careful physical examination enables the physician to put the patient and his/her disease into a larger context of the patient's genetic, social, occupational, medical, and personal history. Understanding the patient and his/her disease within this context enables the physician to direct diagnostic evaluations and to tailor therapy and expectation to the patient's unique situation.

Some diagnoses (e.g., chronic bronchitis) are based totally on history, and in the practical management of patients with COPD, many decisions are made on the clinical information—primarily the history and physical examination—rather than laboratory tests. The major goal of therapy in these patients is to achieve symptomatic relief. Thus, evaluation of the symptoms as an indication for therapy and continuing evaluation to follow the response to therapy are the most important determinants of therapeutic decisions.

There should be an attempt to relate the history and physical examination to pulmonary function abnormalities, but there are real limitations in these correlations that should be clearly recognized, especially with dyspnea. On the other hand, the limitations or lack of correlation may provide clues to mechanisms that lead to those particular symptoms. For example, a patient with marked carbon dioxide retention and little dyspnea may have a major component of blunted ventilatory drive that results in this clinical picture.

On physical examination, the presence of airflow obstruction can be detected by the presence of wheezing or prolonged airflow and can be roughly quantified by the forced expiratory time. Other physical findings associated with COPD are usually the result of phenomena secondary to airflow obstruction, such as hyperinflation and abnormal patterns of the use of respiratory muscles. Careful attention to these epiphenomena results in a more complete and directed evaluation and treatment of the patient with COPD.

References

1. Ashutosh K, Gilbert R, Auchincloss JH Jr, et al: Asynchronous breathing movement in patients with chronic obstructive pulmonary disease. Chest 1975;67:553–557.
2. Gilbert R, Ashutosh K, Auchincloss JH Jr, et al: Perspective study of controlled oxygen therapy: Poor prognosis of patients with asynchronous breathing. Chest 1977; 71:456–462.
3. Austen FK, Carmichael MW, Adams RD: Neurological manifestations of chronic pulmonary insufficiency. N Engl J Med 1957;257:579–590.
4. Pardee NE, Martin CJ, Morgan EH: A test of the practical value of estimating breath sound intensity: Breath sounds related to major ventilatory function. Chest 1976; 70:341–344.
5. Nairin JR, Turner Warwick M: Breath sounds in emphysema. Br J Dis Chest 1969;63:29–37.
6. Lal S, Ferguson AD, Campbell EJM: Forced expiratory time: A simple test for airways obstruction. Br Med J 1964;1:814–817.
7. Godfrey S, Edwards RTH, Campbell EJM,

et al: Clinical and physiological associations of some physical signs observed in patients with chronic airways obstruction. Thorax 1970;25:285–287.
8. Robertson AJ, Coope R: Rales, rhonchi and Laënnec. Lancet 1957;2:417–423.
9. American College of Chest Physicians, American Thoracic Society: Pulmonary Terms and Symbols. Chest 1975;67:583–593.
10. Marini JJ, Pierson DJ, Hudson LD, et al.: The significance of wheezing and chronic airflow obstruction. Am Rev Respir Dis 1979;120:1069–1072.
11. Hudson LD, Conn RD, Matsubara RS, et al: Rales—diagnostic usefulness of qualitative adjectives, abstracted. Am Rev Respir Dis 1976;113:187.
12. Nath AR, Capel LH: Inspiratory crackles—early and late. Thorax 1974; 29:223–227.
13. Nath AR, Capel LH: Inspiratory crackles and mechanical events of breathing. Thorax 1974;29:695–698.

Additional References

Forgacs P: The functional basis of pulmonary sounds. Chest 1978;73:399–405.

Godfrey S, Edwards, RTH, Campbell EJM, et al: Repeatability of physical signs in airways obstruction. Thorax 1969;24:4–9.

LABORATORY EVALUATION OF PATIENTS WITH COPD

RONALD B. GEORGE
WILLIAM M. ANDERSON

Laboratory tests remain an essential part of the management of patients with asthma, chronic bronchitis, and emphysema. While the presence of chronic obstructive pulmonary disease (COPD) is often evident from the history and physical findings, the quantitation of the disease and evaluation of its response to therapy are based on objective data. Just as patients with hypertension are followed with serial blood pressure determinations, patients with COPD should be followed with simple objective tests such as spirometry or peak flow measurements, even when their disease appears stable. Arterial blood gas analysis, chest radiographs, sputum examination, and other tests may be indicated during exacerbations. This chapter discusses tests available for the documentation and management of patients with COPD and their indications.

Since pulmonary function tests and arterial blood gas analysis are used along with the history and physical examination to identify the various disease syndromes (asthma, chronic bronchitis, or emphysema) and their severity, these tests are discussed first. We will then cover chest radiographs, examination of sputum, complete blood count, serum electrolyte levels, and the electrocardiogram, which are especially useful during exacerbations of COPD. The discussion includes certain specialized tests indicated for selected patients with COPD: sleep studies, exercise studies, specialized radiographic techniques, skin tests, serologic tests, determination of serum protease levels, and biopsies. Finally, we will consider the costs of these tests in relation to their usefulness to clinicians and their patients.

PULMONARY FUNCTION TESTS

Routine spirometry provides the clinician with the basic pulmonary function assessment needed for screening, diagnosis, and evaluation of prognosis and therapy in patients with obstructive pulmonary disease. Spirometry along with the history and physical examination determines the need for other common tests (lung volumes, diffusing capacity, blood gases) or specialized ones (inhalation challenge, exercise, polysomnographic) of pulmonary function. Indications for performance of routine tests in patients with obstructive lung disease include: (1) initial evaluation of the patient with symptoms suggestive of pulmonary disease, (2) preoperative evaluation for thoracic and nonthoracic surgery, (3) evaluation of response to therapeutic interventions, (4) progressive neuromuscular disease or kyphoscoliosis, and (5) periodic evaluation of workers in high-risk occupations.

Spirometry

Spirometric testing is inexpensive and can be easily performed in the physician's office. Table 4–1 outlines the standards for acceptable office spirometers.[1] The most important physiologic measurements derived from spirometry are the forced vital capacity (FVC), the forced expiratory volume in one second (FEV_1), and the forced expiratory flow over 25% to 75% of the FVC ($FEF_{25-75\%}$). Each measurement should always be compared to a predicted

Table 4–1. **Office Spirometer Standards***

1. Measure FVC, FEV_1, and $FEF_{25-75\%}$ and provide a permanent graphic record
2. Capable of measuring a minimum volume of 7 L with accuracy of ±3% of volume compared with an accepted laboratory standard
3. Record FEV_1 and $FEF_{25-75\%}$ to ±5% against this system
4. Record air flow for at least 6 seconds (preferably 10 seconds for severe COPD)
5. A "back extrapolation" method of flow curve analysis should be allowed in devices that do not record the initial portion of the spirogram.
6. Calibrated to body temperature and atmospheric pressure, completely saturated with water vapor at body temperature (BTPS) at 25°C
7. Cost less than $1000
8. Weight less than 35 lb

*Modified from the American College of Chest Physicians Committee Statement on Clinic and Office Pulmonary Function Testing: Office spirometry in clinical practice. *Chest* 74:298, 1978, with permission.

Table 4–2. **Examples of Restrictive Lung Disease That May Affect Spirometry Testing in COPD**

Intrinsic	Extrinsic	Muscular Disorders
Interstitial diseases:	Obesity	Guillain-Barré syndrome
Collagen vascular disease	Kyphoscoliosis	Myasthenia gravis
Interstitial pneumonitis	Pleural effusion	Myxedema
Pneumoconiosis	Pneumothorax	Eaton-Lambert syndrome
Pulmonary fibrosis	Tumor or enlarged lymph	Myositis
Pulmonary edema	nodes	
Hypersensitivity	Paralyzed diaphragm	
pneumonitis		
Infiltrative diseases:		
Granulomatous		
Neoplastic		

normal value based on the patient's age, sex, and height. Predicted values that are usually reported represent studies of white subjects and should be decreased by 10% to 15% for blacks.[2]

The FVC is the lung volume expired from maximum inspiration, i.e., total lung capacity (TLC), to maximum expiration, i.e., residual volume (RV), with the patient exhaling as rapidly as possible. Airway obstruction is inferred from a reduction in the FEV_1. To avoid the effects of superimposed restrictive lung disease (Table 4–2), the FEV_1 is compared to the total FVC and expressed as a percent ($FEV_1/FVC \times 100$). With superimposed restrictive disease, the $FEV_1/FVC\%$ may appear normal or inappropriately high for the degree of

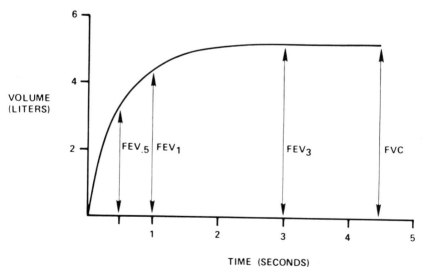

Figure 4–1. A typical forced expiratory spirogram showing the timed volumes obtained from the tracing. $FEV_{.5}$, FEV_1, and FEV_3 represent the forced expired volumes at 0.5, 1.0, and 3.0 seconds, respectively. Forced vital capacity (FVC) is the maximum volume that can be forcefully exhaled. (From Conrad SA, George RB: Clinical pulmonary function testing, in George RB, Light RW, Matthay RA (eds): *Chest Medicine.* New York, Churchill Livingstone, 1983, p 168, by permission.)

reduction in the FEV_1. Expressing the FEV_1 as a percent of FVC also has the advantage of comparison between individuals of different body size. Other values measured from the spirogram include the FEV in 0.5 seconds ($FEV_{.5}$) and in 3 seconds (FEV_3), but whether they add to the information obtained from FEV_1, FVC, FEV_1/FVC, and $FEF_{25-75\%}$) is questionable (Fig. 4–1).

Forced expiratory flows (Fig. 4–2) are sometimes measured along with or instead of forced expiratory volumes. The $FEF_{200-1200}$ measures flow in the initial segment of expiration (200 to 1200 ml) and correlates with peak flow measurements. When the FEV_1 is normal, the $FEF_{25-75\%}$ has been shown to correlate with other tests of small airways dysfunction and with early pathologic findings of chronic bronchitis and emphysema.[3, 4]

Flow-Volume Loops

An alternative way of expressing spirometric measurements is by simultaneous recording of volume and flow during inspiration and expiration to produce a flow-volume loop. Although not necessary for routine spirometric testing, this technique may provide information concerning obstruction of the upper airways (larynx, trachea, and mainstem bronchi) that may complicate COPD (Fig. 4–3).[5] The flow-volume loop also offers the advantage of

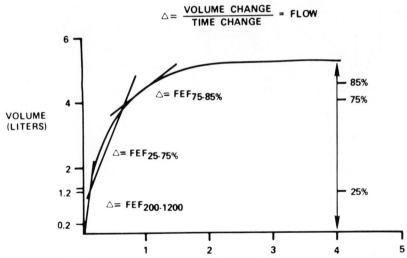

Figure 4–2. A typical forced expiratory spirogram showing the time-averaged flows obtained from the tracing. The flow between 200 and 1200 ml exhaled air ($FEF_{200-1200}$) is taken at a high lung volume near TLC. The average between 25% and 75% of exhaled vital capacity ($FEF_{25-75\%}$) measures flow in the midportion of the exhaled vital capacity. The average flow between 75% and 85% of exhaled vital capacity ($FEF_{75-85\%}$) measures flow at a low lung volume, when small airway resistance is dominant. (From Conrad SA, George RB: Clinical pulmonary function testing, in George RB, Light RW, Matthay RA (eds): *Chest Medicine.* New York, Churchill Livingstone, 1983, p 169, by permission.)

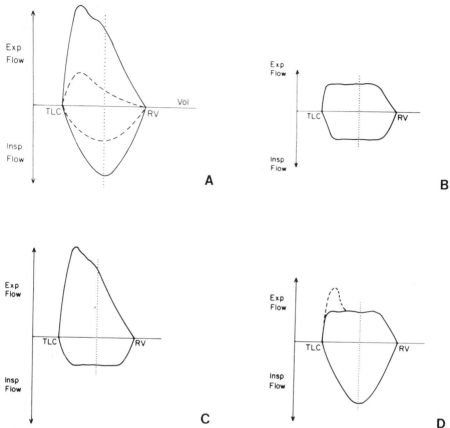

Figure 4–3. *A,* Maximal inspiratory and expiratory flow-volume curves in normal subjects (solid line), and those with COPD (dashed line). The stippled line represents 50% of vital capacity. *B,* Fixed intra- or extrathoracic obstruction. *C,* Extrathoracic variable obstruction. *D,* Intrathoracic variable obstruction; dashed line represents a flow transient occasionally observed just before the plateau in intrathoracic obstruction. (Modified from Kryger M, Bode F, Antic R, et al: Diagnosis of obstruction of the upper and central airways. *American Journal of Medicine* 61:85, 1976, by permission.)

instantaneous determination of peak flow and the ability to separate the early effort-dependent from the later effort-independent portions of expiratory flow.

When spirometry reveals airway obstruction, a repeat study after inhaling a bronchodilator aerosol helps to separate bronchospastic disorders such as asthma and some cases of chronic bronchitis from more irreversible disease (i.e., emphysema). If the FEV_1 improves $\geq 15\%$ after an inhaled bronchodilator, this is evidence for a bronchospastic disorder.[6] While the FVC and $FEF_{25-75\%}$ may also increase after bronchodilator therapy, the FEV_1 remains the best test of reversibility because it has less inherent variability.[7] In the patient who does not respond to bronchodilators, the physician should consider a trial period of days to weeks of bronchodilator therapy to assess subjective and objective (spirometric) improvement. Even "irreversible" airway obstruction has been shown to improve after a two-week trial of corticosteroids. In the absence of objective improvement in spirometry, steroid therapy is not warranted because of related complications.

In assessing the degree of airway obstruction, variability exists in the interpretation of what to consider mild, moderate, and severe obstruction as shown in Figure 4–4.[8–12] We consider the FEV_1 as related to the predicted normal values, provided FVC is normal. If there is associated restrictive disease, this will decrease all the measured lung volumes, including the FEV_1. In this case, a decrease in FEV_1/FVC to less than 75% indicates airway obstruction. A ratio of less than 75% but greater than 60% is interpreted as mild obstruction; 40% to 60% indicates a moderate obstruction, and less than 40% indicates severe obstruction. This method of using a fixed percentage range to represent the expected variation of individuals within a group has been criticized. Error may be introduced either by setting the limits too widely at high values or within too narrow a range at low values. The use of 95% confidence intervals about the predicted regression line has gained increasing acceptance (Table 4–3).[13] While the FEV_1/FVC criteria are useful for excluding the effects of restriction, with severe functional impairment the extent of involvement may correlate better with FEV_1 than the ratio.[12]

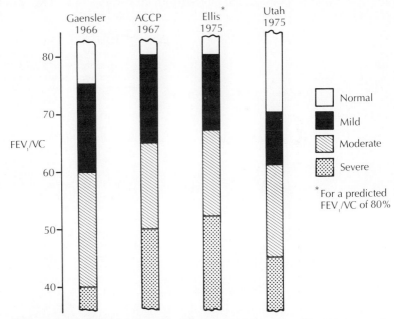

Figure 4–4. Variation in obstructive disease categories using FEV_1/VC ratios. The criteria of Ellis and colleagues are presented as percentages of a predicted FEV_1/VC ratio of 80%. (Modified from Cary J, Huseby J, Culver B, et al: Variability in interpretation of pulmonary function tests. *Chest* 76:389, 1976, by permission).

Table 4–3. **Interpretation of Degree of Obstruction from the Forced Expiratory Spirogram***

| | | 95% Confidence Interval Method of Predicted Value Minus Measured Value (%)† | |
Category	Fixed Percent Method (%)	*Women*	*Men*
Normal	>75	<9.1	<8.3
Mild	61–75	9.1–18.1	8.3–16.5
Moderate	40–60	18.2–36.3	16.6–33.1
Severe	<40	≥36.4	≥33.2

*Modified from Morris AH, Kanner RE, Crapo RO, Gardner RM: *Clinical Pulmonary Function Testing—A Manual of Uniform Laboratory Procedures*, ed 2. Salt Lake City, Intermountain Thoracic Society, 1984, p 22.

†The airway obstruction category by this method is determined by the differences between the predicted and measured values of $FEV_1/FVC\%$.

Lung Volumes and Diffusing Capacity

Measurement of lung volumes is indicated in patients suspected of having restrictive impairment on the basis of spirometry, physical findings, or chest radiographs. In such patients, a two-stage vital capacity can eliminate the effects of air trapping on the vital capacity (Fig. 4–5). The functional residual capacity (FRC) is measured by gas dilution or body plethysmography, and the residual volume (RV) is calculated from this value. The FRC is measured

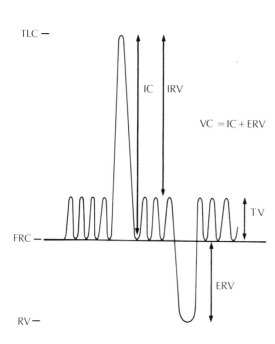

Figure 4–5. Spirometer tracing from a two-stage vital capacity maneuver, showing the lung volumes and compartments measured from the tracing. The tracing is obtained by having the subject breathe quietly for a brief period of time, a maximal inspiration follows, and then a return to tidal breathing for three or four breaths. The subject then makes a slow maximal expiration and returns to tidal breathing. Total lung capacity (TLC), functional residual capacity (FRC), and residual volume (RV) are shown for orientation. Measurements include tidal volume (TV), inspiratory reserve volume (IRV), expiratory reserve volume (ERV), inspiratory capacity (IC), and vital capacity (VC). This separation of vital capacity into two phases reduces air trapping in patients with obstructive lung disease. (From Conrad SA: Lung volumes, in Conrad SA, Kinasewitz GT, George RB (eds): *Pulmonary Function Testing: Principles and Practice*. New York, Churchill Livingstone, 1984, p 11, by permission.)

because of its reproducibility, since it is the baseline volume from which the patient normally inspires. Gas dilution techniques may underestimate FRC in obstructive lung disease because of incomplete mixing of the test gas caused by areas of trapped gas. Burns and Scheinhorn have recently shown that the helium dilution technique may underestimate TLC in moderate and severe obstruction 22% and 38%, respectively, requiring correction equations.[14] Extending the time allowed for gas dilution permits improved mixing within poorly ventilated air spaces.

In severe obstructive lung disease, even though the FVC may be reduced, the total lung capacity is usually increased because of air trapping with a marked increase in the FRC, RV, and RV/TLC ratio. An increased TLC in a stable patient usually indicates the presence of emphysema. Combined obstructive and restrictive disorders are inferred when spirometry reveals moderate to severe obstruction while TLC and the RV/TLC ratio are normal.

The diffusing capacity for carbon monoxide (DL_{CO}) indirectly measures the ability of oxygen to transfer from the alveolar gas to pulmonary capillary blood. Carbon monoxide is used as the test gas because it has similar membrane diffusion properties to oxygen, is not normally found in the blood, and has a hemoglobin affinity 200 times greater than oxygen. The measured DL_{CO} is proportional to the total effective surface area available for gas exchange. This value may be helpful in assessing the presence of emphysema in patients with airway obstruction, since the destruction of alveolar walls results in a decrease in surface area for diffusion. The DL_{CO} is usually normal in patients with asthma and bronchitis.

Arterial Blood Gases and pH

Arterial blood gases are essential to the assessment of severity of lung function impairment in patients with moderate to severe COPD. Their indications are shown in Table 4–4. The normal arterial oxygen tension (Pa_{O_2}) in young adults at sea level is approximately 80 to 100 torr. This value normally decreases with age because of a gradual increase in ventilation/perfusion ($\dot{V}/\dot{Q}$) mismatching. Correction for age can be made for both the supine

Table 4–4. **Indications for Arterial Blood Gas Analysis in COPD Patients**

1. Initial assessment of the symptomatic patient
2. Cor pulmonale and left ventricular heart failure
3. Polycythemia
4. Acute deterioration in cardiopulmonary status
5. Arrhythmia
6. Prior to air travel
7. Initial and periodic evaluation of oxygen therapy
8. Altered mental status
9. Evaluation of response to oxygen or other drug therapy
10. Serum electrolyte abnormalities
11. Preoperative evaluation

Table 4–5. Comparison of Arterial Blood Gas Values at Different Levels of Airway Obstruction in Acute Bronchial Asthma*

Degree of Obstruction	Mean FEV$_1$ (% of Predicted)	pH	Pa$_{CO_2}$ (mmHg)	Pa$_{O_2}$ (mmHg)	Bicarbonate (mEq/L)
Mild	59	7.47	25	83	25
Moderate	35	7.45	33	71	22
Severe	18	7.42	39	63	24

*Modified from McFadden ER Jr, Lyons HA: Arterial blood gas tension in asthma. Reprinted by permission of the *New England Journal of Medicine* 278:1029, 1968.

(predicted Pa$_{O_2}$ = 109 − 0.43 × age) and sitting (predicted Pa$_{O_2}$ = 104.2 − 0.27 × age) patient.[15, 16] Normal oxygen saturation (≥94%) is then calculated or measured directly and represents the ability of hemoglobin to bind oxygen. Even though a patient may have a normal Pa$_{O_2}$ and arterial oxygen percent saturation (SaO$_2$), oxygen content (about 20 vol% for normal subjects with a hemoglobin of 15 g/100 ml blood) may be reduced in the presence of anemia, with subsequent reduction in tissue oxygenation. The hemoglobin level is important in evaluating COPD patients, since it is often elevated in the presence of chronic hypoxemia in order to compensate for the reduced oxygen saturation.

The partial pressure of carbon dioxide (Pa$_{CO_2}$) is the best indicator of alveolar ventilation. Certain individuals with COPD become insensitive to arterial Pa$_{CO_2}$ and chronically hypoventilate with resultant hypercapnia, cyanosis, and cor pulmonale. Since the respiratory drive of these patients is often dependent upon oxygen receptors, they may decompensate acutely and develop respiratory failure when given oxygen to breathe. During exacerbations, they must be observed with serial blood gas determinations with careful administration of controlled doses of oxygen. Patients with normal or low Pa$_{CO_2}$ levels (e.g., during acute asthma attacks) generally tolerate inspired oxygen without hypoventilating and do not require serial blood gas determinations.

Arterial blood gas analysis is useful for determining the severity of an acute asthma attack (Table 4–5). Hypercapnia during an attack should be considered a grave prognostic sign, since these patients all require medical intensive care.[17, 18] Arterial blood gas values should be used together with other findings such as spirographic results and physical findings. They have not been found to be predictive of relapse in patients with acute bronchial asthma.

Bronchial Challenge Tests

Bronchial inhalation challenge tests with pharmacologic and antigenic substances were introduced to North America in 1945 and have been extensively evaluated.[19, 20] Bronchial hyperresponsiveness (BHR), defined as an increased response to inhaled methacholine or histamine, may be involved in the deterioration of lung function in some COPD patients. The prevalence of BHR in COPD has been poorly defined. In a recent random population sample, 27 of 59 COPD patients demonstrated BHR when challenged with histamine.[21] Indications for bronchial inhalation challenge are listed in Table 4–6. In COPD patients with abnormalities on routine spirometry, bronchial inhalation challenge adds little to the diagnostic workup except in these specific instances. Most patients with asthma do not need inhalation challenge, and those with moderate or severe impairment should be tested with caution.

The response to inhalation challenge may be immediate, late, or combined. The immediate response develops within minutes after a cumulative dose has been inhaled. The response is quantitated as the dose of inhaled antigen (measured on a logarithmic scale) required to cause a significant decrease in flow rate. For example, the provocation concentration of inhaled agent required to produce a 20% decrease in FEV_1 is called the PC_{20}. Other acceptable changes in pulmonary function tests after bronchial provocation include a decrease of 10% in vital capacity, 25% in the $FEF_{25-75\%}$, and 40% in airway conductance.[19] This is felt to be an IgE-mediated response and occurs at doses much lower than those required to produce a similar response in normal subjects. The late response develops one to six hours after exposure to antigens and occupational materials but not after histamine, methacholine, and carbachol. While the immediate response is felt to be caused by acute bronchospasm, the late response is the result of inflammatory changes, intramural mucus accumulation, and smooth muscle contraction and may be associated with fever and leukocytosis. IgE and IgG mechanisms have been proposed. Reaction to the diluent (80% propylene glycol and 20% water) is the control, and a response to diluent precludes further testing. These studies should be performed by laboratories experienced in the procedure and with resuscitation equipment and an available physician trained in dealing with complications. Technicians performing bronchial challenge testing should be certified in cardiopulmonary resuscitation.

The measurement of FEV_1 is the most widely applied test in evaluation of response to bronchial challenge.[19] When the primary purpose of the test is to establish hyperreactive airways, the challenge may be performed with one

Table 4–6. **Indications for Bronchial Inhalation Challenge Testing**

1. History of wheezing with normal pulmonary function tests
2. Chronic unexplained cough
3. Unexplained dyspnea or exercise intolerance
4. Recurrent pneumonia with no known predisposing factors
5. History of bronchiolitis or other childhood lung injury
6. Elucidation of the role of specific allergens in asthma
7. Evaluation of treatment modalities and blocking agents
8. Pulmonary symptoms associated with occupational exposure

to three doses of bronchoconstricting drugs. Normal subjects do not usually respond to the initial dose, while asthmatics usually do. This abbreviated method is not recommended for antigen challenges.

Exercise is a form of inhalation challenge that may aid in the diagnosis of exercise-induced bronchospasm. Certain patients have increased airway reactivity during exertion, which is felt to be secondary to cooling and drying of the bronchial mucosa. Symptoms may be limited to cough, chest tightness, or mild wheezing during exercise or shortly afterward. FEV_1 measurements taken before and three, five, 10 and 15 minutes after exercise in such individuals help to make a diagnosis of exercise-induced bronchospasm and provide a guide to bronchodilator therapy, allowing them to be physically active.

Exercise Testing

In nonasthmatic forms of COPD, exercise testing has a different role and may be used to evaluate an inappropriate degree of dyspnea in the patient with a mild-to-moderate abnormality on pulmonary function tests. Exercise testing may also be useful to evaluate exercise capacity and the response to exercise training programs, and to assess the need for oxygen. Furthermore, recent studies indicate that preoperative exercise testing may be predictive of post-thoracotomy complications in COPD patients under consideration for surgery.[22]

The normal cardiopulmonary response to mild exercise is to increase cardiac output primarily by increasing heart rate, increase oxygen uptake (as shown by an increase in the arterial-mixed venous oxygen difference), and increase oxygen consumption ($\dot{V}_{O_2}$) and carbon dioxide production ($\dot{V}_{CO_2}$). The $\dot{V}_{O_2}$ maximum ($\dot{V}_{O_2}$max) is a reliable guide to aerobic capacity in normal subjects. Maximum exercise is normally limited by hemodynamic and metabolic factors, since with increasing levels of exercise, blood flow eventually becomes inadequate to maintain aerobic metabolism. At this point, lactic acidosis develops with a disproportionate increase in minute ventilation relative to oxygen consumption; this has been termed the anaerobic threshold (AT). In the dyspneic patient with left ventricular failure, the stroke volume is reduced. With exercise, heart rate increases and the arteriovenous oxygen difference widens more at any given level of $\dot{V}_{O_2}$ than in normal subjects.

The dyspneic patient with COPD is not limited by hemodynamic factors but by ventilatory limitation and abnormal gas exchange. With increasing exercise, these patients are unable to reach their predicted maximal heart rate because of an early achievement of their predicted maximal ventilation (Fig. 4–6). Factors responsible for ventilatory limitation include altered pulmonary mechanics with respiratory muscle fatigue, increased work of breathing, and large dead space ventilation. In addition, limitation of gas exchange may occur secondary to abnormal ventilatory control, cor pulmonale, and shunting. Thus, $\dot{V}_{O_2}$max becomes dyspnea-limited and AT may not be achieved, reducing the usefulness of exercise testing in the diagnosis and management of COPD. Furthermore, motivational influences may limit interpretation of response to rehabilitation. In patients who are unable to perform progressive, incremental exercise to the maximum, a six- or 12-minute walking test (with arterial blood gases or oximetry) may be useful in assessing functional impairment.[23, 24] Other recommended tests include clinical scales of dyspnea and psychophysical scales using visual analogs.[25]

One of the most useful applications of exercise tests is in the evaluation of the patient for oxygen therapy. Oxygen has been shown to improve exercise performance and decrease mortality in hypoxemic COPD patients. Whether oxygen use lowers mortality in COPD patients who have arterial desaturation only during maximal exercise is not known.[26] For a discussion of exercise in pulmonary patients, see Chapter 11.

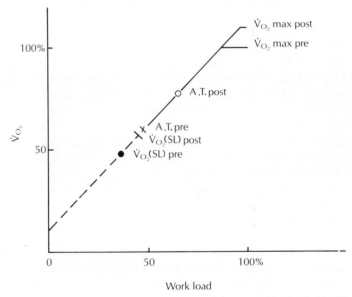

Figure 4–6. Comparison of the $\dot{V}_{O_2}$ max and the anaerobic threshold (AT) in exercise testing in normal subjects and in patients with COPD. In normal subjects the $\dot{V}_{O_2}$ max reaches a plateau that provides an objective endpoint to the test. In addition, the anaerobic threshold is a valuable marker that can be detected at submaximal loads. In normal subjects, the AT increases both in terms of the absolute value and in terms of the percentage of the $\dot{V}_{O_2}$ after training. In patients with COPD, the peak oxygen consumption is symptom-limited ($\dot{V}_{O_2}$ (SL)), and if it increases after training, this could be ascribed to a motivational effect. In this diagram, which is representative of many symptomatic COPD patients, the $\dot{V}_{O_2}$ (SL) occurs below the level at which AT occurs, thus rendering the AT of little value in this setting. (From Belman MJ: Exercise testing and training in patients with COPD. *Pulmonary Clinical Update* 1985; vol. 1, lesson 3, by permission.)

Table 4–7. **Clinical Features of Sleep Apnea Syndrome***

1. Snoring, especially sonorous with intermittent pauses
2. Excessive daytime sleepiness
3. Abnormal motor activity during sleep
4. Apneic periods during sleep
5. Personality or intellectual changes
6. Hypertension
7. Morning headaches
8. Sexual impotence
9. Cardiorespiratory failure:
• Congestive heart failure
• Dependent edema
• Shortness of breath on exertion
• Pulmonary hypertension
10. Nocturnal enuresis

*Modified from Chesson AL: Sleep-related breathing disorders and their monitoring, in Conrad SA, Kinasewitz GT, George RB (eds): *Pulmonary Function Testing: Principles and Practice.* New York, Churchill Livingstone, 1984, p 292, by permission.

Polysomnography (Sleep Studies)

Asymptomatic, presumably normal individuals have been shown to have nocturnal desaturations during sleep, and this appears to correlate with male sex, obesity, the postmenopausal state, and increasing age.[27] Other factors (Table 4–7) should be considered in any patient under evaluation for sleep apnea. For the patient with COPD, sleep may not be a period of rest and recuperation at all but rather a time of considerable stress that may play a role in the progression of the disease.[28] There are three types of sleep apnea: obstructive (absence of airflow despite continued respiratory effort), nonobstructive (absence of airflow and absence of respiratory effort), and mixed (initial absence of airflow and absence of respiratory effort, progressing to active respiratory effort without resumption of airflow). COPD patients show components of all three types, especially the mixed type (Fig. 4–7). Sleep-disordered breathing (SDB) may be more accurate than sleep apnea and is the preferred term.

Routine pulmonary function tests have had poor predictive value in deciding which patients with sleep apnea have significant SDB. However, the daytime waking supine arterial blood gas and SaO_2 does correlate with the mean levels of SaO_2, lowest levels of Pa_{O_2} and highest levels of Pa_{CO_2} during sleep.[28, 29] The clinician should consider obtaining a sleep study in a COPD patient with symptoms of SDB (Table 4–7), and when the resting pulmonary function and arterial blood gases do not explain the presence of pulmonary hypertension, polycythemia, cor pulmonale, or cardiac arrhythmias.

CHEST RADIOGRAPHY

Standard posteroanterior and lateral chest radiographs are useful in the initial evaluation of patients with COPD and may be indicated during acute

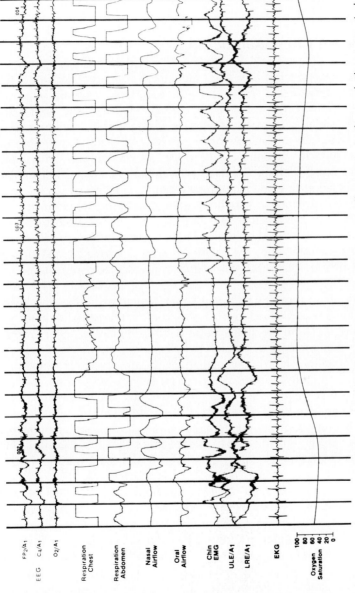

Figure 4–7. In mixed central and obstructive sleep apnea, airflow and respiratory efforts cease simultaneously, but progressively more vigorous respiratory effort occurs before airflow is reinstated. Arousal, reflected by increased EMG activity, is associated with return of effective respiratory effort. Oximetry indicates that maximum oxygen desaturation occurs after resumption of airflow, which reflects the lung-to-periphery circulation delay. EMG artifact is noted in many of the leads. (From Chesson AL: Sleep-related breathing disorders and their monitoring, in Conrad SA, Kinasewitz GT, George RB (eds): *Pulmonary Function Testing: Principles and Practice.* New York, Churchill Livingstone, 1984, p 300, by permission.)

exacerbations. They may detect static abnormalities such as hyperinflation, bullous changes or thickening of bronchial walls, or acute changes such as pneumonia, congestive heart failure, or pneumothorax, which are responsible for exacerbations. They may also detect associated diseases such as lung malignancy.

The Normal Chest Radiograph

A normal posteroanterior (PA) chest radiograph with identification of the normal anatomic structures is shown in Figure 4–8. From an analysis of over 100,000 chest films in a hospital-based population, Sagel and colleagues concluded that routine screening radiographs during hospitalization or prior to surgery are indicated in patients over age 20.[30] A lateral film should be obtained in addition to screening patients over 40 years of age. In patients with COPD, a chest film should be part of the initial evaluation to determine whether hyperinflation or evidence of lung destruction is present and to look for associated abnormalities. The heart size should be determined, the costophrenic angle should be examined for pleural fluid; chest wall structures, including ribs and vertebrae should also be evaluated. Instead of relying on the radiologist's interpretation, the physician who is caring for the patient should personally look at each film, and any disagreements should be discussed.

The mediastinum contains many important structures besides the heart. The trachea should be examined for size and position. Of special significance in patients with COPD are the hilar shadows, consisting of the major bronchi as well as the pulmonary arteries and veins and their branches. Since the hilar areas are common sites of lung malignancies, any change in serial films should be noted carefully.[31] The size of the pulmonary vessels is important because they may be engorged in early left ventricular failure. In pulmonary hypertension, large hilar vessels are seen in association with small peripheral vessels. Hilar lymph nodes are commonly involved in chronic inflammatory diseases, especially granulomas such as tuberculosis or histoplasmosis. In such cases, calcification of the hilar nodes usually indicates that the disease is benign.

Specialized views may be indicated in certain patients if the PA and lateral films suggest an abnormality that is not definitive.[32] Oblique views are especially useful for evaluating the pulmonary hila, and the lordotic view is designed to decrease overlying shadows of the ribs and clavicles to allow the apices of the lung to be more clearly studied. The lordotic view may be useful in patients suspected of having apical tumors or tuberculosis, although conventional tomograms or computerized tomography (CT) may show these areas better. An expiration film may be obtained in patients suspected of having small pneumothoraces. A lateral decubitus film, in which patients lie on their side and the x-ray beam is shot across the table, is useful for defining small pleural effusions. Bilateral decubitus films are usually taken so that both pleural cavities can be studied. The presence of a fluid layer of 10 mm or greater in thickness on the lateral decubitus film suggests a significant pleural effusion and is usually an indication for thoracentesis, unless congestive heart failure is apparent.[33]

Conventional tomograms, CT scans, arteriograms, ventilation-perfusion radioisotope scans, chest fluoroscopy, bronchograms, and esophograms may be useful in specific instances as determined by the routine chest film as well as the history, physical examination, and other clinical findings. These specialized procedures are not indicated for the routine management of patients with COPD. In patients with suspected hilar densities, conventional tomograms taken in the 55° oblique position are useful for analysis of the hilum and its contents.[34] CT is especially useful for evaluation of the mediastinum and chest wall. It is also helpful in analyzing peripheral densities of the lung for cavitation and/or calcification. In patients with metastatic malignancy, CT may identify densities that are not visible on plain films.[35]

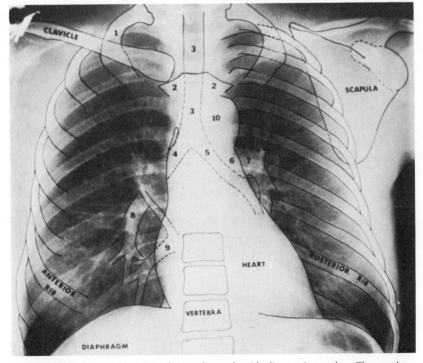

Figure 4–8. Posteroanterior (PA) chest radiograph with diagnostic overlay. The numbers identify the following structures: first rib (1), upper portion of manubrium (2), trachea (3), right main bronchus (4), left main bronchus (5), main pulmonary artery (6), left pulmonary artery (7), right interlobar pulmonary artery (8), right pulmonary vein (9), and aortic arch (10). (From Matthay RA, Sostman HD: Chest radiology, in George RB, Light RW, Matthay RA, (eds): *Chest Medicine*. New York, Churchill-Livingstone, 1983, p 136, by permission.)

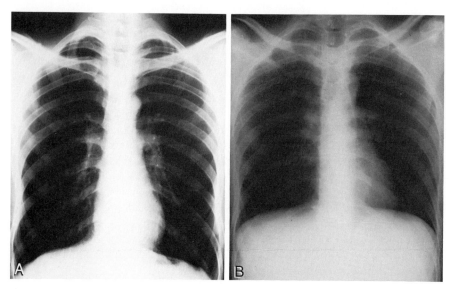

Figure 4–9. Effect of hyperinflation on the chest film during an acute asthma attack. *A,* This PA film, taken at the time of hospitalization of a 32-year-old man for asthma, shows low flat diaphragm shadows, a long narrow cardiac shadow, and wide intercostal spaces. *B,* During recovery 36 hours later, the film is now within normal limits.

The Chest Radiograph in Patients with Asthma

In patients with stable asthma who are not experiencing an acute attack, the chest film is usually normal. During acute exacerbations, marked hyperinflation is usually present, and the film may resemble that of a patient with severe emphysema (Fig. 4–9). Hyperinflation is an important part of the pathophysiology of the acute asthma attack, and the chest radiograph is a relatively easy way to quantitate this phenomenon. Chest films are not indicated in all asthma attacks and are only necessary in severe attacks, usually those requiring hospitalization. If the initial chest radiograph shows no complication, such as pneumothorax or infection, follow-up chest films are usually not required.

The Chest Radiograph in Chronic Bronchitis

In mild chronic bronchitis without complicating disease, the chest radiograph is normal. With progressive disease, the first characteristic finding is increased lung markings. This characteristic pattern of increased lung markings, also called "dirty lungs," is subjective and lacks pathologic correlation (Fig. 4–10).[36] More specific are "ring shadows," which are thickened bron-

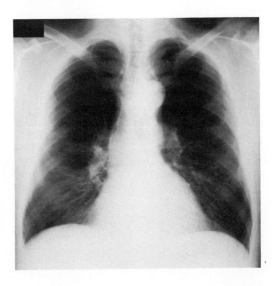

Figure 4–10. PA chest film of a 56-year-old man with chronic bronchitis. The lungs do not appear hyperinflated, and the diaphragm contour is normal. The heart is normal in size, and the pulmonary arteries are enlarged. Peribronchial markings are increased, and interstitial shadows are prominent ("increased lung markings").

chial walls seen on end, and "tram lines," which are parallel branching shadows seen in the right lower lung field in patients with chronic bronchitis.[37] Both ring shadows and tram lines are thought to represent thickened bronchial walls.

Bronchograms of patients with severe bronchitis demonstrate irregular bronchial walls and dilated lumens of the bronchial mucous glands. However, bronchograms are dangerous in these patients since they may cause acute bronchospasm. If bronchiectasis is suspected, CT is a noninvasive way to diagnose it; however, unless the disease is localized, the diagnosis of bronchiectasis has little clinical relevance, since its treatment is similar to that of severe chronic bronchitis. In advanced chronic bronchitis associated with hypoxemia, pulmonary hypertension occurs with dilation of the proximal pulmonary vessels and enlargement of right atrial and ventricular shadows.

The Chest Radiograph in Patients with Emphysema

Although the chest radiograph is usually normal in the milder forms of emphysema, an accurate diagnosis can often be made from the chest radiograph in severe emphysema. The criteria for emphysema include the arterial deficiency pattern (hyperinflation with pulmonary oligemia and the presence of bullae), and the increased markings pattern (overly prominent and irregular vascular markings and enlargement of the pulmonary hila). With hyperinflation, there is an increase in the anterior-posterior diameter of the chest and flattening of the diaphragm, best visualized on the lateral chest film (Fig. 4–11). The lateral view also demonstrates increased width of the retrosternal space. The heart is typically long and narrow because of the

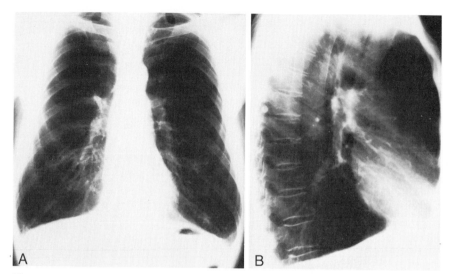

Figure 4–11. PA and lateral chest films of a 62-year-old man with emphysema, taken during hospitalization for pneumococcal pneumonia involving the right upper lobe. *A,* The lungs appear hyperinflated. The areas of consolidation in the upper lobe outline the bullous changes of underlying emphysema. The film superficially resembles that seen with granulomas, with multiple upper lobe cavities. No air-fluid levels are visible. The clinical course is that of pneumococcal pneumonia, and response to antibiotics is rapid, although radiographic resolution may take several weeks. *B,* The lateral film shows the low flat diaphragms and increased retrosternal air space typical of emphysema.

hyperinflation, which lowers the diaphragm and enlongates the pericardium. This is in contrast with the heart shadow in patients with chronic bronchitis, which is usually normal in size or enlarged.

Bullous changes are usually most evident at the apices in patients with emphysema, although they may be more marked at the lung bases in panacinar emphysema. On the lateral view, bullous changes are most prominent in the lung periphery either retrosternally or along the spine, diaphragm, and lung apices. Bullae may become infected and develop air-fluid levels, or they may rupture to produce pneumothorax. These complications usually require prompt therapy because of the severe underlying airways obstruction. Other associated abnormalities that may be evident on the chest film include neoplasms, pneumonia, and chronic infections such as tuberculosis.

Patients with far-advanced emphysema who develop lobar pneumonia may have a distorted pattern of consolidation that resembles granulomatous disease, especially if the pneumonia involves an upper lobe.[38] This pattern of "emphysema pneumonia" was described several years ago and is of interest because its atypical appearance may suggest chronic granulomatous disease (Fig. 4–11). Patients with pneumococcal lobar pneumonia who have emphysema generally respond in the usual manner to antibiotic therapy, although the resolution of abnormalities on the chest film may be delayed. In patients with pneumonia complicating chronic bronchitis or emphysema, complete resolution may be delayed for several months even with effective therapy.[39]

Frequent chest films are unnecessary if their progress is not rapid. If their clinical findings (e.g., cough, fever, and elevated white count) are returning to normal, they can be discharged from the hospital and followed at monthly intervals until resolution is complete.

SPUTUM EXAMINATION

Examination of the sputum is useful during the initial workup, in evaluating acute exacerbations, and when complications such as malignancy or a granuloma are suspected. Proper collection of the specimen is vitally important, since inadequate specimens may yield false information. Coughed sputum specimens are best collected shortly after awakening, since abnormal bronchial secretions tend to accumulate overnight. To reduce contamination with saliva and oropharyngeal organisms, the patient should be instructed to rinse out his mouth and gargle with an antiseptic mouthwash before collecting the sputum. The specimen should be examined promptly because alveolar macrophages and bronchial epithelial cells are broken down rapidly and contaminating organisms from the oropharynx may replace the organisms present in the lower respiratory tract.

During the initial patient evaluation, the sputum may yield clues to the predominant disease process. An attempt should be made to quantitate the daily sputum production, although this is often very difficult. Patients with emphysema generally produce relatively little sputum, while those with chronic bronchitis produce significant quantities, usually 30 cc/24 hours or more. Patients who have asthma may have litle or no sputum during symptom-free periods, but following acute attacks may produce thick, tenacious sputum containing bronchial mucus plugs. Patients with exacerbations of chronic bronchitis, bronchiectasis, or a lung abscess may produce 100 cc/24 hours or more.

The color and consistency of the sputum specimen should be noted. Mucoid sputum from patients with stable chronic bronchitis is translucent and has a viscid, tenacious consistency. During acute infections, the volume increases and it becomes grossly opaque and yellow or green. Yellow sputum may be associated with the presence of either neutrophils or eosinophils, the former suggesting an infectious component and the latter suggesting an allergy. The presence of blood in the sputum, either mixed with the specimen or streaking on the surface, is an important clinical sign suggesting a complication such as malignancy.

Microscopic examination of a wet unstained sputum specimen allows for rapid appreciation of large yeast cells and other cellular elements that may be present. Eosinophils, Charcot-Leyden crystals, Curschmann's spirals, ciliated airway epithelial cells, and alveolar macrophages are readily identified by wet prep evaluation of the sputum.[40]

The first step in the microscopic examination of the sputum is to determine whether expectorated specimens are derived from the lower airways or are contaminated by saliva and oropharyngeal secretions. Wright's stain helps to identify the cell components better if there is doubt after examination of the wet prep. Alveolar macrophages are large round cells with eccentric oval or kidney-shaped nuclei, while squamous epithelial cells are very large and flat and have a round central nucleus. Sputa that contain less than 10 epithelial cells per low-power field ($\times 100$) are representative of lower respiratory tract secretions. If neutrophils are present in significant numbers, a Gram stain should be performed to identify the presence of potentially pathogenic bacteria. While normal patients have sterile lower respiratory tracts, those with chronic bronchitis may harbor potential pathogens such as pneumococci or *Haemophilus influenzae* in their lower respiratory tract secretions. It is important to correlate the results of sputum examination with clinical findings in managing a patient with COPD.

During acute lower respiratory tract infections, a sputum Gram stain performed before any antibiotics are given is a major guide to initial antibiotic therapy. Sputum cultures are less useful since responsible organisms may be overgrown by contaminants.[41] Sputum cultures may be of use, however, if the patient is not responding to appropriate therapy or if a potentially resistant organism, such as gram-negative bacillus, is identified as the predominant pathogen. Thus, sputum cultures may be useful in hospital-acquired infections and in patients who are not responding to initial antibiotic therapy.

Sputum examination is indicated when a complicating granulomatous infection is suspected. At least three first-morning specimens should be examined and cultured for acid-fast bacilli and fungi, although more may be indicated. Special stains for fungi include the methenamine silver, PAS, and fluorescent antibody stains. Sputum specimens should also be examined for malignant cells in the presence of abnormal chest x-ray films or in patients with hemoptysis. The percent of positive sputum cytology in patients with bronchogenic carcinoma ranges from 45% to 90% depending on cell type and location of the tumor.[31] The highest yields are obtained from patients with carcinoma arising in the large proximal airways. False-positive cytologic results are uncommon, occurring in about 1% of cases.[42]

If adequate coughed sputum specimens cannot be obtained during exacerbations of COPD, sputum induction is indicated. This consists of breathing high concentrations of aerosol, usually distilled water, from a nebulizer, followed by vigorous coughing. The procedure may be performed by anyone at the bedside, including the patient's family. The aerosol mixture is usually breathed deeply for 15 to 20 minutes, and the procedure may be accompanied by chest percussion and postural drainage. The sputum specimen should be taken immediately to the laboratory for examination.

Nasotracheal suctioning involves inserting a catheter through the nose into the oropharynx, injecting a small amount of sterile saline, and aspirating through a syringe. This procedure is potentially dangerous, especially in elderly patients and those with inadequate cough reflexes. Since it may be associated with vomiting, hypoxemia, and arrhythmias, it should only be done by knowledgeable personnel, and oxygen should be administered during the procedure. Obviously, the specimens obtained in this manner are contaminated by nasal and oropharyngeal secretions.

A more invasive technique, which samples only lower respiratory tract sections, is transtracheal aspiration, first proposed in the 1950s and popularized by Bartlett in the 1970s.[43] This procedure is potentially dangerous and should be performed only by experienced personnel. After cleansing and sterilization of the skin over the cricothyroid membrane, the area is anesthetized and a needle containing a small catheter is introduced through the membrane into the trachea. The catheter is directed caudally, and a small amount of sterile saline is injected in order to cause the patient to cough. Secretions obtained in this manner are usually not contaminated by oropharyngeal pathogens, although aspiration into the trachea is not uncommon in patients who are ill.

Fiberoptic bronchoscopy with a protected brush catheter may be used to obtain lower respiratory secretions.[44] This procedure is probably less traumatic than transtracheal aspiration and allows collection of specimens from the segment or lobe that is shown to be abnormal on the chest radiograph. Comparison of tracheal secretions with those from the distal lungs in chronically ill patients indicates that tracheal secretions often do not indicate the actual organisms causing the disease process in the lung. Direct needle aspiration of the lung has also been used to obtain secretions and pathogenic organisms; however, this is a potentially dangerous technique and should only be used in critically ill patients in whom an etiologic diagnosis is necessary. It is contraindicated in the presence of a bleeding tendency or if the patient cannot cooperate.

Gastric lavage is a method of obtaining swallowed secretions from the stomach in patients suspected of having tuberculosis or a lung malignancy. This technique has generally been replaced by sputum induction or flexible bronchoscopy; however, in patients who cannot cooperate, such as young children or mentally impaired individuals, a gastric lavage may be indicated. A positive smear for acid-fast bacilli from gastric contents is nondiagnostic since saprophytic organisms may be found there. The diagnosis depends upon the culture of *Mycobacterium tuberculosis* from the specimen.

OTHER DIAGNOSTIC TECHNIQUES

During the initial evaluation of patients with COPD, so-called routine laboratory screening tests are usually obtained. These include a complete blood count, blood chemistries, serum electrolytes, and a urinalysis. The hemoglobin may be elevated in patients who are chronically hypoxemic, and the white blood cell count may be increased in the presence of respiratory infection. The presence of significant eosinophilia in the blood suggests an allergic component to the obstructive airways disease. In patients with COPD and cor pulmonale who are on long-term diuretic therapy, electrolytes should be obtained to rule out a deficiency in potassium, magnesium, or chloride. Hypokalemia and hypomagnesemia may be associated with muscle weakness and easy fatiguability as well as more serious complications such as cardiac arrhythmias. With chronic carbon dioxide retention, the serum bicarbonate normally rises to compensate for the respiratory acidosis, and the serum chloride falls in a reciprocal manner. This is an expected finding in compensated respiratory failure.

Alpha$_1$-Antitrypsin Assay

The severe deficiency of serum alpha$_1$-antitrypsin is a familial disorder associated with early development of emphysema, usually of the panacinar type (Fig. 4–12).[45] The presence of homozygous deficiency can be determined from a serum protein electrophoresis in which the alpha$_1$ peak is low or absent. Most patients with COPD have normal or elevated levels of alpha$_1$ globulin, and only when emphysema occurs at an early age in patients without other risk factors or when a strong familial incidence is present should alpha$_1$-antitrypsin deficiency be suspected. The syndrome of early emphysema occurs only in patients with homozygous deficiency (PiZ pattern), and heterozygotes do not appear to have significant lung disease.[46] If alpha$_1$-antitrypsin deficiency is detected, there is no available therapy at present, although artificial proteases have been developed, and studies are underway to determine their effectiveness. The diagnosis of severe alpha$_1$-antitrypsin deficiency is useful in genetic counseling and in cautioning the patient to avoid other risk factors such as cigarette smoking.

Skin Tests

Skin tests are of two major types, the immediate skin test reaction, which reflects IgE-mediated hypersensitivity to antigens, and the delayed reaction, which reflects a type IV hypersensitivity mediated by T lymphocytes. Immediate hypersensitivity is demonstrated with either scratch tests or intradermal injections of suspected allergens such as pollens, molds, dust, grasses, animal danders, and certain foods. A positive test is manifested by a specific wheal and flare response which occurs within 15 to 30 minutes. Usually a battery of skin tests is performed at one sitting, and their results are used in conjunction with the clinical history in the diagnosis and treatment of allergic diseases such as seasonal rhinitis. In the patient with established COPD, hypersensitivity skin tests are rarely beneficial unless there is a prominent upper respiratory component and the illness is seasonal or associated with specific contacts such as cats or dogs.[47] If seasonal rhinitis is present along with sensitivity to ragweed pollen, desensitization may decrease the sinusitis, postnasal drip, and rhinorrhea.

Among the tests for delayed hypersensitivity, the tuberculin skin test using purified protein derivative (PPD) is the most important. Only the intermediate strength solution (5 tuberculin units) is of diagnostic significance. The standard preparation (PPD-S) prepared from *Mycobacterium tuberculosis* is the only one commonly administered. Patients who have symptoms of chronic illness or abnormal chest films suggesting granuloma and contacts of patients with active tuberculosis should receive a PPD skin test. A dose of 0.1 ml is injected intradermally, and the site is inspected 48 to 72 hours later. The presence of an area of induration 10 mm or greater is a positive test. Smaller areas of induration suggest infection with nontuberculous mycobacteria and are considered nonspecific. In elderly patients who are suspected of having tuberculosis and who have an initial negative PPD skin test, anergy should be excluded by testing other common antigens such as trichophyton, candida, or mumps. Then an intermediate-strength PPD test repeated one week later may yield a booster effect.[48] If the second test is positive, it probably represents an anamnestic response, and remote infection with tuberculosis is likely.

For patients suspected of having coccidioidomycosis, skin tests are available for both the mycelial (coccidioidin) and spherule (spherulin) forms of the organism. Positive skin tests occur in abut 80% of patients with chronic pulmonary coccidioidomycosis. Skin tests are also available for histoplasmosis, but they are of little value in the individual patient and are not recommended. Patients with suspected allergic pulmonary aspergillosis react to intradermal aspergillus antigens in a very large percentage of cases. A positive type III or Arthus reaction to the skin test occurs five to six hours after the test

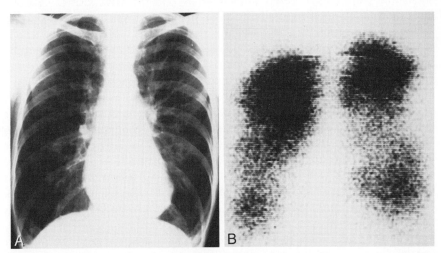

Figure 4–12. *A,* PA chest film of a 38-year-old man with homozygous alpha$_1$-antitrypsin deficiency (PiZ pattern). Emphysematous changes are present—most noticeably in the lower lung zones. The vascular pattern in the upper lobes is relatively well preserved. *B,* Perfusion lung scan performed in the upright position shows the radioactive tracer distributed primarily to the upper lobes. The man died four years later of respiratory failure, and autopsy revealed extensive panacinar emphysema.

is applied and resolves after 24 hours. Patients with invasive aspergillosis usually have negative skin tests.

Serologic Tests

Serologic tests for fungi are occasionally useful in patients with COPD, especially those suspected of having allergic bronchopulmonary aspergillosis (ABPA) or pulmonary histoplasmosis. Complement fixation, immunodiffusion, radioimmunoassay, and enzyme immunoassay have all been used to detect antibodies to *Histoplasma capsulatum*. The complement fixation test suffers from a lack of specificity, while immunodiffusion is frequently negative even in patients with active disease. Serologic tests are less useful in suspected blastomycosis because of the presence of false-negative and false-positive tests.

Allergic bronchopulmonary aspergillosis is associated with markedly elevated total IgE levels as well as increased levels of specific IgE against *Aspergillus fumigatus*. These patients also have positive precipitin reactions to *A. fumigatus*, and serum precipitin levels tend to coincide with the activity of the disease. Serial determination of total IgE levels is useful in adjusting steroid doses during the treatment of patients with ABPA.

Biopsy Techniques

Lung biopsies are rarely indicated in patients with COPD. Specific indications include the possibility of a malignancy or the coexistence of another disease such as pneumoconiosis, which may complicate the course of COPD. The most common method of lung biopsy today is via the fiberoptic bronchoscope. The transbronchial biopsy is a relatively simple technique with an acceptable complication rate.[49] Endobronchial biopsies are indicated if malignancy is suspected, while transbronchial biopsies may be useful in diagnosing sarcoidosis or malignancy involving the lung parenchyma. Percutaneous needle aspiration and biopsy are useful techniques for diagnosing the etiology of peripheral lung masses.[50] These are usually performed under fluoroscopic, ultrasound, or CT guidance. With needle aspiration, a small amount of saline is injected into the density and followed by aspiration. Material should be examined immediately, and if no diagnosis is present, the technique may be repeated. The specimen should always be cultured to rule out the presence of acid-fast bacilli or fungi.

Patients with COPD rarely require open lung biopsy, and if the COPD is severe, they are usually not candidates for thoracotomy. Open biopsy is indicated only for peripheral lung densities that are not diagnosed by other means and for the evaluation of rapidly progressive interstitial lung disease. In patients with severe infections, a lung biopsy may be indicated if fiberoptic bronchoscopy or needle aspiration fails to yield a diagnosis. Lung biopsy for the diagnosis of infections is usually reserved for patients who are immunocompromised and in whom toxic therapeutic agents are being considered.[51] Lung biopsy specimens should always be cultured and submitted for histologic examination. The complication rate for open lung biopsy is low, although the morbidity is significant, especially in the presence of underlying COPD.

SELECTION OF DIAGNOSTIC TESTS

With the current emphasis on controlling the cost of health care, it is becoming increasingly important not to perform a routine battery of diagnostic tests but rather to select only those examinations necessary for proper diagnosis and management. Table 4–8 shows the costs of some common diagnostic procedures, which vary considerably from one institution to another, although they are probably representative. It is easy to see that the cost of laboratory tests can mount rapidly and may become a major item in the expense of caring for these patients.

Chest radiographs should not be taken at regular intervals, but should be ordered only when clinical findings suggest a new abnormality. The relatively slow resolution of pneumonia in patients with COPD militates against frequent radiographs during recovery from acute infections as long as the clinical course is satisfactory.[39] Blood and urine examinations, including complete blood count, blood chemistries, arterial blood gas determinations, and serol-

Table 4–8. **Representative Costs of Laboratory Tests Used in Patients with COPD***

Test	Cost
Complete blood count	$ 27.00
Urinalysis	17.00
Automated blood chemistries	73.00
PA and lateral chest films	64.00
Spirometry	102.00
Complete pulmonary function tests	536.00
Arterial blood gases and pH	64.00
Sputum Gram stain	18.00
Sputum culture for bacteria (with sensitivities)	46.00
Sputum smear and culture for acid-fast bacilli	72.00
Sputum smear and culture for fungi	65.00
Sputum cytology	21.00
PPD skin test	0†
Fungal serology	0‡
Allergy skin testing (routine battery)	80.00
Serum IgE level	33.00
Radioallergosorbent test (per allergen)	10.00
Fiberoptic bronchoscopy with biopsy	413.00
Examination of tissue specimen (biopsy)	113.00
CT of chest without contrast	468.00
CT of chest with contrast	519.00
Bronchography	326.00

*Total costs (technical and professional) at a university hospital in a medium-sized Southern city.
†Performed by nurses, house staff or students.
‡Performed by State Public Health Service laboratory.

ogy, are usually indicated only during acute exacerbations. As the physician becomes more familiar with the patient and the disease, he or she becomes less dependent upon test results.

Some tests, such as spirometry and sputum examination, can be performed rapidly and inexpensively in the outpatient clinic or the physician's office. These procedures are useful in following the course of the disease, making therapeutic changes, and judging response to therapy. They should be performed at regular intervals, and results should be charted on a simple flow sheet so that both interval changes and long-term trends can be assessed easily at each visit. Gross examination of sputum volume and appearance is useful in patients with chronic bronchitis and does not involve additional cost.

References

1. American College of Chest Physicians Committee Statement on Clinic and Office Pulmonary Function Testing: Office spirometry in clinical practice. Chest 1978; 74:298.
2. Rossiter CE, Weill H: Ethnic differences in lung function: Evidence for proportional differences. Int J Epidemiol 1974;3:55–61.
3. McFadden ER, Linden DA: A reduction in maximum mid-expiratory flow rate: A spirographic manifestation of small airway disease. Am J Med 1972;52:725–737.
4. Wright JL, Lawson LM, Pare PD, et al: The detection of small airways disease. Am Rev Respir Dis 1984;129:989–994.
5. Kryger M, Bode F, Antic R, et al: Diagnosis of obstruction of the upper and central airways. Am J Med 1976;61:85–93.
6. Pierson RN Jr, Grieco MH: Isoproterenol aerosol in normal and asthmatic subjects. Am Rev Respir Dis 1969;100:533–541.
7. Light RW, Conrad SA, George RB: The one best test for evaluating the effects of bronchodilator therapy. Chest 1977;512–516.
8. American College of Chest Physicians Committee Statement on Pulmonary Physiology: Grading of pulmonary function by means of pulmonary function tests. Dis Chest 1967;52:270–271.
9. Ellis JH Jr, Perera SP, Levine DC: A computer program for calculation and interpretation of pulmonary function studies. Chest 1975;68:209–213.
10. Gaensler EA, Wright GW: Evaluation of respiratory impairment. Arch Environ Health 1966;12:146–189.
11. Kanner RE, Morris AH (eds): Clinical Pulmonary Function Testing–A Manual of Uniform Laboratory Procedures for the In-termountain Area. Salt Lake City, Intermountain Thoracic Society, 1975.
12. Cary J, Huseby J, Culver B, et al: Variability in interpretation of pulmonary function tests. Chest 1979;76:389–390.
13. Morris AH, Kanner RE, Crapo RO, et al (eds): Clinical Pulmonary Function Testing: A Manual of Uniform Laboratory Procedures, ed 2. Salt Lake City, Intermountain Thoracic Society, 1984.
14. Burns CB, Scheinhorn DJ: Evaluation of a single-breath helium dilution total lung capacity in obstructive lung disease. Am Rev Respir Dis 1984;130:580–583.
15. Mellemgaard K: The alveolar-arterial oxygen difference: Its size and components in normal men. Acta Physiol Scand 1966; 67:10–20.
16. Sorbini CA, Grassi V, Solinas E, et al: Arterial oxygen tension in relation to age in healthy subjects. Respir 1968;25:3–13.
17. Fischl MA, Pitchenik A, Gardner LB: An index predicting relapse and need for hospitalization in patients with acute bronchial asthma. N Engl J Med 1981; 305:783–789.
18. McFadden ER Jr, Lyons HA: Arterial blood gas tension in asthma. N Engl J Med 1968;278:1027–1032.
19. American Thoracic Society Subcommittee Statement on Bronchial Inhalation Challenges. Am Thoracic Soc News Spring 1980, pp 11–19.
20. Boushey HA, Holtzman MJ, Sheller JR, Nadel JA: Bronchial hyperactivity. Am Rev Respir Dis 1980; 121:389–413.
21. Yan K, Salome CM, Woolcock AJ: Prevalence and nature of bronchial hyperresponsiveness in subjects with chronic obstructive pulmonary disease. Am Rev Respir Dis 1985;132:25–29.

22. Smith TP, Kinasewitz GT, Tucker WY, et al: Exercise capacity as a predictor of post-thoracotomy morbidity. Am Rev Respir Dis 1984;129:730–734.

23. Guyatt G, Pugsley SO, Sullivan M, et al: Effect of encouragement on walking test performance. Thorax 1984;39:818–822.

24. McGavin CR, Gupta SP, McHardy GJR: Twelve-minute walking test for assessing disability in chronic bronchitis. Br Med J 1976;3:822–823.

25. Mahler DA, Weinberg DH, Wells CK, et al: The measurement of dyspnea. Chest 1984;85:751–758.

26. Loke J, Mahler DA, Man SF, et al: Exercise impairment in chronic obstructive pulmonary disease. Clin Chest Med 1984; 5:121–143.

27. Block AJ, Boysen PG, Wynne JW, et al: Sleep apnea, hypopnea and oxygen desaturation in normal subjects: A strong male predominence. N Engl J Med 1979; 300:513–517.

28. Phillipson EA, Goldstein RS: Breathing during sleep in chronic obstructive pulmonary disease. Chest 1984;85(suppl): 24–30.

29. Stradding JR, Lane DJ: Nocturnal hypoxemia in chronic obstructive pulmonary disease. Clin Sci 1983;64:213–222.

30. Sagel SS, Evans RG, Forrest JV, et al: Efficiency of routine screening and lateral chest radiographs in a hospital-based population. N Engl J Med 1974;291:1001–1004.

31. Shields TW, Ritts RE: Bronchial Carcinoma. Springfield, Ill, Charles C. Thomas, 1974.

32. Scanlon GT: Use of radiology in the diagnosis of lung disease, in Baum GL (ed): Textbook of Pulmonary Diseases, ed 2. Boston, Little, Brown & Co, 1974, pp 85–102.

33. Light RW, Girard WM, Jenkinson SG, et al: Parapneumonic effusions. Am J Med 1980;69:507–512.

34. Favez G, Willa C, Heinzer F: Posterior oblique tomography at an angle of 55 degrees in chest roentgenology. Am J Roentgenol 1974;120:907–915.

35. Kollins SA: Computerized tomography of the pulmonary parenchyma and chest wall. Radiol Clin North Am 1977;15:297–308.

36. Reid L, Simon G: Pathological findings and radiological changes in chronic bronchitis and emphysema. Br J Radiol 1959; 32:291–305.

37. Fraser RB, Fraser RS, Jenner JW, et al: The roentgenologic diagnosis of chronic bronchitis: A reassessment with emphasis on parahilar bronchi seen end-on. Radiology 1976;120:1–9.

38. Ziskind MM, Schwarz MI, George RB, et al: Incomplete consolidation in pneumococcal lobar pneumonia complicating pulmonary emphysema. Ann Intern Med 1970;72:835–839.

39. Jay SJ, Johanson WG, Pierce AK: The radiographic resolution of Streptococcus pneumoniae pneumonia. N Engl J Med 1975;293:798–801.

40. Epstein RL: Constituents of sputum: a simple method. Ann Intern Med 1972;77:259–265.

41. Barret-Connor E: The non-value of sputum culture in the diagnosis of pneumococcal pneumonia. Am Rev Respir Dis 1971; 103:845–848.

42. Oswald NC, Hinson KFW, Canti G, et al: The diagnosis of primary lung cancer with special reference to sputum cytology. Thorax 1971;26:623–631.

43. Barlett JG: Diagnostic accuracy of transtracheal aspiration. Bacteriologic studies. Am Rev Respir Dis 1977;115:777–782.

44. Wimberley N, Faling LJ, Barlett JG: A fiberoptic bronchoscopy technique to obtain uncontaminated lower airway secretions for bacterial culture. Am Rev Respir Dis 1980;119:377–343.

45. Kueppers F, Black L: Alpha-1-antitrypsin and its deficiency. Am Rev Respir Dis 1974;110:176–194.

46. Mittman C: The PiMZ phenotype: Is it a significant risk factor for the development of chronic obstructive lung disease? Am Rev Respir Dis 1978;118:648–652.

47. Lichtenstein LM: A reevaluation of immunotherapy in asthma. Am Rev Respir Dis 1984;129:657–659.

48. Thompson NJ, Glassroth J, Snider D, et al: The booster phenomenon in serial tuberculin testing. Am Rev Respir Dis 1979;119:587–597.

49. Hanson RR, Zavala DC, Rhondes MD, et al: Transbronchial biopsy via flexible fiberoptic bronchoscope: Results in 164 patients. Am Rev Respir Dis 1976;114:67–72.

50. Zelch JV, Lalli AF, McCormack LJ, et al: Aspiration biopsy in diagnosis of pulmonary nodules. Chest 1973;63:149–152.

51. Bandt PD, Blank N, Castellino RA: Needle diagnosis of pneumonitis. Value in high-risk patients. JAMA 1972;220:1578–1580.

SMOKING CESSATION

IAN A. CAMPBELL

In chronic obstructive pulmonary disease (COPD), the benefits from smoking cessation are clearly established: Symptoms of cough, sputum, and wheeze are reduced; the rate of decline of pulmonary function reverts to normal; the chance of dying from respiratory failure or cor pulmonale is lessened; and the risks of developing lung cancer or ischemic heart disease decline.[1-3] It can be argued that smoking cessation is the most effective step in treating patients with chronic bronchitis and emphysema. Other long-term therapies used in such patients may afford some symptomatic relief, but with the exception of long-term oxygen in certain groups with significant hypoxemia, none has been shown to halt or delay the progression of the disease or to prolong life. Much of the potential symptomatic relief offered by bronchodilators and physiotherapy is negated if a patient continues to smoke. In asthmatics, continued smoking exacerbates the condition, with resulting pressure to escalate therapy. Eventually, the point may be reached when the patient is on regular, systemic corticosteroids in ever-increasing dosage chiefly because he or she will not stop smoking.

Considering the importance of smoking cessation in COPD, there have been remarkably few prospective studies of methods for helping patients to stop smoking. Raw has shown that patients with COPD who were advised by a chest physician to reduce or stop smoking were more likely to do so than those not so advised.[4] In the same study, it was shown that the wearing of a white coat by a clinical psychologist, who interviewed the patients after they had seen the chest physician, increased the number of patients who reduced or stopped smoking. When patients attending a London chest clinic were given simple advice by a physician to stop smoking, 30% to 37% claimed abstinence at six months while 18% to 23% said they had not smoked over the whole six months.[5] Measurements to validate claims of abstinence were not made in these two studies.

The British Thoracic Society has recently conducted a multicenter trial in 1550 new or re-referred hospital patients with smoking-related diseases, over 75% of whom had COPD. In this comparative trial, it was shown that hospital physicians' verbal advice to patients to stop smoking gave long-term results similar to those achieved when that advice was supplemented with a booklet, or with a booklet plus placebo or nicotine chewing gum: One year after entering the study, 10% of patients had stopped smoking and remained abstinent.[6] Among men with COPD, the success rate was 12% while in women it was only 5%.[7] The rates increased with age in both sexes (Fig. 5–1). In the trial as a whole, single or married men were more likely to quit smoking than separated or divorced men, and there was a suggestion that the same was true for women. If the most important other person in the patient's life was a nonsmoker, success was more likely. Cigarette consumption, social class, concern about weight gain, and perceived benefit of stopping smoking

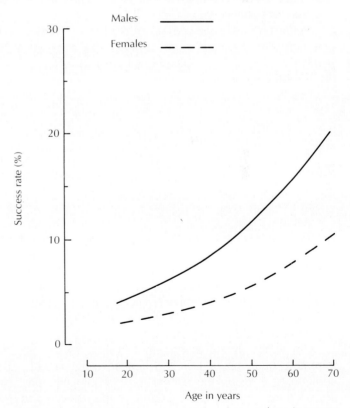

Figure 5–1. Relation between success rate and age and sex in persons who try to quit smoking.

did not relate to success. The successful nonsmokers at one year cited will power as the most important factor in giving up, and the others cited lack of will power most frequently among their reasons for not stopping. Those who failed to give up smoking were more likely to mention worry, anxiety, and tension than those who succeeded. Interestingly, Burns found that patients in a Manchester (England) chest clinic who failed to stop smoking had higher neuroticism scores (as measured by the Maudsley Personality Inventory) than those who claimed to have given up the habit.[8]

It was disappointing to discover that nicotine chewing gum offered so little to patients with COPD, especially after the promise it had shown in smoking cessation clinics.[9–11] Although discouraging, this was not altogether surprising because hospital patients with smoking-related diseases are quite a different population from the highly motivated clients attending smokers' clinics. A further study of nicotine chewing gum came from a smoking cessation clinic in a Swedish hospital.[12] Of the 106 subjects, two thirds had been referred by physicians while one third were self-referrals. The distribution of diagnoses between treatment groups was not described, nor was the influence of diagnosis on the success rate reported. Thus, there is no way of telling whether the overall 29% success rate for nicotine gum in conjunction with group therapy compared with 16% for placebo gum plus group therapy was true for patients with COPD.

Pederson has reviewed other reports of studies concerning smoking cessation among patients with COPD,[13] but these have mostly been retrospective studies with variable follow-up periods often involving small numbers of selected patients and/or physicians and with soft data on cessation. None used carboxyhemoglobin, thiocyanate, or cotinine measurements to verify claims of abstinence. Thus, little weight can be placed on the quoted success rates, but their results tend to support the findings that men do better than women and that success increases with age.

It is not clear why there should be such a sex difference. As death rates among women from COPD, lung cancer, and heart disease rapidly approach the rates among men, this difference must surely be the subject of further urgent research. Not even the most ardent feminist would welcome this sort of equality!

Patients who stop smoking can expect to gain 3 to 6 kg in weight.[7] From a health point of view, stopping smoking is more important than remaining slim, and the vain should be plainly told that a slim, dead partner is decidedly less attractive than a plump, live one.[14] COPD is insidious and does not have the frightening, dramatic impact of heart disease. Weight gain is more apparent to the patient than the damage to the lungs and, in the early stage of COPD, is seen as more of a problem.

Physicians should perhaps not hesitate to describe the protracted and miserable outcome of COPD when advising patients to stop smoking. In addition to advising the patient to stop smoking, physicians should try to persuade the person most important to the patient to stop, too, or at least to advise the patient to take account of this factor. Apart from these measures, and the ploy of involving a white-coated clinical psychologist to reinforce the advice, there is little else of proven benefit. Frequent support sessions in the first few weeks after the advice to stop, perhaps supplemented by nicotine chewing gum, may increase success rates, but this hypothesis must be tested prospectively in those with COPD. If such sessions are shown to boost long-term success, manpower resources may limit their widespread adoption.

Postal support and encouragement is presently the subject of further research in Britain, as is the effect of signing a simple contract to try to give up smoking. Anxiolytics could have a place in preventing relapse and are worthy of further investigation. Pulmonary physicians have a duty to direct substantial research efforts into the field of smoking cessation among patients with COPD. Future studies should be prospective and contain control groups treated with the best currently available treatment—the advice of a physician. Success should be measured as abstinence for at least six, but preferably 12, months. Claims of abstinence should be validated by objective measurements.

Specialists should stimulate and support research by primary care physicians for better ways of reducing smoking among their patients. Advice from general practitioners has already been shown to have a definite effect.[15, 16] All doctors should aid national campaigns to reduce smoking, bring pressure to bear on governments to educate people about the hazards of smoking, and support increasingly restrictive legislation in relation to smoking and to relentlessly tax the habit out of existence. Above all, they must remember to advise their patients to stop smoking.

References

1. Fletcher CM, Peto R,Tinker C, Speizer FE: The Natural History of Chronic Bronchitis and Emphysema. London, Oxford University Press, 1976.
2. Doll R, Peto R: Mortality in relation to smoking: 20 years' observations on male British doctors. Br Med J 1976;2:1525–1536.
3. Tashkin DP, Clark VA, Coulson AH, et al: The UCLA population studies of chronic obstructive respiratory disease, VIII. Effects of smoking cessation on lung function: A prospective study of a free-living population. Am Rev Respir Dis 1984;130:707–715.
4. Raw M: Persuading people to stop smoking. Behav Res Therapy 1976;14:97–101.
5. Williams HO: Routine advice against smoking—a chest clinic pilot study. Practitioner 1969;202:672–676.
6. British Thoracic Society report. Comparison of four methods of smoking withdrawal in patients with smoking related diseases. Br Med J 1983;286:595–597.
7. British Thoracic Society report. Smoking withdrawal in hospital patients: Factors associated with outcome. Thorax 1984; 39:651–656.
8. Burns BH: Chronic chest disease, person-ality, and success in stopping cigarette smoking. Brit J Prev Soc Med 1969;23:23–27.
9. Jarvis MJ, Raw M, Russell MAH, Feyerabend C: Randomised controlled trial of nicotine chewing-gum. Br Med J 1982; 285:537–540.
10. Nicotine chewing gum (editorial). Lancet 1985;I:320–321.
11. Raw M: Does nicotine chewing gum work? (editorial). Br Med J 1985; 290:1231–1232.
12. Hjalmarson AIM: Effect of nicotine chewing gum in smoking cessation. A randomized, placebo-controlled, double-blind study. JAMA 1984;252:20;2835–2838.
13. Pederson LL: Compliance with physician advice to quit smoking: A review of the literature. Pre Med 1982;11:71–84.
14. Royal College of Physicians. Obesity. J R Coll Physn Lond 1983;17:5–65.
15. Russell MAH, Wilson C, Taylor C, Baker CD: Effect of general practitioners' advice against smoking. Br Med J 1979;2:231–235.
16. Jamrozik K, Vessey M, Fowler G, et al: Controlled trial of three different anti-smoking interventions in general practice. Br Med J 1984;288:1499–1503.

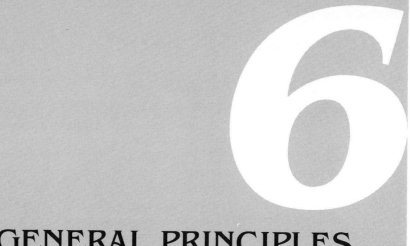

GENERAL PRINCIPLES OF CARE

MITCHELL L. RHODES

Patients with impaired lung function need an individualized approach to care from the physician and health care team. Many factors influence the management of a given patient, including the severity of the lung disease; coexisting medical problems; the patient's occupation, hobbies, family, and social support structure; cultural and educational backgrounds; and his or her motivation to maintain as active and normal a lifestyle as the lung impairment permits. Therefore, no one set of rules apply equally for all patients, but certain general principles should be considered in the care of most patients with chronic obstructive pulmonary disease (COPD).

IMMUNIZATION AGAINST RESPIRATORY INFECTIONS

The common viral and bacterial pathogen can represent a potentially lethal hazard to patients with COPD because of their lack of pulmonary reserve. The episode of acute bronchitis or influenza that might cause a few days loss of work for an otherwise healthy individual might precipitate an episode of acute respiratory failure in the patient with emphysema or chronic bronchitis. Prophylaxis with the use of vaccines should be considered in all these patients. Two vaccines, influenzal and pneumococcal, have been proven safe and efficacious in the general population.

Influenza is particularly hazardous to the patient with COPD, both as a primary infection and of greater concern because of the secondary bacterial respiratory infection that often follows. These patients should receive a yearly influenza immunization each fall because of the annual changes in the antigenic nature of the influenza virus. With improved purification procedures, the incidence of local and systemic reactions to the vaccine are minimal. Epidemiologic surveillance of vaccinated patients has not revealed an increased incidence of Guillain-Barré syndrome, a concern raised after the swine flu epidemic in the 1970s. During the peak of influenza epidemics, patients with COPD should use caution and avoid exposure to crowds and to youngsters, who may have no natural immunity to these viruses from prior exposure.

The commonest bacterial cause of pneumonia in this country remains *Streptococcus pneumoniae*. A polyvalent vaccine has been available since November of 1977. The original vaccine contains capsular polysaccharides from 14 serotypes of *S. pneumoniae*. The original 14 serotypes were responsible for 80% of the clinical cases of blood-culture–positive pneumococcal pneumonia in this country. In 1983, a new formulation containing 23 serotypes, accounting for at least 90% of blood-culture–positive pneumococcal infections, was released for use. It has been shown to be effective in reducing the incidence of pneumonia from those serotypes by 60% to 65%. A recent article has questioned the use of the pneumococcal vaccine in all patients with COPD because of the lack of studies on its effectiveness in that specific patient population.[1] General recommendations favor its use in the elderly and in patients with underlying cardiac and pulmonary disease.[2] Significant antibody levels are maintained for at least five years after vaccination, and current recommendations are to vaccinate adults only once. Repeating the vaccination increases the risk of local and systemic reactions. Six out of 10 patients who are hospitalized with pneumococcal pneumonia had been hospitalized for other reasons at least once during the prior five years. Immunizing COPD patients with the pneumococcal vaccine prior to discharge for any hospitalization appears to be a reasonable approach. Both the influenza vaccine and pneumococcal vaccine can be given at the same time in opposite arms with no interference in the efficacy of either vaccine. Other bacterial vaccines are being studied, but none are currently recommended for routine use.

PROMPT TREATMENT OF INFECTIONS

Acute respiratory infections typically aggravate airways obstruction in patients with COPD and may precipitate acute respiratory failure. An acute exacerbation may be marked by fever, increased cough and sputum production, and a change in sputum color from clear to yellow or green. In some patients, however, because of the increased airways obstruction, sputum production may actually decrease. A change in sputum color to a purulent appearance may be due to allergy or inflammation rather than infection. Examination of the sputum in an allergic condition should reveal large numbers of eosinophils, whereas "polys" predominate in infection. Prompt institution of oral antibiotics to prevent clinical deterioration is important. In the absence of pneumonia, cultures of the sputum are usually of little value. Initiation of broad-spectrum antibiotics such as tetracycline, ampicillin, erythromycin, or trimethoprim and sulfamethoxazole is usually effective. The responsible patient can be given a prescription for these antibiotics and advised to initiate therapy at the first sign of an infection. Depending on the rapidity of response, the antibiotic regime should be continued for seven to 14 days. An extensive literature on the optimal approach to antibiotic therapy is available.[3]

NUTRITION

Maintaining adequate nutrition can be a major problem for the patient with moderate to severe COPD. About 40% to 60% of COPD patients have significant weight loss during some period of their disease. Studies have indicated there is a loss of both fat and lean body mass. The cause of the weight loss is often unclear. Some feel that the increased work of breathing from the impaired lung function leads to an increased metabolic rate. Many patients with COPD become more dyspneic while eating and therefore tend to reduce their caloric intake. Epidemiologic studies have shown that undernourished patients with COPD have poorer survival statistics than those who are at near-normal body weight. The loss of protein from muscle during chronic weight loss can lead to a weakening of the respiratory muscles, and general malnourishment can impair the normal defense mechanisms against infection. So, while obesity should be avoided because of the additional stress it places on the respiratory mechanism, an attempt should be made to maintain a near-ideal body weight. Attention should be given to medications that might cause nausea and aggravate the weight loss. Large meals, by causing gastric distention and elevation of the diaphragm, might impede breathing. Multiple small meals might be better tolerated. Care should be given to patients with a history of gastroesophageal reflux since meals taken within two to three hours of bedtime may lead to aspiration and bronchoconstriction. The use of oxygen or an increase in the flow rate of those chronically on oxygen may help prevent the hypoxemia and dyspnea associated with eating.

The composition of the diet is important since metabolized food is broken down to water and carbon dioxide. An attempt to increase caloric intake in a patient with COPD may lead to an increase in carbon dioxide production, which the patient with impaired lung function may not tolerate well. When patients being weaned from ventilators are given a high carbohydrate load intravenously, their arterial carbon dioxide levels may rise and impede the weaning process. Even the stable patient with moderate to severe COPD may be adversely affected by a high carbohydrate meal.[4] After patients consumed a meal with nearly 1000 calories of carbohydrate, their exercise tolerance (as measured by an exercise bicycle test or ability to walk on the level) was decreased for a period of two to three hours. Special nutritional supplements for patients with COPD have been developed that are high in fat and low in carbohydrates, but these may confer a risk in those with cardiovascular disease. High carbohydrate intake did not adversely affect stable patients at rest. A reasonable approach, then, would be to avoid heavy exercise immediately after meals.

Adequate fluid intake for patients with COPD has been stressed as a means of avoiding thickening of airway secretions. While dehydration should be avoided, there is no evidence that overhydration helps to clear secretions. Patients with COPD, particularly if they are hypercapnic tend to retain fluid even in the absence of cardiac decompensation. Avoidance of excess fluid and salt is important in this population. Some patients report that dairy products increase their sputum production while others report that ingestion of any cold liquid increases cough, sputum production, and dyspnea. Patients with COPD have an increased incidence of peptic ulcer disease, and the inadvisability of alcohol and caffeine ingestion should be discussed with them because of their potentiating role in ulcer disease.

CONTROL OF THE ENVIRONMENT

A number of environmental factors may aggravate the symptoms of chronic airways obstruction. For those who cannot escape to the Sun belt, the cold dry, outside air of winter can provoke severe respiratory difficulties, particularly in those with an asthmatic component. Cold, dry air has been shown to cause the release of inflammatory mediators from mast cells.[5] Cold-weather masks made of soft foam allow heating and humidification of air around the patient's nose and mouth and may reduce dyspnea when walking outside. Another problem occurs when cold, dry, outside air is heated and put through a forced-air furnace system. The relative humidity indoors may fall to extremely low levels. Because water is added to this air as it passes over the nasal and bronchial mucosa, drying of secretions in the upper and lower respiratory tract commonly occurs.

To maintain patient comfort and normal viscosity in nasal and respiratory tract secretions, moisture must be added to the indoor environment. Humidification can be accomplished by vaporizers that blow air over the surface of water in a reservoir and evaporate it. This type of humidifier is common and built into many furnaces. The other approach is by nebulization. In nebulization, water is dispersed as a fine mist that is delivered into the room in an aerosol form. Cool mist vaporizers have been popular as a means of humidifying individual rooms, such as a bedroom. Nebulizers can become easily contaminated with bacteria or mold, which is then aerosolized into the room and can lead to respiratory infections. Recent reports indicate that a new type of home humidifier that uses ultrasonic nebulization significantly reduces the aerosolization of live bacteria or mold. The organisms may be disrupted by the ultrasonic waves before they're dispersed into the air. These units are quiet and can be obtained in sizes that will humidify from one to several rooms. Care must still be taken to insure frequent and adequate cleaning. Aerosolization of nonviable organisms can still lead to allergic responses in some patients, even though the risk of infection is reduced. Indoor relative humidity should be maintained at between 30% and 50%. The newer ultrasonic units have humidistats built in that cycle the units on and off to maintain a given humidity level.

Hot, humid weather in the summer can also stress the patient with COPD. A central air-conditioning system can dehumidify the air as well as cool it and may help control dyspnea. A variety of air cleaners are now available for home use to remove dust, pollen and other particulates from the indoor environment. The typical fiberglass filter used in most forced-air systems is relatively inefficient for removing anything other than large particles of dirt and lint. High-efficiency particulate air (HEPA) filters are available in room console size or can be attached to the main forced-air heating and cooling systems. These filters trap the very small as well as the larger (visible) particulates. Many also contain activated charcoal filters that trap the gaseous components of indoor pollution. Electrostatic filters built into the furnace can be effective in removing small particulates, but they may produce ozone, which is a respiratory irritant. Some electrostatic filters release previously trapped particulates as the filter becomes clogged. A new type of filter is available that is installed in the furnance and creates a static charge from the action of air moving past plastic rods within the filter. There is no external electric source to create ozone, and as long as the furnace is on to create air movement, these filters seem to be highly efficient in clearing both large and small particulates. They are economical because they can be cleaned by rinsing them under water and then replaced in the furnace. These air-cleaning systems have become more important as homes have become more energy-efficient with improved caulking, insulation, and elimination of air leaks. A variety of respiratory irritants can become concentrated in indoor air from sources such as kerosene heaters; toluene diisocyanate from varnishes, adhesives, and polyurethane foams; and formaldehyde from urea-formalde-hyde insulation. Attention must be given to adequate air exchange to prevent this indoor pollution.

The hazards of outdoor pollution to patients with COPD and asthma have been highly publicized. Sulphur dioxide, oxides of nitrogen, and carbon monoxide can lead to bronchoconstriction and impairment of oxygen-carrying capacity, a major threat to the patient with COPD. Most COPD patients are adversely affected by others smoking in the home or workplace, and an attempt should be made to create a smoke-free environment.

HIGH ALTITUDE

Exposure to high altitude by traveling through mountainous areas or by flying on commercial aircraft can worsen the hypoxemia of patients with COPD. In some, the use of oxygen or an increase in their usual oxygen flow may be necessary to prevent acute problems. The cabin pressure in most commercial airlines during flight varies between 567 and 692 mmHg, depending on the altitude of the plane. The lower barometric pressure is equivalent to an altitude on land of about 8000 feet. Patients with COPD during air travel have been shown to have a decrease in their PaO_2 of 15 mm Hg or more. The degree of hypoxemia that an individual may develop during air travel can be predicted by having him or her breathe a hypoxic gas mixture of 17.2% oxygen and drawing an arterial blood gas sample.[6] If arranged beforehand, supplemental oxygen can be provided to the patient during the flight by most airlines. Traveling through mountainous areas can also present a hazard to these patients.

The author and his colleagues have arranged for patients to take their home liquid oxygen systems with them during travel and to get refills at medical oxygen facilities along the way. Patients have been able to vacation in mountainous areas if arrangements were made for them to receive oxygen at their high-altitude destination. Respiratory therapy departments can work with patients in mapping out their route and prearranging the oxygen refill points before their trip. This type of cooperation has been consistent with the effort to encourage COPD patients to lead as active and normal a life as possible.

DRUGS OF POTENTIAL HAZARD TO THE PATIENT WITH COPD

Patients with COPD who have airway hyperreactivity may be at risk from certain medications. Narcotics must be used with great caution because of their potential depression of both the hypoxic and hypercapnic drives. Pentazocine (Talwin), which was initially reported to have little effect on respiratory drive, has the potential to cause significant respiratory depression. Minor tranquilizers such as diazepam (Valium) when given intramuscularly or intravenously can also depress both the hypoxic and hypercapnic drive. The more severe a patient's hypoxemia, the greater the respiratory depressant effect. Nonselective beta-blocker drugs must also be used with great caution in patients with COPD because of their tendency to increase airway resistance. Even the relatively cardioselective beta-blockers, if given in high enough doses, can lead to bronchoconstriction. Topically applied beta-blockers such as timolol eye drops, used in the treatment of glaucoma, can have sufficient systemic absorption to lead to acute bronchospasm.

Vasoactive drugs such as nitroglycerin can lead to changes in the lung's ventilation-perfusion balance with a significant drop in PaO_2 in some patients.

Their use needs to be monitored closely. Finally, a small group of patients with airways obstruction develop a worsening of their symptoms when exposed to aspirin or other nonsteroidal anti-inflammatory drugs. Exposure can bring on acute, severe bronchospasm. These patients may also be sensitive to tartrazine (yellow dye no. 5), an additive used in many foods and drugs including some bronchodilators. Patients may not relate the worsening symptoms to the medication they took for cold symptoms or aches and pains but assume the cold or flu also aggravated their shortness of breath. Patients with sensitivity to these drugs and the yellow dye tend to be those with adult-onset asthma who also have nasal polyps, and they need to be carefully educated because so many over-the-counter drugs contain one of the offending agents.

References

1. Williams JH Jr, Moser KM: Pneumococcal vaccine in patients with chronic lung disease. *Ann Int Med* 1986; 104:106–109.
2. LaForce FM, Eickhoff TC: Pneumococcal vaccine: The evidence mounts. *Ann Int Med* 1986; 104:110–112.
3. Brashear RE, Rhodes ML: *Chronic Obstructive Lung Disease: Clinical Treatment and Management.* St. Louis, MO: The CV Mosby CO, 1978, p 82.
4. Brown SE, Winer S, Brown RA, et al: Exercise performance following a carbohydrate load in chronic airflow obstruction. *J Appl Phys* 1985; 58:1340–1346.
5. Togias AG, Naclerio RM, Proud D, et al: Nasal challenge with cold dry air results in release of inflammatory mediators. *J Clin Invest* 1985; 76:1375–1381.
6. Schwartz JS, Bencowitz HZ, Moser KM: Air travel hypoxemia with chronic obstructive pulmonary disease. *Ann Int Med* 1984; 100:473–477.

7

PHARMACOLOGIC THERAPY OF COPD

IRWIN ZIMENT

The pharmacologic therapy of chronic obstructive pulmonary disease (COPD) is directed mainly at relieving bronchospasm, with secondary drugs being given to loosen mucus. Additional drugs are used for related complications, including cough, bacterial infection, hypoxia, and cor pulmonale. Associated complaints such as anxiety, insomnia, dyspepsia, and hypertension require careful management to avoid troublesome or hazardous drug interactions.

Although bronchodilator therapy is used as the keystone, the benefits may not be readily discernible or demonstrable.[1, 2, 3] In COPD, unless there is an asthmatic component, the obstruction may not show reversibility after either acute or chronic therapy on standard pulmonary function testing. Nevertheless, most clinicians believe there are subtle benefits even in those cases that lack objective improvement, and sympathomimetic bronchodilators, methylxanthines, and steroids may contribute more by enhancing mucociliary clearance than by simply relaxing the bronchial musculature.

SYMPATHOMIMETIC AGENTS

Sympathomimetic beta-adrenoreceptor stimulators are generally used as the first-line therapy in COPD.[4] Currently, there appears to be worldwide agreement that metered-dose aerosol delivery of sympathomimetic beta-stimulators should be the preferred modality for all COPD patients.[5] In contrast, there is less confidence invested in the oral preparations of sympatho-mimetic drugs, since they do not produce a significantly higher peak effect or longer persistence of bronchodilation.[4, 6] Moreover, the relatively large dose required and the unpredictable bioavailability in the bowel results in a marked liability to side effects when compared to aerosolization of an equally effective dose of the same drug.

1. Sympathomimetic Aerosols

The older sympathomimetic agents, epinephrine and isoproterenol, are rarely used for therapy because they offer only short-lasting bronchodilation accompanied by a high incidence of side effects. Isoetharine has less cardio-stimulatory activity and is preferred by those outpatients who like to use their metered-dose inhalers every three or four hours, since the drug is well tolerated and effective on this dosing schedule. Similarly, isoetharine's short half-life may be deemed an advantage for inpatient nebulization therapy when frequent treatments are demanded by an anxious, bronchospastic patient.

Metaproterenol is the standard bronchodilator in many hospitals, and the newer agents, albuterol and terbutaline, do not offer marked advantages. Thus, each of these aerosol drugs is usually required three or four times a day, and their potency and accompanying side effects are comparable.

When self-administered from a metered-dose inhaler (MDI), optimal technique must be used to maximize aerosol deposition in the bronchial tree, and physicians must be assured that patients can use the devices with competence (Table 7–1). Subjects who have difficulty coordinating their breathing pattern with the actuation of the inhaler should benefit from the use of a large volume reservoir (spacer) interposed between the MDI and the mouth.[7, 8] This can improve the aerosol delivery to the lower lung, while decreasing deposition in the oropharynx from where the drug can be absorbed into the systemic circulation.

The Dosages of aerosols recommended in the manufacturers' product literature are extremely conservative, and there is a marked difference between the amounts entering the lungs from a standard treatment with an MDI and an inhalant solution (Table 7–2). Either technique results in an average of less

Table 7–1. **Use of Metered-Dose Inhaler**

1. Hold inhaler with mouthpiece downwards.
2. Shake the container several times.
3. Breathe out normally.
4. Open mouth widely, let mouthpiece touch lip.
5. Start to inhale slowly, then squeeze cartridge to release spray.
6. Continue to inhale as deeply as possible, then hold the breath for approximately ten seconds, if possible.
7. Wait a minute or so before taking a repeat dose.
8. If there is difficulty following these steps, the addition of a spacer may help.

Table 7–2. Oral and Aerosol Dosages of Bronchodilators

	ORAL			AEROSOL					
	Tablets	Solution		MDI				Inhalant	
	Total dose per day								
	mg	mg	mg/ml	mg/puff	Puffs/day	%	ml	mg	Treatments/day
Epinephrine (e.g., Adrenaline, Primatene Mist*)	—	—	—	0.16–0.30	2–3 q2–4 hr	0.1–1.0	0.3–1.0	0.3–10	NA†
Isoproterenol (e.g., Isuprel, Medihaler-Iso)	10, 15	NA	NA	0.08–0.13	2–3 q2–4 hr	0.25–1.0	0.1–0.5	0.25–5	NA
Isoetharine (e.g., Bronkometer, Bronkosol)	—	—	—	0.34	2–4 q3–6 hr	0.1–1.0	0.25–0.5	0.25–5	4–10
Metaproterenol (e.g., Alupent, Metaprel)	10, 20	15–80	2.0	0.65	2–4 q4–8 hr	5.0	0.2–0.3	10–15	4–6
Terbutaline (e.g., Brethaire, Brethine, Bricanyl)	2.5, 5	3.75–15.0	—	0.20	2–4 q4–8 hr	0.1	0.2–0.5	0.2–0.5	3–4
Albuterol (e.g., Proventil, Ventolin)	2, 4	4–16	0.4	0.09	2–4 q4–8 hr	—	—	—	—
Bitolterol (e.g., Tornalate)	—	—	—	0.37	2–3 q6–8 hr	—	—	—	—
Fenoterol (e.g., Berotec)‡	(2.5)	(7.5–10)	—	(0.18)	(1–3 q8–12 hr)	—	—	—	—

*Many of these agents are now available as generic products, e.g., as unit dose inhalant solutions.
†NA = Not advised for routine therapy.
‡Not approved by FDA.

than 10% of the dose being deposited in the lungs; this amount is a small fraction of the dosage that enters the systemic circulation following oral ingestion of the same agent.[9, 10] Furthermore, the alleged half-life of each drug is based on an average population of patients with moderate asthma. In practice, milder disease requires infrequent aerosol therapy, whereas in status asthmaticus, each dose of the drug produces relief for only a few minutes. As a rough guide, the effective half-life of a bronchodilator is inversely proportional to the severity of the bronchospasm.

These considerations emphasize the need to titrate aerosol treatments to individual requirements. In more severe obstructive states, or in less responsive patients, it may be reasonable to prescribe several times the standard number of inhalations for each treatment, e.g., six inhalations rather than two. Often, the side effects, such as tremor, nervousness, and palpitations, are less severe if the drug is introduced at a low dosage with gradual increase over the course of a few weeks.

Treatment for COPD with aerosol bronchodilators should start with the introduction of an MDI, using any of the popular prescription products. The initial dose should be two to three puffs, three or four times a day, and patients must be instructed in appropriate technique and the need for compliance even if no immediate benefit is perceived. When the patient's technique for inhaling the aerosol remains suboptimal, a reservoir spacer may be prescribed.[8] The response should be assessed after a few days, and if no significant side effects are noted, the dosage can be increased if clinically indicated: As many as 16 to 24 puffs a day may be needed. However, patients who require such high dosages may obtain better relief by using oral sympathomimetics or some other pharmacotherapy.

Inpatients, and selected outpatients, may obtain greater benefit by taking the sympathomimetic drug as an inhalant solution given by a powered nebulizer or even by intermittent positive pressure breathing: The improved coordination of inhalation with such devices can help, but the larger aerosol dosage provided is of greater relevance (Table 7–2). When an inhalant solution is used, the manufacturer's recommended dose is usually selected, and sufficient diluent is added to provide at least 2 ml of solution in the device. Patients must be encouraged to use slow, deep inhalations, and it should be recognized that, if a device is used that only nebulizes during inhalation, a much greater total dosage can be delivered. The frequency of treatments should be individually determined, and if tolerated, nebulization of isoetharine or metaproterenol can be given every two to four hours to patients suffering from an exacerbation of bronchospasm, rather than every four to six hours as generally recommended. Terbutaline, when available as an inhalant, can be given as often as every three to five hours for severe bronchospasm.

When patients fail to respond, the cause may be obvious, such as poor technique or lack of compliance. However, gross overuse of an aerosol bronchodilator may result in diminished response, a phenomenon sometimes known as tachyphylaxis.[4] In some cases, it may be worth changing to another bronchodilator aerosol, but it may be better to stop using all aerosols and to rely on other drugs until the patient improves. However, the phenomenon of tachyphylaxis is not understood well, and it is not always clear why responsiveness to therapy declines.

2. Oral Sympathomimetics

In many patients with COPD, it is customary to give oral sympathomimetic bronchodilators alone or as a supplement to an aerosol. The appropriate dose for each agent is one to two low-dose (or one high-dose) tablets three or four times a day, according to the individual patient's needs and tolerance. Tremor and other side effects are usually more severe with oral therapy, and the physician should consider whether improved therapy with less toxicity could be obtained by using either an aerosol or theophylline instead. In Europe, long-acting, slow-release sympathomimetics seem to be effective and well tolerated when given twice a day.

3. Parenteral Sympathomimetics

Patients with COPD can suffer an acute bronchospastic reaction that may respond to subcutaneous epinephrine or terbutaline. The latter is longer-lasting and should not be given more often than every two to four hours. By contrast, 0.1 to 0.25 ml of 0.1% epinephrine can be given every 20 minutes for four doses, and the resulting side effects may be no more severe than those produced by 0.25 to 0.5 ml of the 0.1% solution of terbutaline. Occasionally, long-acting subcutaneous and intramuscular preparations of epinephrine are used; these formulations are less popular currently.

In many countries, sympathomimetic bronchodilators are available for intravenous administration,[4] but in the United States, only isoproterenol has been given by this route. Patients with a bronchospastic exacerbation of COPD are unlikely to tolerate intravenous isoproterenol, since the agent is liable to produce a serious arrhythmia.

THEOPHYLLINE

In the United States, theophylline is a favored bronchodilator,[11] whereas many European authorities regard it as a secondary agent. More recently, the availability of reliable, slow-release theophylline products in Europe has resulted in renewed interest in the drug.[12] The success of the slow-release formulations has displaced the rapidly absorbed products into playing a minor role in therapeutics.

Theophylline has numerous disadvantages, including relatively poor solubility in water. To make it suitable for intravenous injection, the drug is

Table 7–3. **Long-Acting Theophyllines***

Product	50	60	65	75	100	125	130	200	250	260	300	400	500	Formulation
Aerolate			+				+			+				capsules
Bronkodyl					+			+						capsules
Constant-T								+			+			tablets
Duraphyl					+			+			+			tablets
Elixophyllin-SR						+			+					capsules
LaBID									+					tablets
Lodrane							+			+				capsules
Quibron-T/SR											+			tablets
Respbid									+				+	tablets
Slo-bid Gyrocaps	+				+			+			+			capsules
Slo-Phyllin Gyrocaps		+				+			+					capsules
Somophyllin-CRT					+			+	+		+			capsules
Sustaire					+						+			tablets
Theo-24					+			+			+			capsules
Theobid							+			+				capsules
Theobron SR						+			+					capsules
Theoclear L.A.							+			+				capsules
Theo-Dur					+			+			+			tablets
Theo-Dur Sprinkles	+			+	+		+							capsules
Theolair-SR								+	+		+		+	tablets
Theophylline-SR					+			+			+			tablets
Theophyl-SR						+			+					capsules
Theospan-SR							+			+				capsules
Theo-Time					+			+			+			tablets
Theovent						+			+					capsules
Uniphyl								+				+		tablets

Notes: Tedral SA tablets contain immediate-release (90 mg) and slow-release (90 mg) theophylline with ephedrine (48 mg) and phenobarbital (25 mg). Long-acting aminophylline preparations include Aminodur Duratabs (300 mg tablets) and Phyllocontin (225 mg tablets). Long-acting oxitriphylline preparations include Choledyl SA (200, 400, and 600 mg tablets).
*Information based on (1) Huff BB (ed): *Physicians' Desk Reference*. Oradell NJ, Medical Economics Co, 1985 and (2) Boyd JR (ed): *Drug Facts and Comparisons*. St. Louis, Facts & Comparisons Div, JB Lippincott Co, 1986.

dissolved in ethylenediamine to yield aminophylline: This alkaline product is irritating to tissues and, when injected intravenously, must be given over the course of 15 to 30 minutes to avoid severe cardiovascular reactions. The relative insolubility has, however, also been an advantage, since the oral preparation can readily be formulated for slow release in the bowel, thereby permitting adequate blood levels to be attained by dosing twice a day. These popular sustained-action products result in a smoother therapeutic effect, improved compliance, and better prophylaxis of bronchospasm during sleep.[12]

The range of long-acting preparations is shown in Table 7–3. Other oral theophylline products are not listed, since these products tend to undergo change from year to year. However, rapid-acting formulations are marketed as tablets, chewable tablets, capsules, liquids, syrups, and elixirs. These may be more convenient for geriatric patients—as is the long-acting "sprinkle" preparation, which can be readily added to drinks or applesauce to facilitate its administration to noncompliant subjects.

Mode of Action of Theophylline

In the last few years, concepts regarding the action of theophylline have changed dramatically.[11, 13] Formerly, it was taught that the methylxanthines were inhibitors of phosphodiesterase and that theophylline prevented the breakdown of cyclic 3'5'-AMP by this enzyme. However, not enough c-AMP is generated by this effect to explain the resulting bronchodilation, and it is now thought that theophylline has other major actions such as antagonism of natural bronchoconstrictors including adenosine and prostaglandins. Perhaps, it also has a favorable effect on the intracellular movement of calcium.

Theophylline has gained in reputation recently with the finding that it can stimulate the diaphragm and diminish its liability to fatigue. Although this might suggest that the drug would be especially useful in emphysema and bronchitis, there is insufficient clinical evidence to support this concept. Similarly, there is no clinical proof that theophylline is superior to sympathomimetic drugs in the treatment of COPD.[14]

Theophylline has some beneficial effects on the heart, in that it can increase cardiac output by its inotropic effect on both ventricles and by reducing pulmonary artery hypertension.[15] Moreover, it is less likely to cause palpitations and tachycardia than even the selective beta$_2$-adrenergic bronchodilator drugs. Since theophylline also has a diuretic action, it can be particularly useful in cor pulmonale, but clinical studies do not demonstrate it to have significant superiority over the sympathomimetic agents.

Unfortunately, therapeutic doses of theophylline can cause toxicity. The earliest complaints are usually nervousness, insomnia, palpitations, and nausea. Tremor, vomiting, gastrointestinal bleeding, and arrhythmias can follow as the serum level of theophylline increases. Although theophylline causes less disturbance of cardiac rhythm than sympathomimetic bronchodilators given in customary dosages, serious arrhythmias such as multifocal atrial tachycardia can occur with therapeutic levels of theophylline.[16] In the intensive care unit, the combination of aminophylline, sympathomimetic bronchodilators, and anxiety result in a very high incidence of tachyarrhythmias and premature beats. However, the most dreaded toxic effect is convulsions, since these can be relatively intractable and may be fatal. At present, more deaths are likely to occur from theophylline toxicity than from adverse responses to sympathomimetic bronchodilator therapy.

Dosages of Theophylline

Studies have shown that most asthmatic patients benefit optimally from a serum theophylline level of 10 to 20 μg/ml.[11, 13] Although this is widely regarded as an absolute serum range beyond which the patient should not stray, some subjects do quite well with a level of 5 to 10 μg/ml, particularly if they are using sympathomimetic drugs concurrently. A minority of patients

Table 7–4. **Maintenance Dosages of Theophylline***

Increased Needs		Decreased Needs	
	mg/kg/day		mg/kg/day
Age 10–15	14–18	Hepatic insufficiency	<5
Age 16–20	12	Heart failure	5–8
Smoker	12–18	Cor pulmonale	5–8
Marijuana user	12–15	Therapy with:	
Therapy with:		Cimetidine	5
Phenytoin	10–15	Troleandomycin	5
Rifampin	10–15	Estrogen	7.5
Barbiturates	12	Erythromycin	7.5
Dietary factors:		Allopurinol	7.5
High protein	12		
Low carbohydrate	12		
Barbecued food	12		

*Average adult needs 10 mg/kg/day. In obesity, dose should be based on ideal body weight. For aminophylline, increase dosages by 20%.

both require and tolerate levels in the range of 20 to 25 µg/ml, especially during a severe exacerbation of bronchospasm.

Another complexity is that, although bronchospasm often shows progressive improvement as the serum level of theophylline increases, a point is reached where no further improvement occurs and any additional increase in the serum level just adds to the risk of toxicity. For many patients, this plateau effect occurs within the "therapeutic range" of 10 to 20 µg/ml, and since susceptible people can develop marked toxicity in this range, it is possible to harm rather than help the patient with theophylline levels well below 20 µg/ml. Thus, serum levels alone are an inadequate guide to therapy, and clinical judgment must always be used synergistically.

When initiating oral therapy with theophylline, a relatively low dose should be selected on empirical grounds. For a younger adult of normal size and relatively good health apart from bronchospasm, a daily dose of 600 mg would be reasonable; for an older, frail patient in poor general health, 400 mg is advisable. More precise guidelines can be used to calculate the dosage accurately, taking into account the patient's age, associated diseases, concurrent drugs, smoking, and environmental exposures (Table 7–4).

The liability to toxicity is much greater if liver function is impaired. This problem is common in exacerbations of COPD, and toxicity can be minimized by assuring adequate oxygenation of the patient. Since overdosage is far more hazardous in COPD than underdosage, the maximum recommended increase in dosage should be avoided initially, and upward adjustments made if this is warranted by the clinical response of the individual patient.

The appropriate initial maintenance dosage for theophylline for an average nonsmoking, nonobese, relatively healthy adult is 10 to 12 mg/kg/day. For a 70 kg patient, a total of 800 mg a day can be given in two doses of a slow-release product, i.e., 400 mg every 12 hours. After three days of therapy, an adjustment can be made on clinical grounds or by using a theophylline serum level as a guide. Further adjustment may be needed after a few more days to reach the optimal dosage. If the patient has any of the modifying factors listed in Table 7–4, the appropriate reduction or increase in dosage should be made.[17] Rather than simply increasing the theophylline dosage in a smoker, greater efforts should be made to persuade the patient to quit—although one should be aware that the need for a higher dose may persist for many months after quitting. If a patient requires more than 900 mg/day of theophylline, it is advisable to give the long-acting preparation in three equal dosages. Some newer long-acting preparations may be adequate when given once a day, but they are only reliable when required at a lower dosage for patients who have milder bronchospasm. One potential problem with the once-a-day dose preparations is that taking them close to breakfast can result in faster absorption, higher-than-optimal blood theophylline levels during the day, and inadequate levels at night.[18, 19]

Dosages of Aminophylline

Aminophylline contains about 80% theophylline, and it is therefore appropriate to give dosages that are 20% greater. In general, aminophylline is only used as an intravenous drug for patients experiencing an exacerbation of COPD with severe bronchospasm. In such cases, a loading dose is infused over the course of 30 minutes. The amount required can be calculated from basic pharmacokinetic principles, or more simply and empirically, one can give 5 to 7 mg/kg. If no theophylline has been taken recently, such a dose would be expected to produce a mean peak serum level of about 10 to 14 μg/ml, although the actual levels in a mixed population can vary over a much wider range, e.g., 5 to 20 μg/ml. If it is known that there is already theophylline in the patient, the loading dose should be reduced to a half or a third of the standard; an initial serum level should always be obtained as a guide if possible.

If a higher serum level (e.g., 20 μg/ml) is known to be necessary for an individual patient, an increase in loading dosage could be made, e.g., up to about 9 mg/kg. If the patient is a smoker, 10 to 12 mg/kg aminophylline may be justified, although in practice it is safer to give 50% to 75% of this amount and then to consider giving a second loading dose one or two hours later if the response, or a serum level taken half an hour after completing the infusion, is inadequate. Obese patients should be given a loading dose calculated from their actual weight.

Maintenance therapy with aminophylline should be given on a similar basis to therapy with oral theophylline, using a 20% larger dose. In general, a dose of 0.5 to 0.6 mg/kg ideal body weight should be infused every hour (in the average, nonsmoking adult), and a check on the serum level taken after 24 hours. Doses as high as 1.2 mg/kg/hr may be required for heavy smokers, but it is advisable to avoid such large doses initially; if necessary, the dose can be gradually increased to this level using the clinical response and the serum level for guidance. The infusion is usually continued for several days, and further determinations of the serum level should be made as clinically indicated and when the patient is switched to oral theophylline therapy. Since serum levels can now be obtained relatively inexpensively, additional checks on levels should be obtained whenever clinical symptoms need to be evaluated or if any change in dosage is contemplated. Recently, intravenous theophylline preparations have become available, and these should be infused at a dosage equivalent to about 80% that used for aminophylline.

STEROID THERAPY

The anti-inflammatory corticosteroids have been in use for nearly 40 years, and it has become clear that both their value and their dangers in the treatment of pulmonary disease have been exaggerated. Although they have become part of the established regimen in the management of severe asthma, their possible benefits in other forms of COPD continue to be a source of dispute.

Numerous studies over the years suggest that steroids are only of benefit in COPD when there is a component of asthma.[20, 21] Perhaps 10% to 15% of all COPD patients with moderate to severe incapacity show a worthwhile improvement on chronic steroid therapy. If it is decided to initiate a trial of steroids, the patient should be carefully observed for 10 to 20 days, and if objective evidence of benefit is not discernible, the drug should then be discontinued.

Steroid Preparations

Although numerous steroids are available (Table 7–5), most physicians only need to employ two or three in the management of their COPD patients.

For an acute exacerbation with severe wheezing that responds inadequately to sympathomimetic or theophylline therapy, an intravenous steroid can be given. Methylprednisolone (MP) is often preferred, since it has less salt-retaining effect than hydrocortisone. An appropriate dose of MP would be 0.3 mg/kg as a loading dose followed by 0.1 to 0.2 mg/kg/hr; the larger dose is used in steroid-dependent patients or, perhaps, in extremely severe disease. After a day or two, oral therapy can usually be initiated, using prednisone 40 mg a day. This dose should be weaned by 5 to 10 mg every one to two days to a maintenance dose of 7.5 to 10 mg/day.

Judgment is required to determine whether the prednisone should be further reduced or stopped, continued chronically, or switched to alternate-day therapy using a regimen of 5 mg on odd days and 15 to 20 mg on even days. Aerosol steroids have not been shown to be of benefit in the majority

Table 7–5. **Main Corticosteroid Preparations for COPD**

| | Formulations | | | Equivalent Oral or IV Dose (mg) | Effective Half-Life (hours) |
	Oral (mg)	IV (mg/ml)	MDI* (mg/puff)		
Hydrocortisone	5, 10, 20	50		20.0	8–12
Prednisone	1, 2.5, 5, 10, 25, 50			5.0	12–30
Methylprednisolone	2, 4, 8, 16, 24, 32	40, 125, 500, 1000		4.0	15–30
Triamcinolone	1, 2, 4, 8, 16		0.10	4.0	18–48
Dexamethasone	0.25, 0.5, 0.75, 1.5, 2, 4, 6	4, 10, 20, 24	0.084	0.75	36–54
Beclomethasone			0.042		6–12
Flunisolide			0.25		12

*MDI = metered dose inhaler

of patients with COPD, and their use cannot be advocated at this time unless the patient has a major component of asthma. Beclomethasone is given as two to four puffs three or four times a day, triamcinolone as two to four puffs three or four times a day, and flunisolide as two to four puffs twice a day. It is an advantage to aerosolize MDI steroids with a reservoir spacer interposed between the mouthpiece and the mouth; this not only improves delivery to the lungs but also markedly reduces the oropharyngeal deposition of the drug and thus eliminates irritation and candidiasis as complications.

Side Effects

Short courses of intravenous or oral steroids given for 10 to 14 days have no significant side effects in most patients, although sodium retention and potassium loss could be a problem in the critically ill when using large doses of prednisone or hydrocortisone. There is an exaggerated concern that short-term steroids can create a potential for stress-induced adrenal insufficiency for many months afterwards. This very rarely occurs in practice but has been reported after prolonged therapy or when converting abruptly from chronic therapy with large oral doses to an aerosol steroid.

Prolonged therapy carries several risks in COPD patients. Weight gain can be a major problem, and this may cancel out the beneficial effect of the steroid on the airways. Moon facies, posterior subcapsular cataracts, ecchymoses, and osteoporosis are other frequent complications. Peptic ulcer is rarely induced, but steroids and theophylline have an additive irritant effect on the stomach and may necessitate antacid therapy. The risk of significant complications is very low if no more than 10 mg/day of prednisone is taken, whereas the incidence is much higher if doses greater than 20 mg/day are used.

When a patient with COPD is scheduled for elective surgery, steroid coverage is advisable if steroid therapy has been given during the previous few months.[22] A suitable regimen to prevent bronchospasm in such a patient would be hydrocortisone 50 mg intravenously the night before surgery, 100 mg preoperatively, and 100 mg every six hours until the condition is stable or until oral prednisone can be initiated at a dose of 40 to 60 mg/day followed by gradual dose reduction.

OTHER ANTIMEDIATOR DRUGS

Although there has been a huge increase in knowledge about the biochemical events involved in the pathogenesis of bronchospasm, airway inflammation, and mucus production, new drugs that might act favorably on the cyclo-oxygenase and lipoxygenase pathways have not emerged. None of the additional antimediator drugs that have been used for asthma are of general use in COPD.[23]

Cromolyn is a mast-cell stabilizer and is of greatest value in allergic asthma and exercise-induced bronchospasm. No oral derivative of this drug has been introduced into therapeutics, but the powder-form of cromolyn is now available as a solution for nebulization. The preparations are not recommended for use in COPD, unless there is a need for prophylaxis of specific asthmatic episodes such as those that can occur with exercise.

Antihistamines are of benefit in some allergic syndromes associated with asthma but are of no specific value in COPD. In some patients, the sedative effect of antihistamines may help alleviate cough and improve sleep. Although there is a theoretic concern that these drugs could increase the viscosity of the sputum, this is usually not a problem in clinical practice.

Ketotifen is an antimediator drug with antihistaminic properties. It has been introduced in Europe and is reported to be of minor value in asthma. It is not indicated for the management of COPD.

Calcium-Channel Blockers currently in use include verapamil, nifedipine, and diltiazem. Although studies have shown that these agents can be of some benefit in asthma, their effects are very limited.[24] The main use of such therapy appears to be in the prophylaxis of exercise-induced bronchospasm. These drugs have not demonstrated any effect on mucociliary transport, and their overall value in COPD is likely to be disappointing. Future calcium antagonists may have more specific actions on bronchial smooth muscle and mast cells, but their role in COPD will probably be minor.

ANTICHOLINERGIC AGENTS

Since vagal activity is involved in both bronchospasm and mucus production, antiparasympathetic therapy can be of value in COPD.[23] Since vagal control appears to be more active in bronchitis than in asthma, anticholinergic therapy is of greater benefit in bronchitis. In the United States only atropine sulfate is generally available and can be given as a 1% solution by aerosol. The dose is 0.1 to 0.5 ml (1 to 5 mg) every four to six hours. It should be given in combination with an aerosol bronchodilator, since there is a synergistic effect. It does not impair expectoration when given topically, although it could do so if administered systemically. Atropine can cause tachycardia and a dry mouth and may induce mydriasis. It should be reserved for acute exacerbations of bronchospasm and is generally neither effective enough nor sufficiently tolerated to be given as part of a chronic regimen. In Europe, atropine methonitrate and ipratropium (Atrovent) are available. These agents are better tolerated, more effective, and particularly useful in the treatment of chronic bronchitis.[25]

MUCOKINETIC AGENTS

Mucostasis is a major problem in asthma and bronchitis, but no improvements in therapy have appeared in recent years in the United States.[26] It is generally accepted that water is the most important mucokinetic agent, but clear evidence is not available for dogmatic advice regarding either the optimal route of delivery or the amount to be taken. Thus, patients with advanced COPD must often strike a balance between adequate water intake and avoidance of edema, with diuretic therapy interposing a further variable into the balance. Aerosolized water, or saline solutions, are often prescribed for patients, but there is no proof that this therapy improves mucokinesis, and the aerosolized particles can provoke bronchospasm.

Adequate humidity is important, although excess can induce bronchospasm in susceptible patients. In the critically ill, water is given intravenously as well as by aerosol, but the primary concern is usually drug delivery and not mucokinesis. Indeed, in many of these patients mechanical methods, including endotracheal intubation and suctioning, are more relevant than either hydration or pharmacotherapy for removing excessive secretions.

It is fortunate that both sympathomimetic drugs and theophylline stimulate mucociliary clearance, while steroids may improve mucus viscosity. Thus, routine therapy for COPD can improve mucokinesis. Most of the popular mucokinetic drugs (such as salt solutions, guaifenesin, and terpin hydrate) are of lesser value. The potent mucolytic agent acetylcysteine is sometimes employed in both acute and chronic therapy since it can be helpful for breaking up very viscous secretions. Acetylcysteine can be given in a dose of 2 to 4 ml of the 10% solution, diluted with 2 ml of 5% sodium bicarbonate. A standard bronchodilator should be added, and the mixture can be administered by nebulization or instillation every three to eight hours.

The major oral mucokinetic agents are listed in Table 7–6. In practice, many pulmonologists favor using iodide (e.g., saturated solution of potassium iodide) for a maximum of four to six weeks at a time, whereas other oral expectorants are prescribed without much conviction that they are of any value whatsoever. Disadvantages of SSKI include the development of hypothyroidism in patients after sustained use, skin rash, and upset stomach—but over 90% of patients tolerate the drug for as long as six weeks.

Table 7–6. **Major Oral Expectorants**

Agent	Marketed Products	Dosage Give 3–4 times/day
Guaifenesin	Breonesin,* Robitussin,* etc.	200–600 mg
Ammonium salts	Various*	300–1000 mg
Hydriodic acid	Hydriodic Acid Syrup	15–45 ml
Potassium iodide	Pima	300–1000 mg
	SSKI	10–20 drops
Calcium iodide	Calcidrine†	300–1000 mg
Iodinated glycerol	Organidin	30–60 mg
Potassium citrate	Citra Forte,† etc.	0.4 mg/kg
Sodium citrate	Tussar-2,† etc.	1.0 gm
Syrup of ipecac	Various mixtures	0.5–2.0 ml

*Available without prescription.
†This product contains additional agents.

ANTIBIOTICS FOR OUTPATIENTS

Exacerbations of COPD cause the patient to experience increased dyspnea, cough, and difficulty in expectorating the mucus, which becomes more viscous and may change color to yellow or green. Although the patient's temperature and white blood count may not increase, the change in symptoms is generally assumed to be an indication for antibiotic therapy. It may be difficult to prove that there is an infectious process causing the problem, and it is equally difficult to prove that antibotics help.[27, 28] However, the clinical impression is that antibiotic therapy is indicated when symptoms appear, and many physicians advise their patients to initiate a seven- to 14-day course of treatment for each clinical exacerbation. In more severe cases, some physicians advise prolonged therapy or routine courses of antibiotics to be taken every few weeks.

All common agents that cover *Diplococcus pneumoniae* and *Haemophilus influenzae* are acceptable, and it may be advisable to use a different antibiotic for each successive exacerbation. Favored agents include tetracycline, ampicillin, or amoxicillin, erythromycin, and trimethoprim-sulfamethoxazole. For occasional patients, cefaclor (the oral cephalosporin effective against *Haemophilus*) may be worth trying; however, Augmentin (amoxicillin in combination with clavulanic acid) is preferrable in most situations. Sputum culture is rarely of value in exacerbations of COPD unless there are systemic signs of infection or severe deterioration in pulmonary status with a new radiographic infiltrate in the lungs. A Gram stain and culture of secretions can help in the choice of a specific antibiotic if there are signs of overt infection.

ANTITUSSIVE AGENTS

Many patients with COPD have irritating coughs that produce little or no sputum and cause work or sleep disturbances or family problems. In such

cases, it may be worth trying a non-narcotic antitussive in lov
increasing the dose to the maximum if necessary. The most |
drugs is dextromethorphan. Benzonatate, caramiphen, and
used less often (Table 7–7).

If the cough is troublesome, the advantages of suppress
outweigh the concerns about respiratory center or central n
depression, particularly if the patient has untreatable lung canc
terminal weeks of COPD. If non-narcotics are ineffective in su
of the narcotic agents may be justified. Codeine and hydr
relatively safe, but morphine and hydromorphone can only be   ider
strict supervision when hospice-type therapy is indicated. In so   patients,
small doses of sedatives or tranquilizers (such as a benzodiazepine, e.g.,
oxazepam 7.5 to 10 mg) can relieve anxiety and may decrease the sense of
breathlessness, without depressing respiratory drive. Not infrequently, antidepressants are required and may be useful in low doses. However, patients
with COPD must be carefully followed and evaluated whenever such agents
with the potential for respiratory center depressant effects are prescribed.

Chapter 12 presents psychopharmacologic agents that may be useful in
COPD patients.

Many over-the-counter preparations contain dextromethorphan or nos-
capine in combination with antihistamines, vasoconstrictors, drying agents,
or expectorants.[29] Patients should be cautioned to avoid such mixtures since
their side effects could be detrimental in severe COPD. The physician should
counsel patients about avoiding viral infections, and yearly vaccination against
influenza should be encouraged. If a patient does contract the flu during an
influenza A epidemic, amantadine 100 to 200 mg two times a day can be
given for about 10 days to reduce the severity of the illness. A similar
prophylactic measure is to provide pneumococcal vaccine for patients with
COPD. It is currently recommended to administer the vaccination once only,

Table 7–7. **Important Antitussive Drugs**

	Marketed Products	Dosage
Narcotic Agents		
Codeine	Various products	5–20 mg q3–6 hr
Hydrocodone	Dicodid, Hycodan,[a] Tussionex,[b] etc.	5–10 mg q4–8 hr
Hydromorphone	Dilaudid	1–2 mg q3–4 hr
Morphine		2–4 mg q4–6 hr
Non-Narcotic Agents		
Benzonatate	Tessalon Perles	1–2 (100–200 mg) q4–8 hr
Caramiphen	Tuss-Ornade[c]	10–20 mg q4–6 hr
Dextromethorphan[d]	Delsym, DM cough, Romilar, etc.	10–30 mg q4–8 hr
Noscapine[d]	Tusscapine, etc.	15–30 mg q4–6 hr

[a]Each tablet or 5 ml of liquid contains hydrocodone 5 mg and homatropine 1.5 mg.

[b]Each long-acting tablet, capsule or 5 ml suspension contains hydrocodone 5 mg and the
antihistamine phenyltoloxamine 10 mg.

[c]Each long-acting capsule contains caramiphen 40 mg and phenylpropanolamine 75 mg.
Each 5 ml liquid contains caramiphen 6.7 mg and phenylpropanolamine 12.5 mg.

[d]Various products are available without prescription.

since repeat administration enhances the potential for adverse effects from the vaccine.

References

1. Hudson LD: Management of COPD. State of the art. *Chest* (supp) 1984; 84:76S–81S.
2. Make B: Medical management of emphysema. *Clin Chest Med* 1983; 4:465–482.
3. Tattersfield AF: Diseases of the respiratory system. Chronic bronchitis and emphysema. *Br Med J* 1978;1:1123–1125.
4. Van As A, Avner BP: Beta agonists, in Flenley DC, Petty TL (eds): *Recent Advances in Respiratory Medicine, Number 3.* New York, Churchill Livingstone Inc, 1983.
5. Newhouse MT: Principles of aerosol therapy. *Chest* (supp) 1982;21:39S–41S.
6. Popa VT: Clinical pharmacology of adrenergic drugs. *J Asthma* 1984;21:183–207.
7. Konig P: Spacer devices used with metered-dose inhalers. Breakthrough or gimmick? *Chest* 1985;88:276–284.
8. Sackner MA, Kim CS: Auxillary MDI aerosol delivery systems. *Chest* (supp) 1985;88:161S–170S.
9. Lewis RA: Therapeutic aerosols, in Cumming G, Bonsignore G (eds): *Drugs and the Lungs.* New York, Plenum Press, 1982, pp 59–86.
10. Newman SP: Aerosol deposition considerations in inhalation therapy. *Chest* (supp) 1985;88:152S–160S.
11. Weinberger M, Hendeles L: Methylxanthines, in Weiss EB, Segal MS, Stein M (eds.): *Bronchial Asthma. Mechanisms and Therapeutics*, ed 2. Boston, Little, Brown & Co, 1985.
12. Hendeles L, Iafrate RP, Weinberger M: A clinical and pharmacokinetic basis for the selection and use of slow release theophylline products. *Clin Pharmacokinet* 1984;9:95–135.
13. Jenne JW: Theophylline use in asthma. Some current issues. *Clin Chest Med* 1984;5:645–658.
14. Dull W, Alexander M: Theophylline in stable chronic airflow obstruction: A reappraisal. *Arch Intern Med* 1984;144:2399–2401.
15. Matthay RA: Effects of theophylline on cardiovascular performance in chronic obstructive disease. *Chest* (supp) 1985; 82:112S–117S.
16. Levine JH, Michael JR, Guarnieri T: Mul-tifocal tachycardia: A toxic effect of theophylline. *Lancet* 1985;1:12–14.
17. Baumann JH, Lalonde RL, Self TH: Factors modifying serum theophylline concentrations: An update. *Immunol Allerg Pract* 1985;7:259–269.
18. Karen A, Burns T, Wearley L, et al: Food-induced changes in theophylline absorption from controlled-release formulations. Part 1. Substantial increased and decreased absorption with Uniphyl tablets and Theo-Dur Sprinkle. *Clin Pharm Therapeutics* 1985;38:77–83.
19. Hendeles L, Wubbena P, Weinberger M: Food-induced dose dumping of once-a-day theophylline. *Lancet* 1984;2:1471.
20. Rudd R: Corticosteroids in chronic bronchitis. *Br Med J* 1984;288:1553–1554.
21. Sahn SA: Corticosteroid therapy in chronic obstructive pulmonary disease. *Pract Cardiol* 1985;11(8):150–156.
22. Ziment I: Perioperative pharmacologic management. *Respir Care* 1984;29:652–666.
23. George RB, Payne OK: Anticholinergics, cromolyn and other occasionally useful drugs. *Clin Chest Med* 1984;5:685–694.
24. Ahmed T, Abraham WM: Role of calcium-channel blockers in obstructive airway disease. *Chest* (supp) 1985;82:142S–151S.
25. Pakes GE: Anticholinergic drugs, in Buckle DR, Smith H (eds): *Development of Antiasthma Drugs.* London, Butterworths, 1984.
26. Ziment I: Hydration, humidification and mucokinetic therapy, in Weiss EB, Segal MS, Stein M (eds): *Bronchial Asthma. Mechanisms and Therapeutics*, ed 2. Boston, Little, Brown & Co, 1985.
27. Sachs FL: Chronic bronchitis, in Pennington JE (ed): *Respiratory Infections: Diagnosis and Management.* New York, Raven Press, 1983, pp 113–124.
28. Ziment I: Prophylactic and therapeutic management of chronic obstructive pulmonary disease, in Ziment I (ed): *Practical Pulmonary Disease.* New York, John Wiley and Sons, 1983.
29. Ziment I: *Respiratory Pharmacology and Therapeutics.* Philadelphia, WB Saunders Co, 1978.

RESPIRATORY THERAPY TECHNIQUES

THOMAS L. PETTY

Respiratory therapy techniques are fundamental to the long-term care of patients with all stages of chronic obstructive pulmonary disease (COPD). These approaches to therapy include nebulization of bronchodilating agents, oxygen therapy, and mechanical ventilation. The discussion of mechanical ventilation for acute respiratory failure is beyond the scope of this chapter, which focuses on methods of nebulizing inhaled bronchodilators and principles of prescribing home oxygen therapy.

NEBULIZED BRONCHODILATORS

The regular and systematic inhalation of beta agonist aerosols improves air flow in a substantial number of patients with all stages of COPD. In addition, anticholinergics are rapidly being appreciated as offering additional advantages to some patients.[1] Bronchodilating aerosols can be delivered by hand-bulb, pump-driven, or metered-dose inhaling devices. These techniques have replaced intermittent positive-pressure breathing (IPPB), particularly in the home, since there is no demonstrable advantage of using an inhaled beta agonist with an IPPB device.[2]

Hand-bulb and pump-driven nebulizers using bronchodilator solutions

Table 8–1. **Metered-Dose Inhalers Used in North America**

Generic Drug	Product Name
Albuterol or salbutamol	Proventil, Ventolin
Bitolterol	Tornalate
Fenoterol*	Berotec
Isoetharine	Bronkometer
Isoproterenol	Isuprel
Metaproterenol	Alupent, Metaprel
Racemic epinephrine	Vaponefrin
Terbutaline	Brethaire

*Available in Canada and Mexico; soon to be released in the United States.

such as isoproterenol, isoetharine, metaproterenol, or racemic epinephrine can provide effective bronchodilation. These agents are also known to increase mucociliary clearance.[3] Greater amounts of medication are delivered by these devices than by metered-dose devices. Hand-bulb nebulizers are difficult to use by many people, particularly those with arthritis or hand weakness, and thus pump-driven nebulizers have become much more widely used. This type of nebulization therapy, however, usually does not provide any greater bronchodilation than that achieved with a metered-dose inhaler (MDI).[4]

The MDI is rapidly emerging as the most practical and convenient way of delivering a bronchodilator aerosol. Metered-dose agents in common use are listed in Table 8–1. Proper use of this inhaler has recently been learned through systematic studies. There must be an opportunity for large particles coated with propellant to flash, i.e., evaporate into smaller particles that can impact in large airways or reach smaller airways through the process of gravitational sedimentation. All of this takes time. The necessary steps in the proper use of an MDI are listed in Table 8–2; these permit optimal nebulization, distribution, and deposition in the lungs in order for the drug to reach both the large and small airways.

HOME OXYGEN

Home oxygen is now established as beneficial for large numbers of patients with advanced chronic lung diseases and hypoxemia. Two landmark studies, the Nocturnal Oxygen Therapy Trial (NOTT)[5] and the British Medical

Table 8–2. **Proper Use of Metered-Dose Inhalers**

- Open mouth.
- Place device 2–4 inches in front of mouth or use spacer.
- Actuate and inhale slowly.
- Pause for up to 10 seconds.
- Exhale slowly.

Research Council (MRC) Multicenter Trial[6] have clearly shown that oxygen improves survival in selected patients with advanced COPD. In brief, the British study compared 15 hours of oxygen including nighttime use with no oxygen, and the American study compared more continuous oxygen with 12 hours of nighttime oxygen. Both studies enrolled patients with advanced COPD with significant hypoxemia when patients were in a stable state and otherwise receiving good treatment for airflow obstruction. Figure 8–1 summarizes the outcome of these studies and shows the survival curve of patients on no oxygen, 12- or 15-hour oxygen, and 24-hour oxygen. Thus, in selected patients with advanced COPD, living without oxygen represents a significant risk of premature death (MRC controls). By contrast, oxygen administration for approximately 50% of the time including the hours of sleep greatly improved survival (MRC-O$_2$ and NIH-NOT), but the very best survival occurred in patients who received continuous oxygen (NIH-COT), allowing for the oxygen cost of breathing, ambulation, and other activities of daily living.

In addition, quality of life and brain function[7] were better in the American study when continuous ambulatory oxygen was employed and hospitalizations were somewhat reduced compared to only nighttime oxygen.[5] Accordingly, there appears to be substantial benefits from ambulatory oxygen given in a continuous or nearly continuous fashion compared to less continuous oxygen delivery from stationary sources which, although beneficial, do not offer the most desirable outcome.

Many primary care physicians are beginning to ask about principles and guidelines of prescribing oxygen. In addition, recent proposals from third-party payers, including the Health Care Financing Administration, will probably mandate very specific prescriptions and a justification for either stationary or portable oxygen delivery systems. Thus, this section offers current oxygen prescribing principles and gives examples of prescriptions that can be tailored

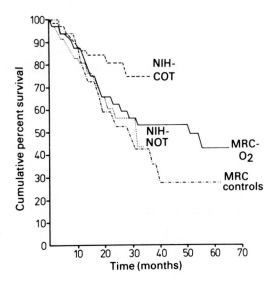

Figure 8–1. Comparison of survival in COPD patients receiving no oxygen (MRC controls), 12 or 15 hours of oxygen (NIH-NOT, MRC-O$_2$), or nearly continuous oxygen (NIH-COT).

Table 8–3. **General Guidelines for Prescribing Home Oxygen for Patients with Advanced COPD**

A. Patient Selection Criteria
1. Stable course of disease on optimum medical therapy, e.g., bronchodilator, antibiotics, or corticosteroids (if indicated).
2. At least two arterial blood gas determinations while breathing air for at least 20 minutes.
3. Room air P_{O_2} consistently ≤55; or consistently 56 to 59 plus cor pulmonale clinically diagnosed and/or hematocrit ≥55%.
4. Normoxic patients where less dyspnea and increased exercise is demonstrated with oxygen.

B. Oxygen Dose
1. Continuous flow by double or single nasal cannulae (see text), or
2. By demand system with demonstration of adequate oxygen saturation.
3. Lowest liter flow to raise P_{O_2} to 60 to 65 or oxygen saturation to 90% to 94%.
4. Increase baseline liter flow by 1 L/min during exercise and sleep.

to each patient's needs. It is likely, however, that prescribing guidelines will be continually revised and updated.

Prescribing Criteria for Home Oxygen

So far, all controlled clinical trials dealing with outcome from long-term home oxygen have dealt with the problem of advanced COPD. Guidelines for prescribing home oxygen in COPD patients, based on the nocturnal oxygen therapy trial are listed in Table 8–3. These include a significant level of hypoxemia (a P_{O_2} of 55 or less for three weeks or more when the patient is in a clinical stable state, i.e., free from exacerbations of bronchitis or congestive heart failure). Supplementary criteria were also used in the NOTT trial when the P_{O_2} was between 55 and 59 while the patient was in a stable condition. These were evidence of pulmonary hypertension as judged by electrocardiogram criteria with a right axis and so-called pulmonale, i.e., P waves in standard leads II and III and AVF greater than 2.5 mmHg. It would also be reasonable to include an enlarged pulmonary outflow tract and prominent major pulmonary arteries, as judged from standard chest x-ray films (PA and lateral) as additional clinical evidence for pulmonary hypertension. Any clinical evidence of right heart failure with elevated jugular venous distention, liver engorgement, and peripheral edema could also be taken as evidence of cor pulmonale. Evidence of secondary polycythemia with a hematocrit 55% or more could also be used as a supplementary criterion. These latter two clinical states, cor pulmonale and secondary polycythemia, are taken as signs of an adverse response to the presence of hypoxemia.

Oxygen Dosage

The Nocturnal Oxygen Therapy Trial (NOTT) established the fact that the great majority of patients with advanced COPD and hypoxemia as described above can be managed with oxygen delivered by nasal cannulae at 1–2 L/min. Less than 10% of individuals with COPD required 3 L/min at rest. Studies during the conduct of NOTT indicated the need for an additional 1 L/min during the stress of exercise and while sleeping. This increased oxygen flow requirement is probably due to the increased metabolic demands of exercise and a modest degree of hypoventilation and/or an additional degree of oxygen transport abnormality during sleep. Thus, with the patient's baseline liter flow at rest, if it takes two liters to bring the oxygen tension within the range of 60 to 65 or the oxygen saturation within 90% to 94%, the same individual will require three liters while exercising or during the hours of sleep.

Should All Patients with Po_2 of ≤ 55 be Prescribed Home Oxygen?

The answer to this question is obviously no. Were this the case, virtually every adult in Leadville, Colorado, (elevation 10,000 feet) would be a candidate for oxygen, since a Po_2 of 55 is normal in older individuals at this altitude. Normal patients are able to compensate for moderate or even severe degrees of hypoxemia through an increase in cardiac output and by modest elevations in red cell mass.

By contrast, patients with pulmonary disease often have little or no ability to adapt to even moderate degrees of hypoxemia. Thus, the ravages of insufficient oxygen supply occur in these patients, and reactive pulmonary hypertension, cor pulmonale, and secondary erythrocytosis, as well as other organ system damage, is the result. Clinical counterparts include mental impairment and reduced renal function. In each instance cited, long-term home oxygen has been shown to improve the specific organ system function and to improve the overall survival and quality of life of most patients. Accordingly, oxygen should be prescribed not only on the basis of blood gas criteria as a first consideration but also in the context of clinical evidence of harm to the patient.

Is Oxygen Ever Useful in Patients Who Do Not Demonstrate Daytime Hypoxemia?

The answer to this question is emphatically yes. The point here is that hypoxemia may not be present when patients are awake, alert, and upright, but the patient may be suffering substantial hypoxemia at other times. Such is the case during the hours of sleep in patients with sleep-disordered breathing.[8, 9] Nocturnal pulmonary hypertension and cardiac arrhythmias have been documented during sleep-related hypoxemia.[10] Nocturnal hypoxemia could be the forerunner of life-threatening cardiac arrhythmias[11] and pulmonary hypertension resulting in cor pulmonale.[12] Accordingly, patients who are symptomatic as a result of hypoxemia or who demonstrate any hint of occult hypoxemia, such as unexplained erythrocytosis or early evidence of pulmonary hypertension, should be studied during the hours of sleep with simple noninvasive oximetry in order to determine if nocturnal hypoxemia, is present.[13]

In addition, other patients may have significant hypoxemia while exercising, and this can be identified by treadmill studies using oximetry or applying an oximeter immediately after walking in corridors and/or on stairs. If it is demonstrated that exercise-induced hypoxemia drastically limits exercise or is accompanied by excessive tachycardia or cardiac arrhythmias, the use of oxygen only during ambulation appears warranted.

Finally, at least one study with an adequate scientific design shows that even normoxemic "pink-puffing" emphysema patients have better exercise tolerance with oxygen than with air.[14] How oxygen is helpful in these situations is not known, but the most likely reason is that it prevents exercise-related hypoxemia and impaired tissue oxygen delivery caused by a fixed low cardiac output or provides extra oxygen for the high work of breathing in states of relative hyperventilation.

What Type of Oxygen System Should Be Prescribed?

Beginning historically, compressed gas high-pressure cylinders, liquid systems, and stationary oxygen concentrators are available for home use by a physician's prescription. The advantages and disadvantages of each are listed in Table 8–4. Certain comments about each system are appropriate. Stationary systems are preferable for patients who are essentially housebound. These individuals can still be ambulatory about the home, using long (50-foot) tubing. Ambulatory patients, including those able to work, should have a portable system, either a transfilling gaseous system or a liquid system.

Liquid systems are preferable for those who require the greatest range away from their stationary source. Primary candidates are people who can work several hours each day away from home in their office and patients participating in a pulmonary rehabilitation program. Today, the weight of evidence indicates that exercise is important therapy for COPD. Thus, if patients who require long-term oxygen are able to ambulate, they should be given portable systems. If their level of activity can be restored or maintained at a high level, the liquid systems are preferable from an overall therapeutic point of view.

A recent conference on the state of the art in home oxygen therapy has been published by the American College of Chest Physicians.[15]

Recently, criteria for Medicare coverage of oxygen services in the home have been proposed, which will become guidelines or requirements for prescribing home oxygen.[16] In general, the guidelines for selection of patients

Table 8–4. **Advantages and Disadvantages of Available Home Oxygen Systems**

	Liquid Portable	Concentrators	Compressed Gas
Advantages	1. Light weight	1. Lower cost	1. Lower cost in general (cost may equal liquid in continuous use situations)
	2. Long-range portable canister	2. Convenient at home	2. Widespread availability
	3. Most practical ambulatory system	3. Attractive equipment	
	4. Valuable for pulmonary rehabilitation	4. Widespread availability	
	5. 100% oxygen at all flow rates		
Disadvantages	1. More expensive than concentrators used alone	1. Electricity required	1. Multiple tanks necessary for ambulation unless transfilling can be done at home
	2. Not available in small or rural communities	2. May need back-up tank system	2. Frequent deliveries needed
		3. Not portable; does not assist in ambulation or pulmonary rehabilitation	3. Heavy and unsightly tanks; not as effective in pulmonary rehabilitation
		4. Noise	

for home oxygen are consistent with those derived from the NOTT and MRC studies as summarized in Table 8–3. In brief, these guidelines call for the use of home oxygen and oxygen equipment under the durable medical equipment benefit (§1861 (s)).[16] Oxygen will be considered "reasonable and necessary *only* for patients with significant hypoxemia who meet (certain) medical documentation, laboratory and health conditions." These are briefly summarized in Table 8–5.

Table 8–5. **Medical, Laboratory, and Health Conditions***

1. Evidence that alternate therapy has been tried to correct hypoxemia, e.g., antimicrobials, bronchodilators, corticosteroids (when indicated), and physical therapy.
2. A diagnosis requiring home oxygen, e.g., COPD, emphysema, or cor pulmonale. Other diagnoses suitable for home oxygen include bronchiectasis, cystic fibrosis, and interstitial fibrosis.
3. Oxygen flow rate requirement and daily duration of use.
4. Laboratory evidence (while patient is stable and breathing room air), e.g., blood gases PO_2 ≤ 55 or pulse oximetry O_2 sat. $\leq 85\%$.
5. Portable oxygen systems may be used alone or to complement a stationary oxygen system. Proper documentation of the activities or exercise routine is required as well as a prescription *and* evidence of clinical benefit by an increase in the patient's ability to exercise and perform various activities.

*Necessary documentation for prescribing home oxygen.

SUMMARY

Our knowledge about inhaled bronchodilators has been materially increased by numerous studies that focus on the various techniques of aerosol administration. At this writing, it appears that metered-dose inhalers are as effective as any other method of bronchodilator aerosol administration. Certainly, intermittent positive-pressure breathing does not offer an advantage to most patients.

The state of the art of oxygen delivery in the home has evolved remarkably in the past 20 years. Oxygen therapy is established as not only safe but effective in selected patients with advanced COPD. Oxygen has clearly been shown to improve the length as well as the quality of life in many patients. Hospitalizations can be reduced, and this appears to be most likely in ambulatory patients receiving long-term oxygen by portable liquid systems. It is likely that further advances will make oxygen more suitable, acceptable, and perhaps less costly for a growing number of patients with progressive chronic respiratory diseases where significant hypoxemia and organ system damage are present.

References

1. Gross NJ, Skorodin MS: Role of the parasympathetic nervous system in airway obstruction due to emphysema. N Engl J Med 1984;311:421–425.
2. The IPPB Trial Group: Intermittent positive pressure breathing therapy in chronic obstructive pulmonary disease. Ann Intern Med 1983;99:612–620.
3. Pavia D, Bateman JRM, Clarke SW: Deposition and clearance of inhaled particles. Bull Eur Physiopathol Respir 1980;16:335–336.
4. Cushley, MJ, Lewis RA, Tattensfield AE: Comparison of three techniques of inhalation in the airway response to terbutaline. Thorax 1983;38:908–913.
5. Nocturnal Oxygen Therapy Trial Group: Continuous or nocturnal oxygen therapy in hypoxemic chronic obstructive lung disease. Ann Intern Med 1980;93:391–398.
6. The Medical Research Council Working Party: Long-term domicilliary oxygen therapy in chronic hypoxic cor pulmonale complicating chronic bronchitis and emphysema. Lancet 1981;1:681–686.
7. Heaton, RK, Grant I, McSweeney AJ, et al: Psychologic effects of continuous and nocturnal oxygen therapy in hypoxemic chronic obstructive pulmonary disease. Arch Intern Med 1983;143:1941–1947.
8. Douglas NJ, Calvenley PMA, Leggett RJE, et al: Transient hypoxemia during sleep in chronic bronchitis and emphysema. Lancet 1979;1:1–4.
9. DeMarco FJ Jr, Wynne JW, Block AJ, et al: Oxygen desaturation during sleep as a determinant of the "blue and bloated" syndrome. Chest 1981; 79:621–625.
10. Boysen PG, Block AJ, Wynne JW, et al: Nocturnal pulmonary hypertension in patients with chronic obstructive pulmonary disease. Chest 1979;76:536–542.
11. Trilapur VG, Mir MA: Nocturnal hypoxemia and associated electrocardiographic changes in patients with chronic obstructive airways disease. N Engl J Med 1982;306:125–130.
12. Block AJ, Boysen PG, Wynne JW: The origins of cor pulmonale, a hypothesis. Chest 1979;75:109–110.
13. Kryger MH, Mezon BJ, Acres JC, et al: Diagnosis of sleep breathing disorders in a general hospital. Arch Intern Med 1982;142:956–958.
14. Woodcock AA, Gross ER, Geddes DM: Oxygen relieves breathlessness in "pink puffers." Lancet 1981;1:907–909.
15. Fulmer JD, Snider GL: American College of Chest Physicians, National Heart, Lung, and Blood Institute, National Conference on Oxygen Therapy. Chest 1984; 86:234–242.
16. Federal Register. 1985;50:3–4 (April 5).

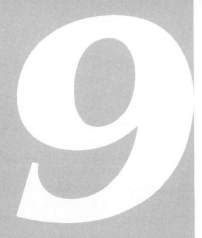

RELAXATION TECHNIQUES AND BIOFEEDBACK

DOROTHY L. SEXTON

The increased use of relaxation techniques and biofeedback therapy has sparked renewed interest in a holistic approach to the management of physical illness. Many have addressed the need for a new "biobehavioral" model that views health and illness as components of an individual's behavioral repertoire and response to daily living.

Implicit in behavioral medicine is the assumption that clients will assume considerable responsibility for their own care. This concept is consistent with an increasing trend in medicine. While some individuals are pleased by this development, others may not relish assuming a more responsible role.[1]

Until recently, individuals with chronic obstructive pulmonary disease (COPD) were considered to be poor candidates for rehabilitation because of the progressive nature of the illness. However, the success rate of cardiac rehabilitation programs has led health care providers to take a second look at rehabilitation programs for individuals with pulmonary disorders.

Relaxation and biofeedback techniques may serve as the nidus that fosters and maintains acceptance of individual responsibility for health and illness.

RELAXATION TECHNIQUES

Relaxation techniques are represented by such approaches as progressive relaxation, autogenic training, hypnosis, yoga, and transcendental meditation. Many of these techniques have their roots in Eastern and Western cultural and religious traditions. However, the relaxation response is not unique to any specific technique or religious practice.

There are a wide variety of procedures for achieving a state of relaxation. While relaxation therapy usually involves a multifaceted program, a relaxation technique is a relatively simple procedure that can be taught without difficulty and performed daily in the individual's home. Simple relaxation techniques bypass the usual complexities of modern technology and may specifically focus on calming the mind by using repetitious and soothing sounds or phrases.[2] Relaxation techniques that focus primarily on reducing muscle tension can, in turn, reduce anxiety simply as a product of muscle relaxation.

The stress reaction is described as an increase of sympathetic nervous system activity and the relaxation response as a decrease of this activity. Complete muscular relaxation is associated with changes that reflect decreased sympathetic nervous system activity, including decreased respiratory rate, oxygen consumption, heart rate, and blood pressure. Relaxation techniques can have a profound effect upon the autonomic nervous system activities associated with the stress response. Through relaxation techniques, the patient may be able to learn conscious control over these involuntary reactions.[3] Table 9–1 summarizes the physiologic, cognitive, and behavioral changes that occur with relaxation.

Relaxation techniques have been studied in a variety of stress-related conditions, such as headaches, hypertension, anxiety, insomnia, and premature ventricular contractions. The findings of the studies support the use of relaxation techniques in stress-related conditions.

Table 9–1. **What Happens When We Relax?**

Physiologic Manifestations	Cognitive Manifestations	Behavioral Manifestations
Decreased pulse	Altered state of consciousness, usually alpha level	Lack of attention or concern for environmental stimuli
Decreased blood pressure		
Decreased respirations	Heightened concentration on single mental image or idea	No verbal interaction
Decreased oxygen consumption		
Decreased carbon dioxide production and elimination	Receptivity to positive suggestion	No voluntary change of position
Decreased muscle tension		Passive movement easy
Decreased metabolic rate		
Pupil constriction		
Peripheral vasodilation		
Increased peripheral temperature		

Adapted from Graves HH, Thompson EA: Anxiety: A mental health vital sign, in Longo DC, Williams RA (eds): *Clinical Practice in Psychosocial Nursing Assessment and Intervention.* New York, Appleton-Century-Crofts, 1978.

Most relaxation techniques start with slow rhythmic breathing. As the muscles relax, the breathing pattern becomes slower and shallower and less oxygen is consumed. The rhythmicity of the breathing itself characterizes relaxation. The relaxation response manifests itself through physical changes experienced by the individual, who blocks out all external phenomena and most internal thoughts by sitting with his or her eyes closed in a relaxed position in a quiet environment.[2]

Benson and others[3] identified four essential components of a successful relaxation procedure:

1. A quiet environment.

2. A mental device such as a word or a phrase that is repeated in a specific fashion over and over again.

3. The adoption of a passive attitude, which is perhaps the most important of the elements.

4. A comfortable position.

A fifth factor that could have been listed is the principle of classic conditioning. The individual is encouraged to use the same technique (that has been successful) over a period of time in the hope that the relaxation response becomes conditioned to certain stimuli associated with the selected procedure (e.g., a repetitive phrase or a focus on breathing slowly).

In 1938, Jacobson described his technique of progressive relaxation. He posited that, when the body is in a state of relaxation, it is impossible to be in a state of stress. The mind and body function as a unit, and relaxation of the skeletal muscles promotes mental relaxation and vice versa. In short, relaxation has both physical and mental components that interact continuously.[4]

Progressive relaxation exercises involve tensing and relaxing specific groups of muscles while concentrating on the feelings of tension versus relaxation. Specific body postures are recommended during progressive muscle relaxation. Sitting or reclining are postures conducive to relaxing. Figure 9–1 shows the recommended posture during relaxation. Whichever posture is selected, the body should be well supported by a chair or bed. Small, soft pillows may be used at the neck or behind the knees to provide support. The position should be balanced to avoid straining of muscles. Tense muscles and discomfort interfere with achieving the relaxation response. It is recommended that relaxation be practiced for 20- or 30-minute sessions twice a day.

The directions for progressive muscle relaxation are:

1. Select a quiet, dimly lit environment with few distractions.

2. Assume a comfortable posture so that muscular tension is minimal (e.g., recline in a lounge chair or lie down on a bed with pillows under your head and knees).

3. Loosen all restrictive clothing and remove shoes.

4. Note your breathing. Is it fast, slow, deep, or shallow? Adjust your breathing pattern to slow, abdominal breathing. Count to six—inhale on one and two, exhale on three to six. Take several slow, deep breaths, and exhale through pursed lips.

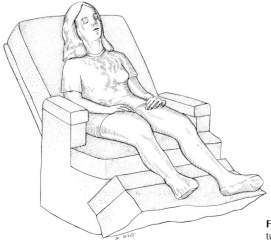

Figure 9–1. Recommended body posture for relaxation.

5. Do not worry about the degree of muscular relaxation being achieved. The following relaxation technique is based on the principle that maximum relaxation follows maximum contraction.

Feet

Tighten all the muscles in your foot and toes (one foot at a time). Curl toes and point them toward the floor. Hold them tense for five seconds. Then relax and feel the tension leave your foot. Let your foot become heavy and limp.

Legs

Tighten all the muscles in your leg (one leg at a time) and raise it from the surface. Hold leg tense for five seconds. Relax and let your leg return to the surface. Let the tension leave your leg so it becomes limp.

Pelvis

Tighten the muscles in your abdomen and buttocks. Hold your muscles tight and concentrate on the tension for five seconds. Then let go and relax. Feel the tension leave your muscles.

Chest

Slowly take in a full breath. While holding your breath, tighten all the muscles in your chest and back for three seconds. Exhale slowly and completely through pursed lips. Exhale the tension. Feel your muscles loosen up.

Arms

Hold your arm out straight (one arm at a time), tighten your muscles, and make a tight fist. Hold your arm and hand tense for five seconds. Relax and let your arm gradually fall to the chair or bed. Feel the muscles from your shoulder to your fingers loosen.

Shoulders

Shrug your shoulders and tighten the muscles. Hold your muscles tight and concentrate on the tension for three seconds. Let go and relax.

Neck

Bring your chin down to your chest as tightly as possible. Hold your neck tense for three seconds. Let go and relax. Roll your head from side to side in a relaxed manner. Stop when your head and neck assume a comfortable position.

Face

Squeeze your eyes tightly, furrow your brow, and clench your jaw. Hold your muscles tight and concentrate on the tension for five seconds. Let go and relax.

Savor the relief from tension and the calm feeling.

When you are ready to end the relaxation period, count to ten, gradually open your eyes, and slowly stretch as if awakening from a deep sleep. Start activities slowly afterwards. Some people relax so thoroughly that they cannot coordinate the movements of their arms or legs for a short time after relaxation.

Certain aspects of relaxation training are particularly important in retaining the skill of eliciting the relaxation response. For example, patients must learn *not to try* to relax. That is, rather than striving, they must learn to "let go," after which an internal quieting occurs.

Although the procedure for relaxation is relatively easy to learn, it involves much practice to become skillful. The learning process is facilitated by trained instructors in live sessions rather than taped instructions.

Music

Music can serve as a background for relaxation procedures. Soft, slow music is soothing and tends to calm physiologic responses. Instrumental music seems to have more of a calming effect than vocal arrangements.

Classical music is particularly conducive to relaxation because its rhythms and harmonic structures are often perceived as soothing. When people listen to classical music, they tend to let their thoughts wander away from their present concerns to more pleasant topics.[5]

The slow movements (often the second movement or the adagio) from a number of classical selections are appropriate for use:

- Pachelbel's Cannon in D Major.
- Mozart's Piano Concerto No. 21 in C Major.
- Vivaldi's The Four Seasons and the Six Flute Concerti, op. 10.
- Albinoni's Adagio in G Minor.
- Bach's Goldberg variations.
- Tchaikovsky's Pathétique Symphony.
- Dvořák's New World Symphony.

Table 9–2. **Patient Instructions for Listening to Music**

Once the patient has selected slow, soft, familiar music that he feels relaxes him, he can be given the following instructions:
1. Listen only to the music.
2. Feel the music lifting you upward.
3. Let each measure rhythmically flow through your body and relax the muscles.
4. Let yourself float through the air with the melody.

From McCaffery M: *Nursing Management of the Patient in Pain*, ed 2. Philadelphia, JB Lippincott, 1979, p 150, by permission.

- Brahms' First Piano Concerto (as well as piano concertos by Mozart, Chopin, Beethoven, and Rachmaninoff).
- Debussy's *L'Après-midi d'un faun* and "Petite Suite."
- Ravel's *Le Tombeau de Couperin* and the Piano Concerto in G.[6]

The adagio, larghetto, and largo movements of several composers have rhythms similar to the human heartbeat. When people listen to these movements, their biologic rhythms tend to synchronize themselves with the beat of the music. This is especially true with the slow, restful rhythm of a largo tempo. The result is deeper, more efficient relaxation.[7]

Other selections include:

- Halpern's *Soundscapes*
- Scott's and Yuize's *Music for Zen Meditations*.[8]

Recordings of environmental sounds (e.g., gentle rain, sounds of the sea, or desert birds) are useful. Also, relaxation cassettes with personally chosen selections can be made for patients.

When individuals listen to music, headsets are useful since they intensify the sounds. Table 9–2 lists a set of instructions to follow while listening to music.

Imagery

Our state of consciousness corresponds to our brain waves. The waking alert state is called beta. The level of consciousness in the relaxed state is termed alpha. In the alpha state (between full consciousness and unconsciousness), our thought processes become less logical and more associative. There tends to be a heightened ability to focus on one image. Because of the alpha state, guided imagery may be used effectively with relaxation techniques. Relaxation reduces tension and facilitates concentration on mental imagery.[5]

Imagery is a method often used in conjunction with relaxation techniques to enhance relaxation by actively visualizing suggested scenes.

> [These] images, or internal representations of events that involve the senses, form a bridge between mind and body, and provide a method for mentally and consciously altering body function.[9]

The therapist or coach should use slow, distinct guiding phrases to create a conducive environment for relaxation. An appropriate script may be selected from Kroger and Fezler who have developed 10 standard structured scenes to be used in healing imagery.[10]

In many relaxation techniques, the use of imagery is implicit, such as the instruction to focus on the air moving in and out of the lungs. Some patients not only feel the sensations of breathing but also visualize the air moving in and out of the lungs.

Guided imagery is not used as a substitute for traditional medical treatment but rather as an adjunct to it. For example, imagery may be used to promote sleep since disturbances are a frequent problem for patients with COPD. The patient who practices using a certain type of imagery usually finds it increasingly easy to create mental sensory images.

While the empirical data on the use of imagery are tenuous, clinical data support the continued use and investigation of relaxation and guided imagery. The subjective responses of patients, after using relaxation with imagery, indicate a lessening of stress, renewed self-confidence, and increased feelings of integration and wholeness.

Despite the substantial evidence accumulated over the past 15 years, a few questions still need to be raised. When a patient is practicing a relaxation technique, how does the patient or the therapist know that a relaxed state has been achieved? How does the patient or the therapist determine where the sources of most tension are? The answers to these questions can be found through the use of biofeedback.[11]

BIOFEEDBACK

Biofeedback may be described as a technique that uses equipment (usually electronic) with auditory or visual signals to make individuals aware of changes in some of their internal physiologic processes mediated by the autonomic nervous system. As individuals learn to manipulate physiologic processes (e.g., heart rate, blood pressure, skin temperature, respiratory rate) by mental control, they are apprised of their performance after brief (millisecond) delays in the form of visual or auditory signals. Signal-processing devices provide feedback by causing a light to flash or a tone to vary with the level of the physiologic response. That is, the feedback reflects the success or failure of the patient's efforts.[1, 12]

When an individual is reliably able to produce the desired response, it is said that he or she has learned an *operant*, that is, a means of operating successfully on the environment to produce desired results. Biofeedback is based on the operant conditioning principles described by B. F. Skinner and Neal Miller.

The goal of biofeedback is to gain control over a body function and then to be able to maintain the control in actual life situations.

Biofeedback of muscle activity for the purpose of relaxation is usually done by electromyogram (EMG). Any one of several muscles may be monitored, but some consider the forehead muscle to be particularly crucial. It is thought that if a person can relax the frontalis muscles he or she can usually relax the scalp, neck, and upper body, too.[13]

During biofeedback training, a therapist takes measurements to determine whether EMG activity has decreased or not. When muscle tension has remained high, EMG feedback can be used to shape the patient's response in the desired direction.[11]

When participating in biofeedback training, the patient sits in a separate room watching or listening to repetitive stimuli. This situation is generally conducive to relaxation. To control any body function, the individual must achieve a state of relaxation. Therefore, those who teach biofeedback use various methods for achieving relaxation. For example, therapists use muscle tension techniques, imagery, classical music, or repetitive phrases.

Biofeedback training not only involves the time in the therapy office but also requires that the patient make a commitment to practice the relaxation response at home. The response must become part of his or her habitual response to everyday stress situations. Such learning is not automatic; it must be acquired through diligent practice.

Patients must understand the rationale for their biofeedback training. In order for the training to benefit patients, their cooperation must be elicited. Cooperation evolves as a result of knowing what is to be done and why it should be done. Individuals need to understand both of these before they can be expected to adhere to recommedations.

EMPHYSEMA OR CHRONIC BRONCHITIS

The increased airway resistance characteristic of emphysema and chronic bronchitis is due to structural changes that are generally irreversible. Individuals experience shortness of breath and fatigue on exertion because of a limited respiratory reserve. They fear that any activity might precipitate an episode of dyspnea and, therefore, feel anxious when they must engage in activity. When individuals feel short of breath, they become more anxious and may even panic. Typically, they use accessory muscles instead of the diaphragm and, with frantic gasps, attempt to take in more air. These instinctive responses—to work harder to breathe and to breathe faster—only aggravate the problem. This breathing pattern is maladaptive because both oxygen consumption and the work of breathing are increased. Additionally, high levels of anxiety are associated with increased ventilation, increased energy expenditure, increased oxygen consumption, and skeletal muscle tension. Also body positions assumed to facilitate breathing may create further muscle tension. Tension causes a tightening of the chest wall muscles, thus making breathing even more difficult. Additionally, tense muscles require more oxygen than relaxed ones.

Individuals with emphysema tend to be extremely nervous and tense because of dyspnea and a fear of suffocation. In fact, they have been described as living in a straitjacket.[14] It has been shown that emphysema patients are more anxious than most individuals being treated for chronic anxiety. In fact, when the two groups were compared, emphysema patients had significantly more frontalis and pectoral muscle tension than did chronically anxious patients.[15]

Many individuals—such as those with emphysema—have become so accustomed to such a high state of tension that they have no idea what a relaxed state is like. For improvement to occur, their ineffective behaviors must be corrected. They must be shown which behaviors are maladaptive and what changes are needed to obtain the desired benefits.

Two major components of a treatment program for emphysema patients are to teach them to relax their muscles and to improve the ventilation of their lungs.

Patients with emphysema or chronic bronchitis can be given a biofeedback diagnostic to assess the level of anxiety and the amount of tension in their muscles. By practicing progressive muscle relaxation with the benefit of biofeedback, they can learn the feel of the tensed state and the relaxed state.[16]

Breathing Retraining

Breathing retraining can be improved with the information provided by biofeedback. EMG biofeedback can assist patients in learning to perform diaphragmatic breathing and to relax the accessory muscles. The procedure involves taping small electrodes to the skin overlying the lower rectus abdominal muscle (for teaching abdominal-diaphragmatic breathing) and the sternocleidomastoid muscle (for teaching patients not to use the accessory muscles). EMG biofeedback provides an auditory signal that allows the patient to develop a sense of the movement of the diaphragm. The desired outcome is for the patient to turn on the signal during inhalation and turn off the signal at expiration. When the signal is turned off, patients know they have relaxed their diaphragm. The biofeedback instrument threshold can be increased so that patients must expand their abdomens further to activate the signal.[16]

When emphysema patients have learned to reduce the muscle activity in the upper pectoral and the accessory muscles, they are given EMG feedback simultaneously from both the upper pectoral and the diaphragm (Fig. 9–2). The training goal is to have the patient keep the diaphragm signal on during inhalation and the upper pectoral signal off.

Because of an increased airway resistance, breathing retraining helps emphysema patients develop a slower breathing pattern with prolonged exhalation. Diaphragmatic EMG biofeedback can facilitate the development of a 1-to-4 ratio between inhalation and exhalation. In short, continuous monitoring increases patients' awareness of their breathing pattern.

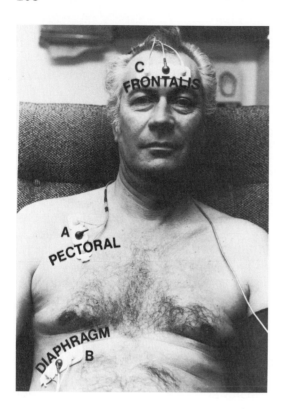

Figure 9–2. Placement of EMG surface electrodes on a patient to obtain EMG feedback from the upper pectoral muscle (*A*), diaphragm (*B*), and frontalis muscle (*C*). (Reproduced with permission from Holliday JE: Biofeedback, in O'Ryan JA, Burns DG (eds): *Pulmonary Rehabilitation: From Hospital to Home.* Copyright © 1984 by Year Book Medical Publishers, Inc., Chicago.)

Muscle Relaxation

While being monitored with EMG biofeedback, patients can be taught to check themselves for tense muscles. After a while, they should be able to identify the areas most likely to be tense. For many, their tension is evident in the muscles of the jaw, neck, or shoulders. Patients can be taught that, when they detect tension, they can initiate a simple technique to promote relaxation. For example, some may find that taking a deep breath or tensing and relaxing the area will help. Signals from the biofeedback instrument tell patients immediately whether they are moving in the right direction. The experience allows emphysema patients to be trained in greater body awareness. Table 9–3 lists the information provided to the patient through biofeedback that can help reduce tension and anxiety and to control dyspnea.

After patients are weaned from the biofeedback instrument, they can continue the development of body awareness and control through the use of progressive relaxation tapes. The body awareness should help them sense the development of muscle tension it might trigger shortness of breath.

The goal of relaxation is to give patients a feeling of control over their body and to help them conquer anxiety and fear and thereby enable them to participate in satisfying activities.

For patients who cannot exert much effort, the suggestion approach developed by Lazarus, which includes muscle flexion and suggestion techniques for relaxation, is appropriate.[14, 17]

ASTHMA

Asthma is characterized by hypersensitivity of the airways to various external and internal stimuli. The diffuse airway obstruction is reversible. While nearly all asthmatics have more reactive airways than nonasthmatics, some asthmatics have airways that are much more hyperreactive than others.[18]

During an attack, thoracic breathing is predominant, and the accessory muscles are often fully contracted. There may be spasmodic contractions or no contractions of the diaphragm. The ventilatory process of asthmatics may be described as uneven.

Many asthmatics have muscle tension throughout the voluntary muscle system. Affected muscles include the frontal area just above the eyes, the neck and shoulders, and the voluntary respiratory muscles. Asthmatics overuse the accessory respiratory muscles—namely, the muscles of the chest wall and neck. In fact, a prominent characteristic of asthma is conditioned compensatory muscle activity. Muscle tension can contribute to the perpetuation of asthmatic symptoms. Whether the etiology of an asthma attack is allergy, infection, exercise, or emotion, anxiety usually occurs during the episode. When a heightened arousal level occurs with attacks, conditioning may cause anxiety to become a significant aggravating factor.[18]

When bronchodilator or corticosteroid therapy is administered, airway obstruction is relieved, and the anxiety accompanying the attack is alleviated. While this protocol tends to be immediate, another component is needed to interrupt the continuing cycle between physical and emotional symptoms.

Recently, attention has focused on anxiety reduction as an adjunct to the medical treatment of asthma. The approaches have included mental and muscular relaxation therapy, systematic desensitization, and biofeedback-assisted relaxation.

It is important to note that two types of anxiety have been described in

Table 9–3. **Information Provided by Biofeedback**

The following information is given to the COPD patient by biofeedback in order to reduce his tension and anxiety and to control his dyspnea.
1. Information on how to relax in general and how to relax specific areas in the body.
2. Information on how to relax during activity.
3. Information on the effect of anxious thoughts on the body.
4. Information on the tension in the body (where it is and when it occurs).
5. Information from the diaphragm, chest, and accessory muscles for breathing retraining.

asthmatics. One type is the anxiety focused directly on the breathing difficulties and is viewed as adaptive. The other, which is unrelated to the illness, is rather characteristic of the individual in various situations. That is, some individuals—asthmatic patients included—tend to feel anxious in many situations and not just during episodes of asthma. Therefore, reduction techniques should address the high characterological anxiety and not the illness-focused anxiety.[18]

Relaxation Techniques for Asthma Patients

Relaxation therapy for asthma patients is based on the theory that emotional stress may trigger or aggravate an asthma attack. Relaxation can be considered the antithesis to stress and may interrupt the continuing cycle between physical and emotional symptoms.

Relaxation requires conscious control over well-established ways of dealing with tension. The reduction of muscular tension and resting the mind can cause the individual to perceive a sense of greater control over the body.

Meditation can serve the same purpose. By having patients concentrate on a single word, perhaps by saying it over and over to themselves, other thoughts, which could be anxiety-producing, are allowed to pass harmlessly through the mind. Asthmatics can learn to use these techniques when they anticipate attacks.

Systematic Desensitization

In the late 1950s, Wolpe developed a technique called systematic desensitization for the counterconditioning of fear responses. Wolpe incorporated a form of Jacobson's progressive muscle relaxation with the imagery of a threatening situation. This technique involves a hierarchical presentation of fear-producing experiences, starting with the least threatening.[19]

The technique of systematic desensitization is based on the notion that deep muscular relaxation is not compatible with anxiety. Patients are taught to relax deeply and then are exposed to a hierarchy of anxiety-provoking situations associated with their asthma attacks. By having such images while relaxed, individuals in effect cause the stressful events to lose their anxiety-producing capability. Thereafter, when patients encounter an anxiety-provoking situation, their response may be one of relaxation instead of bronchospasm.

Data based on case studies and small numbers of subjects suggest that systematic desensitization is effective in reducing the frequency of acute asthma attacks.

Biofeedback

A number of studies involving the use of biofeedback with asthmatics are described in the literature. In nearly all cases, asthmatic children were the subjects, and biofeedback was used to try to correct the basic pulmonary problem—increased airway resistance. Some reports described short-term benefits of biofeedback training;[20-22] however, long-term evidence was seldom obtained. Other studies yielded equivocal findings both immediately after treatment and at one year.[23]

While the data cast uncertainty on the outcome of biofeedback training on airway resistance, there is considerable evidence that patients learn relaxation much faster with biofeedback than with conventional approaches. Biofeedback training requires an investment of time and gives patients a sense of mastery over their body. EMG biofeedback is used as an adjunct to medical treatment.

When the asthmatic learns the relaxation response and practices it, relaxation becomes a conditioned response. With the help of biofeedback-assisted relaxation, the asthmatic can learn to detect tension before it becomes too great and, thereby, prevent the panic/fear reaction. Learning a technique to counter the effects of psychological stress can set the asthmatic on the path to a more tranquil life.

Some clinicians believe that whatever approach helps the patient to function better should be used, even when research data supporting the efficacy of a technique are lacking. Health care providers should discuss their views about the advantages and disadvantages of conventional and newer treatments with the patient and encourage him or her to participate in the decision. This also creates an environment for clinicians and patients to collaborate on an approach that is comfortable and feasible.

References

1. Weiss T: Biofeedback training for cardiovascular dysfunctions. *Medical Clinics of North America* 1977;61(4):913–928.
2. Benson H: *The Relaxation Response.* New York, Avon Books, 1975.
3. Benson H, Kotch JB, Crassweller KD: The relaxation response. *Medical Clinics of North America* 1977;61(4):929–938.
4. Jacobsen E: *Progressive Relaxation.* Chicago, University of Chicago Press, 1938.
5. DiMotto JW: Relaxation. *American Journal of Nursing* 1984;84(6):754–758.
6. Funk DR: Personal communication, October, 1985.
7. Ostrander S. et al: *Superlearning.* New York, Delacorte Press, 1979.
8. Halpern S: *Tuning the Human Instrument.* Belmont, CA, Spectrum Research Institute, 1978.
9. Achterberg J, Lawlis F: Imagery and health intervention. *Topics in Clinical Nursing* 1982;3(4):56.
10. Kroger WS, Fezler WD: *Hypnosis and Behavior Modification: Imagery Conditioning.* Philadelphia, JB Lippincott Co, 1976.
11. Stoyva JM: Guidelines in cultivating general relaxation: Biofeedback and autogenic training combined, in Basmajian JV (ed): *Biofeedback: Principles and Practices for Clinicians.* Baltimore, Williams & Wilkins Co, 1983.
12. Basmajian JV: *Biofeedback: Principles and Practice for Clinicians.* Baltimore, Williams & Wilkins Co, 1983.
13. Budzynski TH, Stoyva JM, Adler C: An instrument for producing deep muscle re-

laxation by means of analog information feedback. *J Applied Behavioral Anal* 1969;2:231–237.

14. Dudley DL, Glaser EM, Jorgenson BN, et al: Psychosocial concomitants to rehabilitation in chronic obstructive pulmonary disease. *Chest* 1980;77(4):413–420, 544–551.

15. Holliday JE, Ruppel G, McDaniels S: Comparison of biofeedback in emphysema patients and chronically anxious patients. *Proceedings of the Fourteenth Annual Meeting of the Biofeedback Society of America* (Denver) 1983;107–110.

16. Holliday JE: Biofeedback, in O'Ryan JA, Burns DG (eds): *Pulmonary Rehabilitation: From Hospital to Home.* Chicago, Year Book Medical Publishers Inc, 1984.

17. Lazarus AA: *Behavior Therapy and Beyond.* New York, McGraw-Hill Co, 1971.

18. Kinsman RA, Dirks JF, Jones NF, Dahlem NW: Anxiety reduction in asthma: Four catches to general application. *Psychosomatic Medicine* 1980;42(4):397–404.

19. Wolpe, J: *Psychotherapy by Reciprocal Inhibition.* Stanford, CA, Stanford University Press, 1976.

20. Vachon L, Rich ES: Visceral learning in asthma. *Psychosomatic Medicine* 1976; 38(2):122–130.

21. Davis MH, Saunders DR, Creer TL, Chai H: Relaxation training facilitated by biofeedback apparatus as a supplemental treatment in bronchial asthma. *J Psychosomatic Research* 1973;17:121–128.

22. Kotses H, Glaus KD, Crawford PL, et al: Operant reduction of frontalis EMG activity in the treatment of asthma in children. *J Psychosomatic Research* 1976;20:453–459.

23. Miklich DR, Renne CM, Creer TL, et al: The clinical utility of behavior therapy as an adjunctive treatment for asthma. *J Allergy Clinical Immunology* 1977;60:285–294.

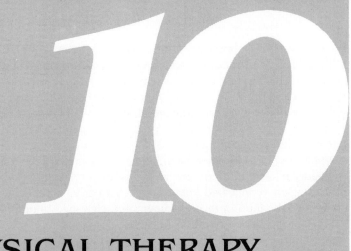

PHYSICAL THERAPY TECHNIQUES

REUBEN M. CHERNIACK

A number of physical therapy techniques are major components of the therapeutic armamentarium utilized in the management of patients with acute and chronic respiratory disorders. Although some are cynical about the efficacy of these procedures and feel that the benefits are too little to warrant the effort required, clear objective and subjective benefits result from application of these techniques, particularly in overcoming some of the secondary effects of chronic airflow limitation.[1-3]

Among the physical therapeutic measures utilized are:

1. Postural drainage and chest percussion.
2. Breathing retraining (diaphragmatic breathing exercises).
3. Pursed-lip breathing.
4. Respiratory muscle training.
5. Exercise reconditioning.

POSTURAL DRAINAGE AND CHEST PERCUSSION

Postural drainage and chest percussion or clapping may be particularly effective in patients who have copious secretions or have difficulty in raising secretions.[4, 5] Properly applied postural drainage techniques appear to be as beneficial as bronchoscopy in clearing lobar atelectasis and, in combination with early mobilization, clearly reduce postoperative complications. The procedure increases the rate of removal of radioactive aerosol deposited in the airways[6] and the volume of sputum expectorated, particularly in patients with cystic fibrosis and bronchiectasis as well as stable chronic airflow limitation.[5] This is particularly true when airways collapse during coughing because diminished lung elastic recoil reduces the effectiveness of mucous elimination. On the other hand, there is no greater elimination of sputum, increase in arterial blood oxygen tension, or improvement in the clinical course of uncomplicated pneumonia.[7] Similarly, no effect has been demonstrated on duration of fever, radiographic clearing, amount of expectoration, arterial blood gases, duration of hospital stay, or mortality in patients with chronic bronchitis or emphysema who develop acute exacerbations.[8]

Technique

The procedure consists of postural positioning combined with chest clapping and vibration.[4, 5] In addition, several other techniques have been proposed to facilitate drainage of secretions. Deep breathing, repeated coughing or forced expiratory bursts during a vital capacity maneuver while the glottis is open (huffing), percussion with rapid vibration, high-frequency ultrasound generation, and an electric percussion vest have all been advocated, but their efficacy has not been determined.[9]

In general, postural drainage should be preceded by inhalation of a bronchodilator and, in some patients, inhalation of heated aerosol.[10] The involved segmental bronchus should be placed in a vertical position so drainage is assisted by gravity. The upper lobes are best drained in the upright position. The right middle lobe and lingular segment of the left upper lobe are best drained in the supine position with the head lowermost and the body tilted at a 45° angle. The superior segments of both lower lobes are best drained in the prone position, and for the remaining segments of the lower lobes, the patient should lie in the Trendelenburg position. In chronic airflow limitation, the most important positions are generally those that drain the lower and middle lobes but, in acute situations, will depend on the area of lung involved.

While postural drainage is being carried out, the chest should be "percussed" or "clapped" with rapid strokes and then vibrated, at least twice a day for 15 to 20 minutes. In some patients, manual compression of the lower thorax and upper abdomen during a slow, full expiration may also facilitate the expectoration of secretions.[1] With each session, the patient should be encouraged to cough and expectorate sputum, and records should be kept of the amount expectorated.

BREATHING RETRAINING

In some patients with chronic airflow limitation, the size and total mass of diaphragmatic muscle fibers may be increased, and in others it may be reduced, probably as a result of poor nutrition.[11, 12] In advanced conditions, there may be excessive use of accessory muscles and asynchronous or ineffective contraction of the diaphragm. In addition, the hyperinflation shortens the fibers of the diaphragm and the intercostal muscles and places them on an inefficient portion of their length-tension curve. The mechanical work and energy cost of breathing of the respiratory muscles are increased, and their capacity to endure the work is diminished.[12, 13] Respiratory failure is thought to result if inspiratory muscle fatigue is present, and it would appear that the ability to avoid respiratory failure depends in good measure on the strength and endurance of the inspiratory muscles.[14]

Breathing retraining is generally applied to patients suffering from chronic airflow limitation—the goal being to slow the respiratory rate and increase tidal volume by increasing diaphragmatic excursion. The slow deep breathing may be associated with a reduction in the work of breathing and energy expenditure, improved distribution of inspired gas, and the matching of ventilation and perfusion at the lung bases and, consequently, gas exchange.[15–17]

Technique

In general, a number of procedures, including relaxation techniques, slowly paced inspiration, pursed-lip expiration, augmented diaphragmatic breathing, and specific respiratory muscle strength and/or endurance training have been applied during breathing retraining. The patient should place his or her hand on the sternum and practice immobilizing the thoracic cage and controlling its movement while inhaling very slowly by sniffing, which is a diaphragmatic function. Exhalation should then proceed slowly through pursed lips while the other hand pushes the abdomen inward and upward.[1, 16] Increased use of the abdominal muscles during expiration has also been advocated, but such expiratory efforts may actually increase the work of breathing.

Mastering this technique may be easier when lying in the head-down position, which enhances the movement of the diaphragm, because it is pushed upward by the abdominal contents.[1] In addition, leaning forward in the upright position helps to relax the accessory respiratory muscles and elevate the diaphragm, which may facilitate diaphragmatic movement during inspiration. Once this breathing pattern is mastered in all positions as well as during exertion, lower costal breathing may be taught and practiced while sitting, standing, and walking.

PURSED-LIP BREATHING

Pursed-lip breathing is frequently adopted spontaneously by patients. When practiced in association with diaphragmatic breathing, it is generally associated with a fall in minute ventilation and respiratory rate, an increase in tidal volume, and improvement of gas exchange.[17–19] Often, there is a reduction in dyspnea and an increase in exercise tolerance and, therefore, the ability to carry out the activities of daily living. Pursed-lip breathing is thought to be effective because it raises the pressure in the airways during expiration, and this, along with the slowed expiration, helps prevent dynamic collapse of the airways so that a fuller expiration and decrease in air trapping is fostered.[18–20] However, simply slowing the respiratory rate without the use of pursed lips may result in similar physiologic benefits.

Technique

In those patients who have not already adopted pursed-lip breathing spontaneously, a full, very slow inspiration by sniffing, while the abdomen is moved outward, should be followed by "whistling" the air away and contraction of the abdominal muscles. In other words, pursed-lip breathing is taught in combination with diaphragmatic breathing.[18, 20]

RESPIRATORY MUSCLE TRAINING

The ability of a muscle to sustain work declines when the work load increases above a critical value (i.e., the fatigue threshold), and it is currently suspected that the respiratory muscles become fatigued in respiratory insufficiency. Respiratory muscle strength can be evaluated fairly accurately as long as patients cooperate by determining maximal inspiratory and expiratory and transdiaphragmatic pressures. Respiratory muscle endurance is reflected to some extent by the maximum voluntary ventilation or the length of time one can breathe against an added resistance.[14]

It has been shown that the respiratory muscle strength and endurance limit can be increased by special exercises.[21] In addition, exercise tolerance has been shown to improve after respiratory muscle training,[22, 23] but the converse is not true following leg and arm exercises.[24] Whether respiratory muscle training and an increase in their strength or endurance is more beneficial than a generalized increase in physical activity, or whether the course of the disease is altered by such exercises is not known.

Technique

Attempts to improve the strength and endurance of the respiratory muscles generally involve sustained hyperpnea into and out of a spirometer at a ventilation of about 40% of the maximum voluntary ventilation for 15 minutes twice a day.[14, 22–26] Some carbon dioxide should be added to the spirometer in order to prevent hypocapnea. Another technique that has been used involves inspiring through a device with adjustable resistance for about 30 minutes once or twice daily and gradually increasing the resistance to air flow.[22, 26]

EXERCISE RECONDITIONING

This subject is covered in Chapter 11 in detail, but since exercise reconditioning is an important aspect of physical therapy,[27] a few aspects are discussed here.

Although excessive physical activity should be avoided during acute illnesses, there is no question that patients with chronic airflow limitation who continue to be active remain in better health and function far more effectively than those who restrict their activities.[28] It is unfortunate that many patients abstain from any physical activity in order to avoid the possibility of dyspnea. Inactivity begets further inactivity, and consequently, patients are generally in poor physical condition. Thus, emphasis must be placed on achieving maximal physical fitness and encouraging patients to gradually increase their exercise tolerance.

The increase in exercise tolerance with exercise reconditioning appears to be due to a training effect on the exercising muscles because the improvement is largely task-specific. Nevertheless, there is no doubt that improving physical fitness through a three- to six-week program of gradual increases of work load while exercising either on a bicycle ergometer or treadmill (or by stair climbing or walking) leads to a significant increase in exercise tolerance and allows patients to function at much higher levels of activity and to carry out daily tasks with more comfort.[28, 29]

The benefit derived from a training program is probably due to a more efficient delivery of oxygen to the tissues.[29] Supplemental oxygen during the exercise training is generally provided for severely limited patients, particularly if they become progressively hypoxemic during exercise.[30] The additional oxygen may allow the patient to increase exercise sufficiently to improve cardiovascular performance and thus to increase the work level at which the delivery of oxygen is limited, i.e., the anaerobic threshold. After the training period, such patients frequently also demonstrate improved exercise performance while breathing air. Whatever mode is used to increase the exercise load, it is important to realize that even markedly abnormal function should not inhibit instituting a graded exercise program, since there is little relationship between the severity of pulmonary function abnormality or gas exchange and the ability to improve exercise tolerance.

Technique

Calisthenics and stretching exercises are probably of little benefit except in limbering up in preparation for exertion. The most practical exercises for most patients are walking and stair climbing. One should begin with walking while leaning forward and using pursed-lip breathing. Someone should be in attendance if there is any evidence of cardiac abnormality or poor coordination during walking. For most patients at home, the prescription should entail a gradual increase in the distance walked, or the number of flights of stairs climbed. If a stationary bicycle or treadmill is utilized to increase exercise load, the exercise program should begin using the lowest possible resistance or work load, and the exercise should be carried out for 10 to 15 minutes several times a day, with the ventilatory and cardiovascular status being assessed at regular intervals. Measurements of pulse (and the cardiogram, if concerned), blood pressure, and respiratory rate during the exercise along with the time required for recovery to baseline levels are important assessments. The work load should be increased gradually, as tolerated by the patient. A chart recording exercise performance while in the training program as well as the continued activity at home, i.e., the distance walked or the number of flights of stairs climbed without dyspnea, should be filled in regularly to determine progress.

References

1. Barach AL: *Physiologic Therapy in Respiratory Diseases.* Philadelphia, JB Lippincott, 1948.
2. Fernandez E, Cherniack RM: Rehabilitation of the patient with chronic airflow limitation, in Simmons D: *Current Pulmonology.* Chicago, Year Book Medical Publishers, 1985, pp 68–89.
3. Lertzman MM, Cherniack RM: Rehabilitation of patients with chronic obstructive pulmonary disease: State of the art. *Am Rev Respir Dis* 1976;114:1145–1165.
4. Gaskell DV, Welsher BA: *The Brompton Hospital Guide to Chest Physiotherapy,* ed 2. Philadelphia, FA Davis Co, 1973.
5. Cherniack RM, Cherniack L: Management of acute respiratory failure. *Respiration in Health and Disease,* ed 3. Philadelphia, WB Saunders, 1983, pp 389–410.
6. Bateman JRM, Newman SP, Daunt KM, et al: Regional lung clearance of excessive bronchial secretions during chest physiotherapy in patients with stable chronic airways obstruction. *Lancet* 1979;1:294–297.
7. Graham WGB, Bradley DA: Efficacy of chest physiotherapy and intermittent positive pressure breathing in the resolution of pneumonia. *N Engl J Med* 1978;299:624–627.
8. Anthonisen P, Rus P, Sogaard-Anderson T: The value of lung physiotherapy in the treatment of acute exacerbations in chronic bronchitis. *Acta Med Scand* 1964;175:715–719.
9. Murray JF: The ketchup-bottle method. *N Engl J Med* 1979;300:1155–1157.
10. Chopra SK, Taplin GV, Simmons DH, et al: Effect of hydration and physical therapy on tracheal transport velocity. *Am Rev Respir Dis* 1977;115:1009–1014.
11. Braun NMT, Rochester DF: Respiratory

muscle strength in obstructive lung disease. *Am Rev Respir Dis* 1977;115:91.

12. Sharp JT, Danon J, Druz WS, et al: Respiratory muscle function in patients with chronic obstructive pulmonary disease: Its relationship to disability and to respiratory therapy. *Am Rev Respir Dis* 1974;100: 154.

13. Cherniack RM: The oxygen consumption and efficiency of the respiratory muscles in health and emphysema. *J Clin Invest* 1959;3:494–499.

14. Roussos CH, Macklem PT: The respiratory muscles. *N Engl J Med* 1982;307:786–797.

15. Campbell EJB, Friend J: Action of breathing exercises in pulmonary emphysema. *Lancet* 1955;268:325–329.

16. Miller WF: A physiologic evaluation of the effects of diaphragmatic breathing training in patients with chronic pulmonary emphysema. *Am J Med* 1954;17:471.

17. Motley HL: Effects of slow deep breathing on blood gas exchange in emphysema. *Am Rev Respir Dis* 1963;88:484–492.

18. Barach AL: Breathing exercises in pulmonary emphysema and allied chronic respiratory disease. *Arch Phys Med Rehabil* 1955;36:379.

19. Mueller RD, Petty TL, Filley GF: Ventilation and arterial blood gas changes induced by pursed-lip breathing. *J Appl Physiol* 1970;28:784–789.

20. Thomas RL, Stoker GL, Ross JG: The efficacy of pursed-lip breathing in patients with chronic obstructive pulmonary disease. *Am Rev Respir Dis* 1966;93:100–106.

21. Leith DE, Bradley M: Ventilatory muscle strength and endurance training. *J Appl Physiol* 1976;41:508–516.

22. Pardy RL, Rivington RN, Despas PJ, et al: The effect of inspiratory muscle training on exercise performance in chronic airflow limitation. *Am Rev Respir Dis* 1981;123:426–433.

23. Pardy RL, Rivington RN, Despas PJ, et al: Inspiratory muscle training compared with physiotherapy in patients with chronic airflow limitation. *Am Rev Respir Dis* 1981;123:421–425.

24. Belman MJ, Mittman C: Ventilatory muscle training improves exercise capacity in chronic obstructive pulmonary disease patients. *Am Rev Respir Dis* 1980;121: 273–280.

25. Andersen JB, Dragsted L, Kann T, et al: Resistive breathing training in severe chronic obstructive pulmonary disease. *Scand J Respir Dis* 1979;60:151–156.

26. Sonne LJ, Davis JA: Increased exercise performance in patients with severe COPD following inspiratory resistive training. *Chest* 1982;81:436–439.

27. American College of Sports Medicine: *Guidelines for Graded Exercise Testing and Exercise Prescription.* Philadelphia, Lea & Febiger, 1973.

28. Cherniack RM, Handford RG, Svanhill E: Home care of chronic respiratory disease. *JAMA* 1969;208:821–824.

29. Pierce AK, Taylor HF, Archer RK, et al: Responses to exercise training in patients with emphysema. *Arch Intern Med* 1964;113:28.

30. Levine BE, Bigelow DB, Hamstra RD, et al: The role of long-term continuous oxygen administration in patients with chronic airway obstruction with hypoxemia. *Ann Intern Med* 1967;66:639–650.

11

EXERCISE TESTING AND TRAINING

JOHN E. HODGKIN

Once exertional dyspnea develops in patients with chronic obstructive pulmonary disease (COPD), a continuous downhill cycle of deconditioning often develops. Figure 11–1 presents the pathophysiology of exercise limitation in COPD patients. Individuals begin to limit their activity to avoid shortness of breath, and this results in worsening muscle weakness and decreased capacity for exercise.[1, 2] All too often, the individual accepts a relatively inactive lifestyle and consequently becomes a "respiratory cripple." There are numerous published studies demonstrating an improvement in work capacity as well as the development of an enhanced sense of well-being in respiratory patients who participate in aerobic exercise training programs.[3–14] Most individuals participating in an exercise training program show an increased ability to participate in activities of daily living and, as a result, are more likely to function as productive members of society.

Exercise training has become common for individuals interested in health promotion and is also used routinely in cardiac rehabilitation programs. However, a structured exercise training program is still uncommon for patients with chronic airways obstruction. While many patients with COPD are unable to achieve the kind of exercise training response exhibited in healthy individuals and even in some patients with cardiovascular disease, exercise conditioning clearly results in significant benefit for most patients with chronic lung disease.

120

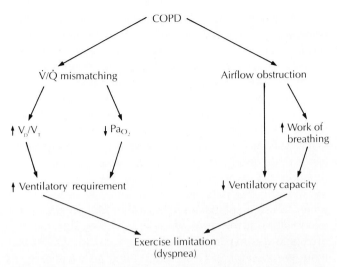

Figure 11–1. Pathophysiology of exercise limitation in patients with COPD. V_D/V_T indicates physiologic dead-space–tidal-volume ratio; $\dot{V}/\dot{Q}$ indicates the ratio of ventilation to perfusion in lung gas exchange units. (From Brown HV, Wasserman K: Exercise performance in chronic obstructive pulmonary diseases. *Medical Clinics of North America* 65:525–547, 1981, by permission.)

EXERCISE TESTING

There are three common reasons for patients with respiratory disease to undergo exercise testing: (1) to help determine the cause of dyspnea, (2) to help evaluate a patient's potential for working in his or her current occupation, and (3) to help outline an exercise training program.

A diagnostic exercise test can be of significant value in attempting to determine the etiology of a patient's sensation of dyspnea.[15, 16] For example, if a patient has a reduced work capacity but reaches the anaerobic threshold at a normal level, i.e., at or greater than 40% of his or her predicted maximal oxygen consumption ($\dot{V}_{O_2}$max), and if the maximal ventilation achieved during the exercise period approximates the patient's maximal voluntary ventilation (MVV), the dyspnea is probably caused by a respiratory impairment. On the other hand, if the patient reaches the anaerobic threshold abnormally early, i.e., at less than 40% of the predicted $\dot{V}_{O_2}$max, a cardiovascular etiology for the exercise limitation and dyspnea is suggested.

An exercise evaluation can help to determine a patient's ability to work at a certain job.[17] It has been shown that a patient will have difficulty in working over an eight-hour period if the oxygen consumption (metabolic equivalent level) of the job exceeds 40% of the patient's maximal achievable oxygen consumption.[18] By determining a patient's achievable $\dot{V}_{O_2}$max, one can then consult a "work dictionary" to determine the metabolic equivalent requirements of various occupations. This can help a vocational rehabilitation counselor to determine if job retraining is necessary or useful.

Most pulmonologists feel that some type of exercise evaluation is indicated before outlining an exercise training program for patients with chronic respiratory impairment. An exercise assessment can determine if the patient is prone to cardiac arrhythmias or angina pectoris and if supplemental oxygen would be useful during exercise training periods.

The type of diagnostic exercise test varies widely among pulmonary laboratories. Pulmonary stress tests may be performed at a submaximal level (either steady-state or a progressive test) or to a symptom-limited or maximal level. Maximal exercise stress tests are recommended if the purpose for the test is to determine the cause of dyspnea or to evaluate the patient's ability to function in various occupations. On the other hand, if the major reason for the exercise test is to help in outlining an exercise training program, many prefer to use a submaximal level of work that approximates the same energy expenditure at the level of exercise during the training periods. The author prefers to use maximal exercise stress tests in COPD patients even when the main purpose for the test is to outline an exercise training program since it provides the following additional helpful information: (1) observation of arrhythmias or ischemic electrocardiogram changes, which might not be noted at lower levels of work; (2) an objective determination of the anaerobic threshold to help determine whether a cardiovascular impairment may exist in addition to the respiratory problem; (3) assistance in developing a target heart rate for many individuals by determining the patient's achievable peak heart rate; and (4) detection of oxygen desaturation, which may not be evident at lower levels of work.

The preference for the mode of exercise selected during an exercise test for pulmonary patients is dependent on the bias of the physician supervising the test. When attempting to determine the cause of dyspnea or the level of a patient's impairment and disability, either an exercise bicycle or a treadmill is reasonable. When the exercise test is being used mainly for outlining and then following the progress of an exercise training program, the author generally selects a treadmill since COPD patients most commonly use walking as their mode of exercise training. For an individual intending to use a bicycle for exercise training, it would make sense to use an exercise ergometer for the initial and follow-up testing. Based on the observation that muscle training is often selective,[19] treadmill testing would accurately detect improvement in a patient's exercise capacity during a walking program, while an exercise bicycle might underestimate it. Some prefer to use a 6- or 12-minute walk test for baseline evaluation and then use follow-up tests of the same duration to determine if the individual is making progress.[20]

An ear oximeter can monitor oxygen saturation and is a noninvasive way of detecting exercise-induced hypoxemia. While many COPD patients show improvement in their blood oxygen level during exercise, a significant number develop oxygen desaturation, which may predispose them to arrhythmias or angina pectoris and can limit the intensity of the exercise that can be achieved during the exercise training period. A comparison of pre- and postexercise arterial blood gases not only detects changes in the PaO_2 and arterial oxygen saturation but also shows if the blood bicarbonate level has dropped significantly, i.e., whether lactic acidosis has developed, which can indicate that the patient achieved a satisfactory work capacity during the test.

Although there are equations that can estimate the $\dot{V}_{O_2}$max,[21] there may be wide variation using such predicted values. The actual measurement of expired air constituents and direct calculation of $\dot{V}_{O_2}$max is preferable, since it provides reliable data.[22, 23]

The remainder of this chapter deals with exercise training in patients with COPD and how exercise testing can be utilized in establishing a safe exercise conditioning program.

EXERCISE TRAINING

An exercise prescription has four basic components: (1) mode of exercise—the type of exercise performed, e.g., walking or bicycling; (2) intensity—how strenuous the exercise should be; (3) duration—the length of time one exercises during a single session; and (4) frequency—how many times during each week the patient should exercise.

The mode of exercise generally selected for COPD patients is walking. However, some patients prefer other modes such as bicycling or swimming. Studies have shown that normal healthy people and cardiac patients, in order to achieve physical fitness, must exercise with an intensity in the range of 60% to 80% of their maximal oxygen consumption (or 70% to 85% of their maximal heart rate) for 20 to 30 minutes at a time, and at least three or four times a week.[24–26]

Although there is little controversy regarding the mode, duration, and frequency of exercise training periods in the pulmonary patient, there is controversy regarding the way to determine the appropriate intensity of exercise. A target heart rate (THR) is often used to determine the intensity of exercise when outlining an exercise training program in healthy individuals and in those with heart disease.[27] While some promote the use of a THR in patients with COPD, others feel it is unreliable in these patients and oppose its use.[28, 29]

There are several ways that a THR can be determined. In healthy individuals, it is usually determined by first calculating the predicted maximal heart rate (Fig. 11–2). A formula commonly used to estimate this is:

$$\text{Predicted maximal heart rate} = 220 - \text{Patient's age}$$

The individual then starts out exercising at about 70% of this predicted maximal heart rate. Since many patients with cardiac or pulmonary disease cannot exercise sufficiently to reach their predicted maximal heart rate, some advocate basing the patient's THR on the maximal heart rate achieved during an incremental stress test rather than on their predicted maximal heart rate.[23]

Karvonen has advocated another technique for determining a THR, which

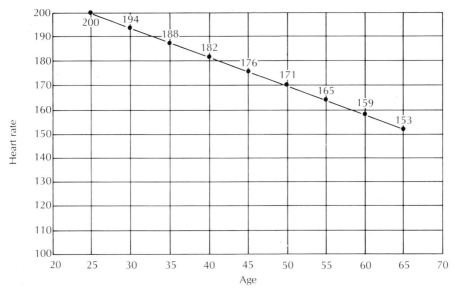

Figure 11–2. The decline of maximum heart rate with age. Adapted from *Physician's Handbook for Evaluation of Cardiovascular and Physical Fitness.* Tennessee Heart Association, Ed 2, 1972, p 39. (From Bell CW, Kass I, Hodgkin JE: Exercise conditioning, in Hodgkin JE, Zorn EG, Connors GL (eds): *Pulmonary Rehabilitation: Guidelines to Success.* Boston, Butterworth Publishers, 1984, by permission.)

is commonly used in cardiac rehabilitation programs.[30, 31] This formula uses a factor for the level of oxygen consumption desired during exercise. If the individual is to exercise at a level approximating 60% of the patient's maximal oxygen consumption, then the THR is determined by multiplying 0.6 and the difference between the peak heart rate (PHR) achieved during maximal exercise and the resting heart rate (RHR), and then adding the RHR to the product:

$$THR = 0.6 \times (PHR - RHR) + RHR$$

The author prefers this formula for determining the THR since it has the advantage of taking both the patient's achievable maximal heart rate and the resting heart rate into account. Another alternative, for those who measure the patient's $\dot{V}_{O_2}$ at each level during an incremental stress test, is to select the heart rate at which the patient's $\dot{V}_{O_2}$ is approximately 60% of his or her $\dot{V}_{O_2}$max as the initial THR.

Some investigators have reported that incremental changes in the heart rate of patients with severe COPD may not accurately reflect their level of oxygen consumption and have recommended that patients simply be encouraged to exercise to tolerance, and not to use a THR.[28]

Frequently, patients with COPD are unable to exercise continuously for 20 to 30 minutes, at least initially. We therefore ask such patients to exercise for shorter periods of time several times per day, e.g., five minutes three or four times a day. The goal is to increase the exercise time to reach the target of 20 to 30 minutes of continuous exercise. Some patients may take from several weeks to several months to achieve this goal, e.g., to gradually increase the time, speed of walking, and distance covered.

Warm-up and cool-down sessions should be used routinely prior to and following exercise training in order to reduce the risk of skeletal muscle injury or sore muscles. Stretching, dance-type activity, and light calisthenics are useful warm-up and cool-down techniques.

Weight training to strengthen arm and shoulder muscles may be a useful adjunct to the usual exercise training program. For example, an arm ergometer for exercise training periods may complement the progress which can be made by an individual using a walking program. The addition of weight training or other resistance-type exercise for patients can improve skeletal muscle strength and endurance.[23]

Studies have shown that the use of supplemental oxygen in patients with significant hypoxemia during training periods not only helps to relieve dyspnea but also increases exercise endurance.[6, 32–37] The use of oxygen during exercise may allow some individuals to participate in exercise training who would not otherwise be able to do so. The author routinely uses oxygen during exercise training periods for those individuals who have at rest or during exercise (i.e., while exercising at the work level to be used during the exercise training periods) a $Pa_{O_2} \leq 55$ mmHg or an oxygen saturation below 88%. Using a nasal oxygen flow rate at a level that results in an oxygen saturation of 90% or above during exercise is recommended.

RESPIRATORY MUSCLE TRAINING

Patients with severe lung disease frequently develop respiratory failure as a result of respiratory muscle fatigue. Some have suggested respiratory muscle training as a helpful adjunct to a rehabilitation program for pulmonary patients. Specific respiratory muscle training can improve the maximal inspiratory and expiratory force that can be developed as well as the maximal sustained ventilatory capacity.[38] Some studies have shown mild improvement in aerobic capacity following respiratory muscle training alone,[39–42] while another study involving young children with cystic fibrosis did not demonstrate such improvement.[43]

While such respiratory muscle training may increase one's exercise capacity, there is no evidence yet that adding such training to an aerobic exercise program adds significantly to the benefits achieved by aerobic exercise alone. The author feels that there is insufficient evidence to justify respiratory muscle training as a routine part of a pulmonary rehabilitation program for all COPD patients. It should certainly be considered for those patients unwilling to participate in aerobic exercise training programs and for those who are unable to perform walking or bicycling because of medical problems, e.g., paraplegia, amputation, or degenerative disease of the hips or knees.

SUMMARY

While there is no uniform agreement about the best way to perform exercise testing or to determine the appropriate intensity for an exercise training program for patients with pulmonary disease, several things seem clear. An exercise test can help determine the appropriate and safe level of exercise and whether supplemental oxygen would be useful during an exercise training program. Patients with COPD should be encouraged to exercise for at least 20 to 30 minutes at least three to four days each week. A THR can be used to help determine the intensity of exercise training in many COPD patients, particularly those with mild to moderate impairment of function. If a THR is not used, as in the case of a patient with severe disease, the patient should be advised to progressively increase the intensity of exercise, and a 12-minute walk test can be used to determine if a higher level of activity is being achieved. Exercise should be an integral part of comprehensive care, since most patients with COPD can achieve a higher level of activity and an improved quality of life through an exercise training program.

References

1. Bell CW: Pulmonary rehabilitation and exercise testing, in Wilson PK, Bell CW, Norton AC (eds): *Rehabilitation of the Heart and Lungs*. Fullerton, CA, Beckman Instruments, 1980, p 54.
2. Miller WF, Taylor HF, Jasper L: Exercise training in the rehabilitation of patients with severe respiratory insufficiency due to pulmonary emphysema: The role of oxygen breathing. *South Med J* 1962;55:1216–1221.
3. Miller WF: Rehabilitation of patients with chronic obstructive lung disease. *Med Clin North Am* 1967;51:349–361.
4. Rusk HA: *Rehabilitation Medicine*, Ed 3. St. Louis, CV Mosby Co, 1971.
5. Woolf CR, Suero JT: Alterations in lung mechanics and gas exchange following training in chronic obstructive lung disease. *Dis Chest* 1969;55:37–44.
6. Pierce AK, Paez PN, Miller WF: Exercise therapy with the aid of a portable oxygen supply in patients with emphysema. *Am Rev Respir Dis* 1965;91:653–659.
7. Bass H, Whitcomb JF, Forman R: Exercise training: Therapy for patients with chronic obstructive pulmonary disease. *Chest* 1970;57:116–121.
8. Barach AL, Bickerman HA, Beck GJ: Advances in treatment of non-tuberculous pulmonary disease. *Bull NY Acad Med* 1952;28:353–384.
9. Pierce AK, Taylor HF, Archer RK, et al: Responses to exercise training in patients with emphysema. *Arch Intern Med* 1964;113:28–36.
10. Woolf CR: A rehabilitation program for improving exercise tolerance in patients with chronic lung disease. *CMA Journal* 1972;106:1289–1292.
11. Paez PN, Phillipson EA, Masangkay M, et al: The physiologic basis of training patients with emphysema. *Am Rev Respir Dis* 1967;95:944–953.
12. Christie D: Physical training in chronic obstructive lung disease. *Br Med J* 1968;2:150–151.
13. Vyas MN, Banister EW, Norton JW, et al: Response to exercise in patients with chronic airway obstruction. I. Effects of exercise training. *Am Rev Respir Dis* 1971;103:390–400.
14. Mertens DJ, Shephard RJ, Kavanagh T: Longterm exercise therapy for chronic obstructive lung disease. *Respiration* 1978;35:96–107.
15. Wasserman K: Dyspnea on exertion: Is it the heart or the lungs? *JAMA* 1982;248:2039–2043.
16. Killian KJ, Jones NL: The use of exercise testing and other methods in the investigation of dyspnea, in Loke J (ed): *Clinics in Chest Medicine*. Philadelphia, WB Saunders Co, March 1984.

17. ATS Position Statement. Evaluation of impairment/disability secondary to respiratory disease. *Am Rev Respir Dis* 1982; 126:945–951.
18. Astrand PO: Quantification of exercise capability and evaluation of physical capacity in man. *Prog Cardiovasc Dis* 1976; 19:51–67.
19. Astrand P-O, Rodahl K: *Textbook of Work Physiology*, ed. 2. New York, McGraw-Hill, 1977.
20. McGavin CR, Gupta SP, McHardy GJR: Twelve-minute walking tests for assessing disability in chronic bronchitis. *Br Med J* 1976;1:822–823.
21. Jones NL, Cambell EJ: *Clinical Exercise Testing*, ed. 2. Philadelphia, WB Saunders Co, 1982.
22. Bell CW, Kass I, Patil KD, et al: Relationship of pulmonary function variables and maximal oxygen consumption rate in the determination of disability in patients with chronic obstructive pulmonary disease (abstract). *Am Rev Respir Dis* 1980; 121:223.
23. Bell CW, Kass I, Hodgkin JE: Exercise conditioning, in Hodgkin JE, Zorn EG, Connors GL (eds): *Pulmonary Rehabilitation: Guidelines to Success*. Boston, Butterworth Publishers, 1984.
24. Hellerstein HK, Hirsch EZ, Ader R, et al: Principles of exercise prescription for normals and cardiac subjects, in Naughton J, Hellerstein HK (eds): *Exercise Testing and Exercise Training in Coronary Heart Disease*. New York, Academic Press, 1973.
25. Pollock ML: The qualification of endurance training programs, in Wilmore JH (ed): *Exercise and Sports Science Reviews*. New York, Academic Press, 1973.
26. American College of Sports Medicine: *Guidlines for Graded Exercise Testing and Exercise Prescription*. Philadelphia, Lea & Febiger, 1973.
27. *Exercise Testing and Training of Individuals with Heart Disease or at High Risk for Its Development: A Handbook for Physicians*. New York, American Heart Association, 1975.
28. Belman MJ, Wasserman K: Exercise training and testing in patients with chronic obstructive pulmonary disease. *Basics of RD* 1981;10:1–6.
29. Spiro SG, Hahn ML, Edwards RHT, et al: An analysis of the physiologic strain of submaximal exercise in patients with chronic obstructive bronchitis. *Thorax* 1975;30:415–425.
30. Karvonen M, Kentala K, Mustala O: The effects of training heart rate: A longitudinal study. *Ann Med Exp Biol Fenn* 1957; 35:307–315.
31. Davis JA, Convertino VA: A comparison of heart rate methods for predicting endurance training intensity. *Med Sci Sports* 1975;7:295–298.
32. Petty TL, Finigan MM: Clinical evaluation of prolonged ambulatory oxygen therapy in chronic airway obstruction. *Am J Med* 1968;45:242–252.
33. Barach AL: Ambulatory oxygen therapy: Oxygen inhalation at home and out of doors. *Dis Chest* 1959;35:229–241.
34. Barach AL: *Physiologic Therapy in Respiratory Diseases*. Philadelphia, JB Lippincott Co, 1948.
35. Hass A, Rusk HA: Rehabiliation of patients with obstructive pulmonary disease: The role of enriched oxygen. *Postgrad Med* 1966;39:612–620.
36. Vyas MN, Banister EW, Morton JW, et al: Response to exercise in patients with chronic airway obstruction: II. Effects of breathing 40 percent oxygen. *Am Rev Respir Dis* 1971; 103:401–412.
37. Miller WF, Taylor HF, Jasper L: Exercise training in the rehabilitation of patients with chronic obstructive lung disease: The role of oxygen breathing. *South Med J* 1962;55:1216–1221.
38. Leith DE, Bradley M: Ventilatory muscle strength and endurance training. *J Appl Physiol* 1976;41:508–516.
39. Sonne LJ, David JA: Increased exercise performance in patients with severe COPD following inspiratory resistive training. *Chest* 1982;81:436–439.
40. Belman MJ, Mittman C: Ventilatory muscle training improves exercise capacity in chronic obstructive pulmonary disease patients. *Am Rev Respir Dis* 1980;121: 273–280.
41. Pardy RL, Rivington RN, Despas PJ, et al: The effect of inspiratory muscle training on exercise performance in chronic airflow limitation. *Am Rev Respir Dis* 1981; 123:426–433.
42. Pardy RL, Rivington RN, Despas PJ, et al: Inspiratory muscle training compared with physiotherapy in patients with chronic airflow limitation. *Am Rev Respir Dis* 1981; 123:421–425.
43. Bell CW, Nielsen SJ, Gibbs GE, et al: Generalized aerobic training versus ventilatory muscle training in the inprovement of aerobic and ventilatory muscle capacity in children with cystic fibrosis (abstract). *Am Rev Respir Dis* 1982;125 (part 2):249.

12

PSYCHOSOCIAL REHABILITATION AND PSYCHO- PHARMACOLOGY

EDWARD M. GLASER
DONALD L. DUDLEY

Especially in its early stages, COPD is a relatively "invisible" disease. Patients, particularly men still in the work force, often minimize and deny the seriousness of the diagnosis because others cannot notice any health problem. Shortness of breath, cough, and sputum production are kept hidden with great effort by the individuals to prevent loss of job and consequently being viewed as lazy or "pension-hungry."

Unlike heart disease, the disabling effects of COPD are not well known to the general public. Furthermore, families often do not know about the progressive nature of COPD or the self-care program that should be initiated early, or the necessity for curtailment of certain activities. Therefore, a physician's contact with the patient should include family members whenever possible.

A unique program to involve family members and help them prepare for the aftercare of certain types of patients was developed at Stanford University Medical Center in the 1970s. This program, initiated by the Division of Physical Therapy, School of Medicine, was called Family Focus. The objective was for the family to learn about and gain skill in the practices and procedures essential to the continuity of care for COPD patients before their discharge and to assist in the patient's transition to everyday living. In a home-like setting on hospital grounds, patients and their families were taught health care skills adapted to their needs with consideration for their interrelations and cultural environment. The program was found to be highly valuable but was discontinued in the 1980s because it could no longer be supported financially. It is mentioned here because the model was demonstrated to be so successful.

Perhaps *the* key to effective comprehensive care for patients with COPD (and for many patients with other chronic or recurring health problems) is individualization of diagnosis and treatment. While a focus is on the patient's obstructed or restricted airways, attention must also be paid to the whole person and his or her reactions to and handling of problems related to the illness. This individualization requires more time spent with each patient and often with the family in order for them to understand the nature of the disease, its implications, its prognosis, and what can be done to cope with it.

The physician concerned with comprehensive management of COPD needs to be aware of the various factors bearing on the patient's illness. The psychosocial history is particularly important. Information about the following health-related personal adjustments and problems should be elicited. (With appropriate training, the psychosocial inquiry can generally be carried out by an office nurse.)

1. Work (if Employed or Potentially Employable) and Social Interaction. What is the nature of the patient's work experience and capabilities? Does he or she feel capable of working now or in the near future? If so, doing what? Fulltime or part-time? If he or she doesn't feel able to work, why? Has the patient's work experience in general been satisfying? If not, in what ways? What does the patient do in his or her spare time? What are the patient's interests? Does he feel he has friends whom he enjoys being with at reasonably frequent times, or does he feel lonely or bored? What is the character of his or her family relationships?

2. Family Origin and Childhood. What are the current and former character of relationships with parents and siblings? What was the patient's father like? Mother? How would the patient characterize or describe himself or herself at major developmental stages, i.e., as a child (including early development and schooling), while growing up into adulthood, and now?

3. Sex. Does the patient have the kind of sexual relations he or she would like to have? If not, what is the nature of the frustrations or dissatisfactions? Does sexual activity induce dyspnea? Does the patient (or the sex partner) give up, or desire re-education that would help meet the particular situation?

4. Economic Problems in Living. How does the patient feel about financial resources in relation to living needs? What are his or her sources of income? If the patient had more income, how would he or she use it?

5. Patient's Perception of His or Her Medical and Stress-of-Life Problems, Along with Future Orientation. How does the patient view the nature and extent of his or her distress, and how might he or she best resolve these problems? What does the patient perceive as his or her strengths, limitations, responsibilities, and coping capabilities? What are his or her main fears, hopes, and expectations?

Much of the information needed to obtain a picture of medical and stress-of-life problems can be elicited by an open-ended question, such as "Would you tell me the things that bother you and what you think may be related to the state of your health?" In general, patients should be encouraged to express themselves and tell their story from the beginning. Questions can be interjected for clarification as needed, and further specific inquiry can be ventured as may seem relevant. But it is important to avoid mechanically going through a set of questions or appearing like a cross-examiner. Summary notes can be recorded under a framework of headings such as suggested above, along with another framework to record medical history and present complaints. The history-taking also should include a detailed account of how patients usually spend their time during the day from waking-up to bedtime.

REFERRING PATIENTS TO A PULMONARY REHABILITATION CENTER

Many medical centers and large hospitals have pulmonary rehabilitation centers to which the primary care physician can refer patients for psychosocial and other COPD-relevant workups. A report is sent back to the primary care physician. Such centers may also be staffed to provide appropriate specialized professional follow-through to help the patient deal more effectively with certain problem areas or stressors revealed in the psychosocial workup. The primary care physicians may not have the specialized knowledge or office resources (or time) to deal with these in an optimal fashion. If such service is deemed by the primary physician to be worthwhile and feasible, the pulmonary rehabilitation center would serve as a consultant to the primary care physician.

Patient Evaluation Instruments

The following instruments may be useful for eliciting life occurrences and assessing various aspects of lifestyle factors, attitudes, stress, and other feelings that have a significant bearing on psychophysiologic reactions. The manual that accompanies each instrument contains information on how to use and interpret the results.

1. The Social Readjustment Rating Questionnaire[1] contains 43 items of two types—those indicating the individual's lifestyle and those indicating stressful life events that occurred around the time of the disease onset. The related Social Readjustment Rating Scale (SRRS) provides a table for quantitatively rating the 43 life events according to their relative degree of necessary readjustment.

2. The Human Service Scale[2] contains 80 items that measure the satisfaction of human needs in seven life areas. It can be used as a diagnostic instrument to identify areas of low need satisfaction and as an evaluation instrument prior to and following rehabilitation services. Computer scoring is available through the University of Wisconsin, Rehabilitation Research Institute.*

3. The Berle Index[3] is designed to measure individuals' social support system, coping ability, and adaptive ability.

4. The Mooney Problem Checklist[4] contains 288 problem statements (such as "feeling tired much of the time") that relate to health, work, family, temperament, and so on.

5. The Evans County Health Department Heart Project[5] contains a useful physical activity and sociologic questionnaire.

6. Older American Research and Service Center (OARS) Social Resource Scale[6] provides a way to assess patients' social relationships with their significant others.

7. Short Portable Mental Status Questionnaire (SPMQ)[7] is a 10-item test designed to assess organic brain deficiency in elderly patients. It can be easily administered.

Goal-Setting

Goal-setting is a practical technique that is often helpful to an emotionally upset COPD patient who needs to regain hope and confidence in his or her ability to cope with this chronic illness after recovery from a frightening exacerbation. These goals should represent reasonable increments from a previously measured (or even subjectively experienced) baseline, progressing through stages toward optimal functional improvement judged possible by the patient in terms of activity level, independence, and self care. A simple form (Table 12–1) can be filled in during a brief treatment-planning and goal-setting discussion between physician and patient. Once a baseline evaluation has been made and a starting point established for each goal, progress can be either measured readily or at least judged subjectively. To accomplish such follow-up, definite appointments need to be made for appropriate periodic checkpoint evaluations.

Another question that may be raised for some patients with COPD is whether to recommend psychological counseling as adjunctive treatment. In a workbook and cassette by Dudley and colleagues,[8] psychotherapy with the COPD patient is discussed as follows:

---

*Contact George N. Wright, Ph.D., Professor, Behavioral Disabilities Department, and Director, Rehabilitation Research Institute, 2605 Marsh Lane, Madison, WI 53706.

Table 12–1. **Assessment Form for Goals Achievement***

Goal Planning for _____ from _____ to _____
                (Patient's Name)   (starting date)   (checkpoint date)

Outcome Value	Ability to walk _____ a day	Ability to engage in _____, X times a week	Additional goals to be worked out on individualized basis for each patient
Most unfavorable treatment outcome thought likely (-2)	Less than at starting date	Unable to engage	
Less than expected success with treatment (-1)	About same	Engaged X $-$ 1 times	
Expected level of treatment success (0)	10% improvement	Did engage X times	
More than expected success with treatment ($+1$)	20% improvement	Engaged X $+$ 1 times	
Best anticipated treatment success ($+2$)	More than 20% improvement	Engaged more than X $+$ 1 times	

Score _____

*Adapted from Kiresuk TJ, Sherman RE: Goal attainment scaling: a general method for evaluating comprehensive mental health programs. *Community Mental Health Journal* 1968;4(6):443–453. (Reprinted by permission from Hodgkin JE: *Chronic Obstructive Pulmonary Disease: Current Concepts in Diagnosis and Comprehensive Care.* Park Ridge, IL, American College of Chest Physicians, 1979.)

Probably the first thing to be discussed is when *not* to attempt psychotherapy. As a general rule, it has been found best not to try to deal with the psychological aspects of the disease *until the patient actually develops a psychological problem.*

In addition, it's usually best not to attempt traditional psychotherapy with patients suffering from truly severe chronic obstructive lung disease—specifically, not to tamper with the denial and repression. To do so would be to risk shattering those defenses a person in such precarious health absolutely needs for survival, shattering them without replacing them with any other form of emotional buttress. By opening such a patient up to all kinds of emotional changes, the therapist might be exposing him to metabolic demands and pulmonary tumult that can drive the patient into respiratory acidosis and cause his death. The best thing to do with these patients is to treat their depression or anxiety or anger in a "subtle" way—that is, with medication. At the same time, give them emotional support and be the good listener they need.

Another thing learned is that emphysema patients generally can't tolerate insight-oriented group therapy; they feel more comfortable as "loners," but they can do quite well in individual therapy tailored to their needs. It has been found that the asthma patient, however, can do well in either group or individual therapy. If emphysema patients do participate in group therapy, the kind of group should be tailored to the degree of insufficiency.

Both types of patients do well in didactic individual or medical treatment groups. (In this context, it sometimes is helpful for the patient to see a psychiatrist or clinical psychologist primarily to assure him that he is mentally stable—if that is essentially true. It also may be constructive to enable the patient to bring out his hostile, angry, depressed, or anxious feelings about his disease. This can be done on an individual or group basis, but preferably the latter to clear the air and help him realize that he is not alone in his problems or common emotional reactions.)

If psychotherapy is not feasible, patients who exhibit maladaptive coping mechanisms or behaviors may be encouraged to examine their own actions and feelings. One useful approach is described by Fink in which patients maintain a diary of their activities and feelings every day and then examine them to determine which are productive and satisfying.[9] While it may be helpful if the physician reviews the activities with the patient, this method may be self-taught.

Biofeedback Training

Before concluding this section, biofeedback might appropriately be mentioned. Biofeedback training uses instrumentation to give the patient immediate and continuing signals on changes in bodily functions, such as fluctuation of skin temperature, blood pressure, brainwave activity, or muscle tension.[10] Theoretically—and often in practice—these signals enable the patient to learn how to control certain involuntary functions.

Although its efficacy in COPD has not been documented by research studies, biofeedback training has been reported as clinically helpful in a number of cases.[11] See Chapter 9 for a discussion of relaxation techniques and biofeedback.

Since the respiratory system is an integration of conscious and unconscious control of function, it should be amenable to such a methodological approach. Control of panic and other cumulatively erosive costs of chaotic respiration have been studied by a number of investigators.[12] This technique is probably most valuable in alleviating the sensation of dyspnea in those COPD patients with reversible airway obstruction; however, its maximal potential in respiratory care must still be determined.

When biofeedback equipment is used, it is important to follow safety guidelines closely.[13] Physicians who desire specific training in biofeedback techniques and application should contact an organized laboratory, preferably at a well-equipped university.[14]

VOCATIONAL AND FUNCTIONAL REHABILITATION

The basic philosophy of rehabilitation is for the COPD patient to return to a role that is as self-sufficient and useful as possible. Questions about the patient's age, the nature and stage of the illness, job market possibilities and retraining opportunities for older patients, and the possibility of precipitating right-side heart failure all enter into this judgment. Once patients have increased their activity level to the optimum within their physiological capabilities, other members of the rehabilitation team, such as the psychologist, vocational or job placement counselor, social worker, and occupational therapist, may be needed for the complex task of restoring patients to their fullest physical, medical, emotional, social, economic, and vocational potential.[15] When appropriate, the earlier in the course of the disease vocational rehabilitation is instituted, the better the prognosis.[16, 17] The ideal time to begin vocational exploration is in connection with taking the psychosocial history—when patients are not in a respiratory crisis and may still be able to retain their job.

Patients are classified into four clinical and vocational rehabilitation groups: (1) those who can return to their previous activity—perhaps under somewhat modified conditions, if necessary, (2) those who should and can be retrained (if desired) for more suitable work, (3) those who can work only in sheltered situations, and (4) those who can be retrained only for self-care.

Proper evaluation and categorization of the patient's capacities are essential to successful vocational rehabilitation.[17–22] Care should be exercised in selecting patients for a vocational rehabilitation program, particularly if they have had a recent significant change in lifestyle and evidence of rapid clinical deterioration, personality change, alcoholism, or inability to mobilize psychologial and social assets.[20, 21]

Physicians must carefully decide whether a patient's cardiorespiratory reserve will enable him or her to return to work on a full- or part-time basis. If the patient's tolerance to work seems to require job modification, the vocational counselor should be alerted.[22, 23] If, as is often the case, physically rehabilitated patients require new vocational skills commensurate with their educational level and reduced pulmonary capacity, they should be trained for a job that is likely to be available in a rapidly changing employment market. Skilled job placement counselors are helpful in determining this.

In some instances, laboratory and clinical evaluations indicate that the patient can function only in sheltered situations or at home.[22] Here, occupational therapists and job placement counselors can help find suitable sources and settings for productive work. Those who are unable to care for their households or for themselves are trained in energy-saving methods by the occupational therapist.

With appropriate assessment and advice, patients can usually accomplish such tasks as housekeeping, shopping, shaving, bathing, or dressing with less dependence on others.

The social worker can assist the physician by (1) helping the family to understand the patient's limitations, (2) guiding the patient and family to appropriate resources, and (3) helping to establish a follow-up program.

Vocational rehabilitation (VR) may be difficult to achieve because of the patient's age, a low degree of psychosocial assets, the progressive nature of the disease, a poor job market, limitations in the ability to retrain patients, or serious respiratory impairment—particularly when associated with heart failure.

A retrospective analysis of a group of patients compared their VR outcome with their intelligence test scores (IQ) and the pulmonary physiologic results.[24] It was determined that the intelligence scores were able to predict the VR outcome with 83% accuracy.

A regression analysis of percentages predicted for the FEV_1 and IQ increased the accuracy of prediction to 90%. Most persons with an IQ greater than 90 and a FEV_1 above 56% of predicted did not appear to require job modification to remain gainfully employed. It was further hypothesized that the difference in job energy requirements among various IQ levels may be the underlying reason for this finding. Estimates of the energy demands of the patient's job supported this hypothesis.

MOTIVATING PATIENTS TO REMAIN IN COMPREHENSIVE CARE PROGRAMS

Where feasible, a community resource using public health nurses, respiratory therapists, social workers, and vocational rehabilitation counselors should be developed, if one is not already available. The personnel can be specially trained in the problems of patients with chronic lung disease and can effectively function as a useful adjunct to the physician, who often does not have the time to commit to the ongoing process necessary for a comprehensive program.

When reconditioning exercises seem appropriate, the following seven interrelated strategies have been found useful in clinical practice for motivating patients to remain in rehabilitation programs at home:

1. Obtain from patients an hour-by-hour description of how they usually spend their day.

2. Describe the recommended program, including the reasons for it and the benefits likely to accrue.

3. Invite patients to discuss all the reasons they can think of for *not* following the recommended program, e.g., inconvenience, difficulties, and possible doubts about benefits.

4. Help patients resolve their negative feelings and find solutions to perceived difficulties. Weigh any remaining objections against the potential benefits of the program, and encourage them to make an appropriate value assessment. If necessary, revise the program on the basis of strongly felt resistances or difficulties.

5. When agreement has been reached, work out a goal attainment chart in the form of a diary that records what is done every day in accordance with the agreed-upon program and how patients feel about the anticipated benefits.

6. If feasible, have the office nurse or a social worker visit the patient's family to discuss the recommended treatment program. If this is not possible, key persons helping to care for patients should accompany them to the physician's office for such a discussion.

7. Arrange for patients to return to the office at appropriate intervals to review their goal-attainment record (Table 12–1), and discuss their treatment progress. Periodically, patients' exercise capabilities should be evaluated on a treadmill or exercise bicycle. This provides the physician with objective data regarding the patient's improvement or maintenance level and helps to determine if the patient is faithfully following the exercise program. The demonstration of improved exercise tolerance can provide needed encouragement to the chronically ill patient. New program and goal-attainment procedures should be worked out during periodic progress review visits.

PSYCHOTROPIC MEDICATIONS

In contrast to psychosocial and psychophysiologic problems and the accompanying emotions that affect most patients with severe COPD, psychiatric disease is probably no more frequent than in patients without COPD.[25] One must be positive about the diagnosis. The medications reviewed below are not substitutes for counseling and psychotherapy. On the other hand, counseling and psychotherapy are not substitutes for psychotropic medications. A strong effort should be made to make a positive diagnosis and then tailor the treatment to the diagnosis and the patient. If one knows what is being treated, the reason for using psychoactive agents should be obvious.

The distinction between psychophysiologic and psychosocial problems and psychiatric disease is critical. As noted above, the treatment of the former can often be done with various psychotherapies, behavioral therapies, and social support systems with medication as adjuncts, when necessary, while treatment of the latter should be initiated with medications.

The role of psychoactive medications in the treatment of COPD patients is of considerable importance since many lack the ability to utilize other treatment techniques. In other words, some patients reject or cannot respond to any treatment of a "psychological" nature, and the clinician is left with the use of medications or nothing. Also, in a number of these patients, counseling and psychotherapy may not be possible because of time limitations, financing, or the physiologic and psychological stage of the disease.

If a patient fulfills the major and minor criteria for depression as indicated in the *Diagnostic and Statistical Manual of Mental Disorders,* third edition (DSM III),[26] an antidepressant is indicated. If counseling or psychotherapy is used, it is an adjunct to the antidepressant medication. On the other hand, if a patient fulfills the DSM III criteria for a traumatic stress reaction, counseling or psychotherapy is indicated, and medications (including antidepressants) are seen as adjuncts. Treatment should be tailored to the patient and the diagnosis.

Some General Guidelines

The patient's age, chronicity of the disease, and individual variations in metabolism determine the dose utilized. Since the metabolism of psychoactive medications can vary up to 30 times among people, one patient may need a dose of 30 mg and another a dose of 900 mg. A good general rule is that the dose of psychoactive medication is inversely related to age and chronicity of disease. It is important to select medications that do not depress, overly stimulate, or interfere with the respiratory center or with respiratory movement. The psychoactive medication should also have little interference with existing pulmonary medications. Blood levels for psychoactive agents are essential for adequate treatment in the COPD patient, particularly when the possible 30-fold difference is considered. Psychoactive agents are usually of great benefit when used discriminately and with awareness of the indications, contraindications and side effects of a given case.[27-32] The same guidelines apply to all medications and other treatments.

Neuroleptics

The neuroleptics (also called major tranquilizers or antipsychotics) are used in the treatment of psychiatric diseases such as schizophrenia, mania, acute psychotic reactions, and delirium (Table 12–2). Similar to the antidepressants, they do not tend to be habit-forming or addictive and are generally well tolerated if their side effects are understood. Neuroleptics and antidepressants are usually seen as being too powerful and dangerous, while the anxiolytic agents are considered innocuous. All three types of medications can have side effects in some patients, and they all should be considered equally powerful. It makes little difference to a patient if breathing is compromised because he or she has been stimulated by an excess of protriptyline, has had the respiratory center reduced by chlordiazepoxide, or cannot move the chest muscles because of a respiratory extrapyramidal reaction secondary to haloperidol.

Two neuroleptics that provide reasonable examples of the benefits and problems of this class of medications are thiothixene and chlorpromazine. Both are considered good neuroleptics—that is, they do the job the psychiatrist needs to have done. Both have side effects that lessen their usefulness in patients with COPD. The major side effects are extrapyramidal symptoms (drug-induced parkinsonism), acute dyskinesias (acute dystonic reactions), akathisias, tardive dyskinesia, and the neuroleptic malignant syndrome.

Regardless of the neuroleptic compound prescribed, about half of the patients experience some kind of side effect that interferes with their functioning. It is important to know the side effects when the agent and dosage are selected. In general, thiothixene has been utilized widely in COPD patients and seems well tolerated. As with other neuroleptics, it is useful orally,

Table 12–2. Examples of Neuroleptics (Major Tranquilizers)*

Specific Medication	Special Properties	Usual Daily Dose	Daily Dose in Moderate to Severe COPD
PHENOTHIAZINES			
Thioridazine HCl (Mellaril)	As chlorpromazine, with the exception that it has been reported to produce pigmented retinitis in doses over 800 mg. Mild D-2, highest alpha-1, moderate alpha-2, and high cholinergic receptor blocking.	Oral: 50–800 mg	Oral: 5–200 mg
Chlorpromazine (Thorazine)	Older dose forms may contain tartrazine and should be avoided if this medication is used in asthmatics. Current dose forms should be free of tartrazine. Can be very sedating. Associated with the production of antinuclear antibodies. Mild to moderate D-2, high alpha-1, moderate alpha-2, high H-1, and high cholinergic receptor blocking effect.	Oral: 50–2000 mg IM: 50–100 mg q30–60 min until symptoms are under control to a total dose of 200 mg	Oral: 5–200 mg IM: 25 mg q30–60 min until symptoms are under control to a total dose of 100 mg
Fluphenazine (Prolixin)	Available in depot form (Prolixin Decanoate or Enanthate) that can be administered to patients who are unreliable or who prefer the convenience of not taking daily medications.	Oral: 2–20 mg Depot form: 12.5 to 75 mg q1 to 3 weeks by IM injection	Oral: 1–10 mg Depot form: 6.25 to 37.5 mg q1 to 3 weeks by IM injection
Trifluoperazine HCl (Stelazine)	Can be activating. Moderate D-2, low alpha-1, low alpha-2, moderate H-1, and moderate cholinergic receptor blocking effect.	Oral: 10–40 mg	Oral: 2–5 mg
DIHYDROINDOLONES			
Molindone HCl (Moban)	Apparent low cardiovascular toxicity. Does not block guanethidine. Mild D-2, low alpha-1, moderate alpha-2, low H-1, and low cholinergic receptor blocking effect. There is little experience with this medication in COPD.	Oral: 30–100 mg	Oral: 10–30 mg
THIOTHANTHENES			
Thiothixene (Navane)	No tartrazine. Low anticholinergic effect. May have significant antidepressant effect. Decreases sensory input. Can be nonsedating or sedating. Strong D-2,	Oral: 5–80 mg IM: 5–20 mg q30–60 min to a total dose of 80 mg	Oral: 2–20 mg IM: 5 mg q30–60 min to a total dose of 40 mg

138

Table continued on opposite page

Table 12–2. **Examples of Neuroleptics (Major Tranquilizers)** *Continued*

Specific Medication	Special Properties	Usual Daily Dose	Daily Dose in Moderate to Severe COPD
	moderate to low alpha-1, moderate alpha-2, high H-1, and low cholinergic receptor blocking effect. (D-2 receptor blocking refers to antipsychotic effect. Higher D-2 blockade is thought to be synonymous with greater antipsychotic effect.)		
BUTYROPHENONES			
Haloperidol (Haldol)	The 1 mg, 5 mg, and 10 mg tablets of haloperidol contain tartrazine. These dose forms should be avoided if this medication is used in patients with asthma. Can be nonsedating. Decreases sensory input. Likely to produce movement disorders that can interfere with chest movement. Moderate D-2, moderate alpha-1, low alpha-2, low H-1 and low cholinergic receptor blocking effect.	Oral: 2–40 mg IM: 5–10 mg q30–60 min to a total dose of 40 mg IV: 2 mg q6–8 hr	Oral: 1–10 mg IM: 2–5 mg q30–60 min to a total dose of 20 mg IV: 2 mg q6–8 hr

*As one goes from thioridazine to haloperidol, extrapyramidal symptoms increase, and moving backward, alpha adrenergic blocking, allergic responses, sedation, atropine-like effects, seizures, and orthostatic hypotension generally increase. For all neuroleptics listed, drowsiness or lack of attention may make operation of machinery dangerous. This is particularly so during initial treatment. Selected patients may need the usual daily dose. Respiratory depression with aggravation or onset of hypoxia and hypercarbia is always a possible complication when the neuroleptics are used in the COPD population.

Neuroleptics in general can alter sexual function and drive. Each medication in this class can produce specific types of problems. For example, thioridazine may contribute to delayed or inhibited ejaculation, and chlorpromazine may contribute to a simple reduction in sexual drive. On the other hand, both may increase sexual drive and performance in specific patients. In addition, sexual dysfunction is so common in patients who need to be treated with neuroleptics that it is often difficult to know what the cause of the change in sexual function is secondary to.

Common Side Effects	Precautions With	Contraindications
Blurred vision	Seizures	Comatose states
Dysuria	Depression	Central nervous system depression
Constipation	Pregnancy	
Nasal congestion	Respiratory disease	Bone marrow depression
Postural hypotension	Cardiac disease	Subcortical brain depression
Photosensitivity	Respiratory depression	Seriously impaired liver function
Drowsiness	May reverse the hypertensive action of medications, such	
Fatigue	as epinephrine, and block	Hypersensitivity
Weight gain	the antihypertensive effect	Uncontrolled epilepsy
Extrapyramidal side effects	of guanethidine	Severe retarded depression
Respiratory depression		
Potential difficulty handling secretions		
Changes in temperature control		

intramuscularly, and intravenously. Although the intravenous route is not recommended or approved by the FDA, it may prove to be the future route of choice in certain patients. Tables 12–3 and 12–4 compare the relative clinical uses of neuroleptics. Using these tables as a guide, thiothixene is the best D-2 blocker—almost nine times more effective than haloperidol. Since D-2 receptor blocking is an indication of antipsychotic activity, it may be the best antipsychotic on the market. A dose of 100 mg of thiothixene is the equivalent of 888 mg of haloperidol in D-2 receptor blocking effect, 0.08 mg of atropine in anticholinergic effect, 254 mg of diphenhydramine in H-1 blocking effect, and 0.8 mg of prazosin in alpha-1 blocking effect.

Similar figures for thioridazine would be 14.0, 13.3, 92.5, and 18.2, respectively. In other words, Tables 12–3 and 12–4 can be used to choose a neuroleptic such as thioridazine that requires a high dose (low D-2 effect) and that has high anticholinergic and high alpha-1 blocking. If a low dose (high D-2 effect) with low anticholinergic activity and relatively low alpha-1 blocking is desired, thiothixene might be chosen. These data have been provided by Richelson[33, 34] and are based on receptor studies done on the human brain. The relationships listed are seen as rough guides. It is recognized that much information of this nature has been published using the rat or other nonhuman brains, and that the technology varies. The particular set of studies

Table 12–3. **Receptor Blocking Properties of Selected Neuroleptics***

	D-2 (Haloperidol)	Cholinergic (Atropine)	H-1 (Diphenhydramine)	Alpha-1 (Prazosin)	Alpha-2 (Yohimbine)
Thiothixene	8.88†	0.00081	2.5373	0.00827	0.0081
Trifluoperazine	1.52	0.00357	0.2390	0.00382	0.0006
Haloperidol	1.00	0.00010	0.0079	0.01455	0.0004
Chlorpromazine	0.21	0.03333	1.6418	0.03455	0.0021
Thioridazine	0.14	0.13333	0.9254	0.18182	0.0019
Molindone	0.03	0.00001	0.0001	0.00004	0.0026
Haloperidol	1				
Atropine		1			
D-Chlorpheniramine			1		
Prazosin				1	
Yohimbine					1

*From Richelson[33] and personal communication.
†The figures for the psychotropic agents in all five columns represent the number of mg of the reference blocking agent effect represented by 1 mg of the psychotropic agent. For example: 1 mg of thiothixene = 8.88 mg of haloperidol in terms of D-2 blocking effect, 0.00081 mg of atropine in terms of anticholinergic effect, 2.54 mg of diphenhydramine in terms of H-1 blocking effect, 0.008 mg of prazosin in terms of alph-1 blocking effect, and 0.008 mg of Yohimbine in terms of alpha-2 blocking effect. Receptors are cellular recognition sites for neurotransmitters and neurotransmitter blockers.They are generally membrane-bound proteins on the outside of the cell and have the ability to recognize specific molecular structures. The names of the receptor recognition sites are usually related to the function of the site. For example, D-1 and D-2 are recognition sites for dopamine. The D-2 site seems to be the one that when blocked decreases psychotic activity. Histamine recognition sites are called H-1 and H-2 sites.The antihistamine action of diphenhydramine and d-chlorpheniramine is secondary to their ability to block H-1 cellular recognition sites. Similarly, there are two subclassifications of alpha-adrenergic receptors called alpha-1 and alpha-2 sites. These sites are found in both the central and peripheral nervous system and play important roles in the regulation of blood pressure. Blocking alpha-1 recognition sites lowers blood pressure while blocking alpha-2 recognition sites increases blood pressure.

Table 12–4. **Receptor Blocking Characteristics of
Six Selected Psychotropic Medications***

	D-2 (Haloperidol)	Cholinergic (Atropine)	H-1 (Diphen-hydramine)	Alpha-1 (Prazosin)
Thiothixene	888.0†	0.08	254	0.8
Haloperidol	100.0	0.01	1	1.5
Thioridazine	14.0	13.33	92	18.2
Doxepin	0.2	2.70	77,500	0.3
Amitriptyline	0.4	10.00	19,250	0.2
Amoxapine	2.8	0.18	380	0.1

*From Richelson[33, 34] and personal communication.
†The figures in all four columns represent the approximate number of mg of the reference blocking agent effect represented by 100 mg of the psychotropic agent. For example: 100 mg of thiothixene = 888 mg of haloperidol in terms of D-2 blocking, 0.08 mg of atropine in terms of anticholinergic effect, 254 mg of diphenhydramine in terms of H-1 blocking effect, and 0.8 mg of prazosin in terms of alpha-1 blocking effect.

was used because they seemed to parallel clinical experience, and the information was translatable in terms of milligrams of standard blocking agents.

Rapid treatment of extrapyramidal reactions is important in maintaining unimpaired respiratory movements. These reactions to neuroleptics can be treated with benztropine mesylate (1–2 mg), or with diphenhydramine hydrochloride (50–100 mg) intravenously in most cases of respiratory impairment. Oral maintenance therapy can be accomplished with any of the antiparkinson medications, such as benztropine mesylate or procyclidine hydrochloride.

Antidepressants

In the treatment of depression, it is helpful to have information on the clinical use of antidepressants that can be used to produce sedation and activation. Since nonifensine has been removed from the market it is hoped that an activating compound such as bupropion might be available and appropriate for patients with COPD.

Doxepin is the antidepressant of choice in agitated, depressed patients with COPD. In addition to its antidepressant characteristics, it is sufficiently sedating to reduce or eliminate agitation. The sedative effect is apparent in minutes or hours, while the antidepressant effect may take days or weeks to be apparent. As with other antidepressants, it appears to have little or no effect on the respiratory center, and it seems to act as a bronchodilator. It should be noted that doxepin and other psychotropic agents have been found to decrease seizures in patients with seizure disorders. A dose of 100 mg of doxepin contains the equivalent of 0.2 mg haloperidol in D-2 blocking, 2.7 mg of atropine in anticholinergic effect, 77,500 mg of diphenhydramine in H-1 blocking, 0.3 mg of prazosin in alpha-1 blocking, and 4.0 mg of phentolamine in alpha-2 blocking (Tables 12–4 and 12–5). Doxepin has relatively low side effects if used for the appropriate indications.

Table 12–5. **Receptor Blocking Properties of Selected Antidepressants***

	H-1 (Diphen-hydramine)	Cholinergic (Atropine)	Alpha-1 (Prazosin)	Alpha-2 (Phen-tolamine)	Serotonin (Methy-sergide)	D-2 (Halo-peridol)
Doxepin	775.0†	0.02708	0.00257	0.040	0.067	0.002
Trimipramine	250.0	0.03542	0.00256	0.065	0.049	0.025
Amitriptyline	192.5	0.11458	0.00236	0.050	0.067	0.004
Maprotiline	25.0	0.00416	0.00067	0.005	?	?
Amoxapine	2.8	0.00208	0.00122	0.017	?	0.028
Nortriptyline	3.5	0.01458	0.00098	0.017	0.042	?
Imipramine	2.5	0.02292	0.00067	0.014	0.015	0.002
Protriptyline	0.7	0.08333	0.00050	0.007	0.014	0.002
Trazodone	0.4	0.00001	0.00171	0.087	?	0.001
Desipramine	0.1	0.01042	0.00045	0.006	0.005	0.001
Diphenhydramine	1					
Atropine		1				
Prazosin			1			
Phentolamine				1		
Methysergide					1	
Haloperidol						1

*From Richelson[34] and personal communication.
†The figures in all six columns represent the approximate number of mg of the reference blocking agent effect represented by 1 mg of the psychotropic agent.

Bupropion is probably the antidepressant of choice in retarded, depressed patients with low drive and motivation. The activating effect can appear in hours and the antidepressant effect in days or weeks. The most common side effects are sleep disturbance, restlessness, and diaphoresis. This medication is to be released for commercial use in 1986, and clinical information must await its use in this country. It reportedly has little or no anticholinergic effect and is not cardiotoxic. There should be a reliable receptor blocking profile available soon.

It is generally inadvisable to utilize doxepin in the morning or bupropion at night. As a general rule, patients will not adapt well to doxepin if it is given during the day, or to bupropion if it is given at night. To obtain optimal therapeutic effect, advantage should be taken of the initial sedation or activating characteristics by prescribing them at times when sedation or activation does not interfere with the patient's life.

In utilizing antidepressants and neuroleptics, it is important to remember that blood levels may have little relationship to oral dose, and cellular levels may be poorly related to either. Since these compounds may have a therapeutic window, above or below which there are no positive clinical effects, optimal blood levels must be maintained. This is particularly true for the antidepressants. The desired clinical response can be associated with a specific blood level and then maintained, which is the preferred method of determining dosage in patients with combined psychiatric and pulmonary disease. Since metabolism varies greatly among individuals, major side effects such as cardiotoxicity can be avoided by the measurement of blood levels and appropriate adjustments in dose.

Although it is important for the clinician to deal with side effects of individual psychoactive agents, it is also important to understand that certain

Table 12–6. **Examples of Heterocyclic Antidepressants***

Specific Medication	Special Properties	Usual Daily Dose	Daily Dose in Moderate to Severe COPD
TRICYCLIC AGENTS†			
Amitriptyline HCl (Elavil)	Information uncertain. May act as a mild bronchodilator and may depress ventilation. Generally not recommended in COPD patients with arrhythmias. Metabolically converted to nortriptyline (Aventyl or Pamelor) thus may begin as sedating and end up in 7–14 days as nonsedating or activating. Low D-2, moderate H-1, high cholinergic, low alpha-1, and moderate serotonin receptor blocking effect.	Oral: 50–300 mg	Oral: 10–100 mg
Doxepin HCl (Adapin, Sinequan)	Adapin contains tartrazine and should be avoided in asthmatics. Some preliminary evidence indicates comparatively low bioavailability for Adapin. Low cardiac toxicity; has little or no effect on respiratory center; may act as a mild bronchodilator. Particularly effective in treatment of panic attacks associated with depression. Antidepressant of choice for agitated/depressed patients. Acts as an antiseizure agent in patients with a seizure disorder. Unlikely to inhibit guanethidine in doses under 150 mg. Initially may be sedating. May produce rapid remission in steroid-dependent intractable asthma. Low D-2, high H-1, low to moderate cholinergic, low alpha-1, and moderate serotonin receptor blocking effect.	Oral: 50–300 mg	Oral: 10–100 mg
Imipramine HCl (Janimine, SK-Pramine, Tofranil)	Tofranil-PM (100 mg and 125 mg dose sizes) and Janimine (10 mg and 25 mg) contain tartrazine and should be avoided in asthmatics. Generally as amitriptyline HCl, but more activating. Metabolically converted to desipramine (Pertofrane or	Oral: 50–300 mg	Oral: 10–100 mg

Table continued on following page

Table 12–6. **Examples of Heterocyclic Antidepressants*** *Continued*

Specific Medication	Special Properties	Usual Daily Dose	Daily Dose in Moderate to Severe COPD
	Norpramin) thus may begin as sedating or activating and end up in 7–14 days as more activating. Low D-1, low H-1, moderate cholinergic, low alpha-1, and low serotonin receptor blocking.		
Desipramine (Pertofrane, Norpramin)	Norpramine (25 mg, 50 mg, 75 mg and 100 mg) contains tartrazine and should be avoided in asthmatics. Metabolic product of imipramine. Clinically less cardiotoxic than protriptyline, but probably not as activating. Low D-1, low H-1, low to moderate cholinergic, low alpha-1, and low serotonin receptor blocking.	Oral: 50–200 mg	Oral: 10–100 mg
Nortriptyline (Aventyl, Pamelor)	Clinically generally as desipramine. Unknown D-2, low H-1, low to moderate cholinergic, low alpha-1, and low serotonin receptor blocking.	Oral: 50–100 mg	Oral: 10–50 mg
Protriptyline (Vivactil)	May stimulate ventilation. Generally the antidepressant of choice for retarded depressed patients with low motivation. Similar cardiotoxicity with amitriptyline. New generation of antidepressants may substitute for this medication. Low D-2, low H-1, moderate cholinergic, low alpha-1, and low serotonin receptor blocking.	Oral: 5–60 mg	Oral: 2.5–20 mg
TETRACYCLIC AMINES			
Maprotiline (Ludiomil)	Generally as protriptyline and desipramine with the exception that it appears to have the highest incidence of seizures of any antidepressant on the United States market. Unknown, D-2, low to moderate H-1, low	Oral: 75–225 mg	Oral: 10–100 mg

Table continued on opposite page

Table 12–6. **Examples of Heterocyclic Antidepressants*** Continued

Specific Medication	Special Properties	Usual Daily Dose	Daily Dose in Moderate to Severe COPD
	cholinergic, low alpha-1, and unknown serotonin receptor blocking.		
TRIAZOLOPYRIDINES			
Trazodone (Desyrel)	Contains tartrazine in the 50 mg and 150 mg dose forms, and these should be avoided in asthmatics. Associated with priapism, and impotence subsequent to treatment of the priapism. Generally sedating. Low D-2, low H-1, low cholinergic, low alpha-1, and unknown serotonin receptor blocking.	Oral: 150–400 mg	Oral: 50–150 mg
DIBENZOXAZEPINE			
Amoxapine (Asendin)	Useful in psychotic, depressed patients (in roughly the group of patients that are treated with combinations of antidepressants and neuroleptics.) Has some of the side effects of the neuroleptics including extrapyramidal symptoms. Generally sedating. High D-2 (for an antidepressant), low H-1, low cholinergic, low alpha-1, and unknown serotonin receptor blocking.	Oral: 75–400 mg	Oral: 25–100 mg
TETRAHYDROISOQUINOLINE			
Nomifensine (Merital)	Activating antidepressant. Removed from the market for unknown reasons.		
MONOCYCLIC AMINOKETONE			
Bupropion (Wellbatrin)	To be released in the United States in the future. Reportedly an activating antidepressant with a half-life of 2 to 4 hours. Other than Nomifensine, which had a similar half-life, the half-life of this compound is roughly 1/10 that of the above compounds. No experience in the country with COPD. It has some dopamine-mimetic properties in humans such as suppression of prolactin levels. Side effects are		

Table continued on following page

Table 12–6. **Examples of Heterocyclic Antidepressants*** *Continued*

Specific Medication	Special Properties	Usual Daily Dose	Daily Dose in Moderate to Severe COPD
	reportedly mild and uncommon, with the most important being restlessness, insomnia, and diaphoresis. Does not have receptor blocking characteristics as of this date.		
BENZODIAZEPINE (TRIAZOLOBENZODIAZEPINE)			
Alprazolam (Xanax)	An anxiolytic with what may prove to be reasonable antidepressant characteristics.	Oral: 0.25–4 mg	Oral: 0.125–2.0 mg

*For all antidepressants listed, drowsiness or lack of attention may make operation of machinery dangerous. This is particularly so during initial treatment. A beneficial side effect of these medications in COPD patients may be mild bronchodilation. Selected patients may need the usual daily dose.

†As one goes from amitriptyline to protriptyline in the tricyclic agents, the initial activation effect generally increases. Initial effects should be distinguished from the antidepressant effect, which takes several days. Initial sedation or activation is present in hours. However, the initial effect is therapeutic and demonstrates to the patient that the condition is responsive to medications. In general, avoid giving a sedating antidepressant during the day or to a patient with a retarded depression. The initial sedation may incapacitate the patient and lead to noncompliance with therapy.

Common Side Effects	Precautions with	Contraindications
Dry mouth	Urinary retention	Acute myocardial infarction
Potential difficulty handling secretions	Cardiovascular disorders	Hypersensitivity
Blurred vision	Narrow angle glaucoma	Acute schizophrenia
Constipation	Organic brain syndrome	Mania
Nausea	Schizophrenia	Monoamine oxidase inhibitors
Heartburn	Mania	
Hypotension	Convulsive disorders	
Weight gain	Thyroid disease	
	Pregnancy	
	Potentiation of sympatho-mimetic amines	
	Blocking guanethidine	

medications are converted to known psychoactive agents in the course of their metabolism in the human body. For example, imipramine is broken down to desipramine, and amitriptyline is broken down to nortriptyline. The metabolite varies from the parent compound by having different receptor blocking characteristics and different side effects (Tables 12–5 and 12–6). The issue is complicated by the fact that once a steady state is reached (in seven to 10 days), the ratio of desipramine to imipramine is about 2 to 1, and the ratio of nortriptyline to amitriptyline is about 1.2 to 1.

Lithium

Understanding lithium therapy has been increasingly important as clinical studies continue to demonstrate its effectiveness in controlling mania, depression, or cyclic swings from mania to depression. Initially mania may be treated by a neuroleptic and depression with an antidepressant. However, lithium should be started concomitantly if mood swings are a serious problem. The starting dose of lithium is generally from 150–450 mg/day. This dose may require modification if the patient is taking theophylline or a diuretic, since theophylline tends to increase excretion of lithium and most diuretics decrease excretion of lithium. In addition, lithium excretion may vary with salt intake, which should therefore be kept stable during lithium administration. A fasting morning level of lithium (nine to 10 hours after the evening dose) of 0.5 to 1.0 mEq/L (or lower) is usually therapeutic in patients with moderate to severe lung disease. It may take three to 10 days to equilibrate at a therapeutic blood level. Lithium usually has a seven- to 10-day lag between the onset of therapy and the therapeutic response. When the maintenance dose is reached, the neuroleptic or antidepressant can often be withdrawn. Note that some COPD patients obtain good therapeutic effects with blood levels of less than 0.5 mEq/L.

Table 12–7. **Examples of Manic-Depressive Agents**

Specific Medication	Special Properties	Usual Daily Dose	Daily Dose in Moderate to Severe COPD
Lithium carbonate* (Eskalith, Lithane)	Reduces or stops cyclic mood swings. Prophylactic against recurrent mania or depression. Often takes 7–14 days for therapeutic effect to be utilized. Give with psychiatric supervision. 20% or more of the population with manic-depressive disease does not respond or has unacceptable side effects, and other agents need to be utilized. Can produce diabetes insipidus.	Oral: 900–1800 mg/day until blood level of 0.8–1.2 mEq/L is attained; dose may have to be reduced to 1/2 to 2/3 of starting dose for maintenance	Oral: Same dose; aim for serum level of 0.6–1.0 mEq/L (stay on low side)
Carbamazepine (Tegretol)	An iminodibenzl derivative with a tricyclic structure similar to the tricyclic antidepressants. For treatment of acute episodes, it is particularly efficacious in mania. It has a growing use in bipolar or schizoaffective patients who do not respond to or tolerate lithium. It has also been used in treatment of	Psychiatric evaluation recommended to help determine appropriate dose.	

Table continued on following page

Table 12–7. **Examples of Manic-Depressive Agents** *Continued*

Specific Medication	Special Properties	Usual Daily Dose	Daily Dose in Moderate to Severe COPD
	lithium-induced diabetes insipidus. Carbamazepine is usually used as an antiseizure agent, but has growing applications as a psychotropic medication. The feared adverse effect of aplastic anemia is rare, but white blood cell count suppression early in treatment is common. Regular hematologic monitoring is recommended. Common side effects are dizziness, ataxia, and clumsiness. Use only under the supervision of those familiar with the medication.		
Valproic acid (Depakene)	Valproic acid is a gaba-ergic drug that is a strong antiseizure agent. Preliminary studies indicate that this medication may have antimanic characteristics. It should be used only by those familiar with its action and with the failure of other methods of controlling manic depressive disease.	Psychiatric evaluation recommended to help determine appropriate dose.	
Lecithin, choline	Lecithin in doses of between approximately 20 and 40 grams has been shown to exert some antimanic activity. Adverse side effects seem to be onset of depression and diarrhea. Choline can produce an unpleasant body smell in about 20% of those who take it and is not recommended for those individuals. Adverse side effects seem to be onset of depression and diarrhea.	Oral: 20–40 gm	Oral: 20–40 gm

*Blocks release of T-4; likely to precipitate depression; contraindicated with brain damage or significant cardiovascular or renal disease. Considerable caution should be used with diuretics since lithium carbonate may be substituted for sodium, and rapidly produced toxic levels of lithium lead to potentially fatal cardiac arrhythmias. Caution should also be used when it is utilized in hot weather or when the patient is losing salt. Contraindicated in patients in comatose states, in the presence of a large amount of CNS depressants, in hypersensitive patients, or those with a history of addiction or habituation.

Patients should be monitored carefully for signs of toxicity (particularly hyperthermia) and an alternate treatment planned in advance. Lithium carbonate occasionally produces a severe depression and, if this occurs, an antidepressant with or without lithium carbonate must be used.

Increasing experience is being gained with carbamazepine, valproic acid, lecithin, and other agents in treating the approximately 25% of patients who cannot tolerate or do not respond to lithium (Table 12–7).[35]

Anxiolytic Agents

These psychopharmacologic agents are often overused. They tend to be given in sympathy for the patients' condition and in recognition of the physician's inability to cure them rather than for specific indications. As with any medication, it is better not to prescribe anxiolytic agents if clinical indications for their administration are unclear. These are potent compounds, and prescribing them indiscriminantly (that is, to patients who may not need

Table 12–8. **Examples of Anxiolytic Agents (Minor Tranquilizers or Sedative Hypnotics)***

Specific Medication	Special Properties	Usual Daily Dose	Daily Dose in Moderate to Severe COPD
BENZODIAZEPINES			
Chlordiazepoxide HCl (Librium)	May be drug of choice in alcohol withdrawal. Poor absorption by intramuscular route.	Oral: 10–200 mg IV: For treatment of acute reactions including seizures and delirium tremens, 0.5 mg/kg at rate of 5 mg/min to a total dose of 50 mg q4–6 hr	Oral: 10–100 mg IV: half the usual dose
Diazepam (Valium)	Good muscle relaxant. Poor absorption by intramuscular route.	Oral: 5–50 mg IV: For treatment of acute reactions including seizures and delirium tremens, 0.1 mg/kg at rate of 1 mg/min to a total dose of 5–10 mg q4–6 hr	Oral: 5–10 mg IV: half the usual dose
Chlorazepate dipotassium (Tranxene)	Antiseizure agent.	Oral: 3.75–45 mg	Oral: 3.75–15 mg
Alprazolam (Xanax)	Often recognized as the medication of choice in panic attacks and similar	Oral: 0.25–4.0 mg	Oral: 0.125–2.0 mg

Table continued on following page

Table 12–8. **Examples of Anxiolytic Agents
(Minor Tranquilizers or Sedative Hypnotics)*** *Continued*

Specific Medication	Special Properties	Usual Daily Dose	Daily Dose in Moderate to Severe COPD
	conditions. Also, noted by some to have antidepressant properties (see above).		
Triazolam (Halcion)	Short half-life of approximately 2.5 hours. Usually well-tolerated sleep medication. Can be utilized in low doses as a temporary treatment for anxiety (0.0625–0.125 mg) with low risk of sedation. Has reportedly been given in a dose of 0.125 mg daily for up to a year without habituation.	Oral: 0.125–0.5 mg	Oral: 0.0625–0.25 mg
DIPHENYLMETHANE DERIVATIVES			
Hydroxyzine HCl (Atarax, Vistaril)	Antihistamine, low abuse potential. Generally not as effective as the benzodiazepines, but known bronchodilator.	Oral: 25–200 mg	Oral: 10–100 mg
GLYCEROL DERIVATIVES			
Meprobamate (Miltown, Equanil)	May have low safety factor with overdose as compared to other anxiolytic agents.	Oral: 400–1600 mg	Oral: 200–800 mg

*Barbiturates produce unacceptable central nervous system depression, sedation, dependency, and addiction risk and have a low safety margin compared to the medications listed, with the exception of meprobamate. For all anxiolytics listed, drowsiness or lack of attention may make operation of machinery dangerous. This is particularly so during initial treatment. Selected patients may need the usual daily dose. Respiratory depression with aggravation or onset of hypoxia and hypercapnia is always a possible complication when the anxiolytic agents are used in the COPD population. In selected patients with high anxiety levels, there may be no effect on respiratory drive, sedation, or habituation, and the primary effects may be symptom-reducing and life-saving.

Common Side Effects	Precautions with	Contraindications
Drowsiness	Glaucoma	Hypersensitivity
Ataxia	Anticoagulants	Porphyria (do not use mepro-
Confusion	Renal impairment	bamate)
Slurred speech	Respiratory depression	Comatose states
Headache	Hepatic impairment	Severe dependency or addic-
Dizziness	Pregnancy	tion
Impaired visual accommoda-	Withdraw slowly after long-	
tion	term use to avoid problems	
Dependency	such as convulsions	
Dry mouth	Breast-feeding moth-	
Potential difficulty handling	ers—medication may be	
secretions	transferred via milk	
	May occasionally produce paradoxical rage or anxiety or depression	

them or who may need some other type of medication, such as an antidepressant or neuroleptic) can be antitherapeutic and even dangerous to the COPD patient. Without a positive diagnosis, the only effect would probably be sedation and potentiation of depression and/or behavioral disorganization that can further aggravate COPD problems. Generally, these agents should be used to attain short-term goals such as overcoming an acute stress reaction. The statement that giving them over long periods of time leads to significant problems with habituation and addiction needs to be studied. In particular, some newly released, not yet released and probably some older compounds in this category may carry roughly the same probability of habituation and addiction as digitalis or hydrochlorothiazide. If an anxiolytic agent has been administered in high dosage over a period of months, withdrawal should not be abrupt but rather carried out by gradual reduction of dosage. A reasonable schedule is to withdraw at the rate of 10% of the current dose each day or each week. In some cases, it may be desirable to replace one type of anxiolytic by another rather than withdraw the medication and experience recurrence of the symptoms it was originally prescribed for. Abrupt withdrawal is not desirable for any medication, and anxiolytic agents are no exception. Sudden withdrawal often results in such symptoms as nervousness, anxiety, tremor, and insomnia. Commonly used anxiolytic agents include diazepam, chlordiazepoxide, chlorazepate, alprazolam, triazolam, and hydroxyzine (Table 12–8).

Anticholinergic Problems

Medications with high anticholinergic properties such as antiparkinson agents, thioridazine, and amitriptyline occasionally lead to an anticholinergic psychosis (delirium). The use of multiple medications increases the probability of the reaction. This is associated with the signs and symptoms of atropine ingestion, including mild temperature elevation, flushed, warm skin, increased heart rate, decreased sweating, mydriasis, and an acute brain syndrome. It is important that this is recognized early, since increasing the dose of the offending agents increases the severity of the psychosis. Treatment with intramuscular or intravenous physostigmine (1 mg) is recommended, if necessary, for the patient's well-being and/or survival. Reversal is rapid (in minutes). Only physostigmine crosses the blood-brain barrier; neostigmine simply produces symptoms of peripheral cholinergic action. Methscopolamine (0.5–1.0 mg intramuscularly) can be used to block the peripheral effects of physostigmine to help avoid respiratory problems, if necessary.

SUMMARY

There are four primary types of medications useful in the treatment of psychiatric disease or sustained emotional upsets in patients with COPD:
1. Neuroleptics, also called major tranquilizers or antipsychotic agents,

are used in the treatment of disorders such as schizophrenia, mania, acute psychotic reactions, and in some cases, delirium and dementia.

2. The heterocyclic antidepressants were previously called tricyclic antidepressants before the introduction of molecular structures that were not tricyclic in origin. They are used in the treatment of both bipolar and unipolar depression (either recurrent or single episodes).

3. Medications are also available for the control of mood swings (from depression to mania, from depression to a normal mood, or from mania to a normal mood). The only medication in this group recognized in the past was lithium carbonate. Increasing evidence indicates that there is a role for carbamazepine, lecithin, valproic acid, and other compounds.

4. Anxiolytic agents can be used for the control of anxiety in conjunction with any of the above compounds. They vary from medications for panic to those for seizures, insomnia, and anxiety. They are safe—if not abused—and generally have little effect by themselves on major psychiatric problems. In this group of people they should be used as an adjunct to the primary neuroleptic, antidepressant, or medication for mood control and are most useful in the person who is acutely or chronically emotionally upset.

With the availability of receptor blocking profiles for many of these agents, the clinician can look up a particular medication and estimate the amount of a specific receptor blocking characteristic present. For example, if one is worried about a possibly harmful anticholinergic effect, one can compare the blocking characteristics of other familiar agents by using the tables in this chapter. This is an area of medicine with several imponderable questions, but the information is undoubtedly useful to clinical medicine.

References

1. Holmes TH, Rahe RH: The social readjustment rating scale. *J Psychosom Res* 1967;11:213–218.
2. Rehabilitation Research Institute, University of Wisconsin: *Human Service Scale.* Madison, WI, Human Service Systems, Inc, 1973.
3. Berle BB, Pinsky RH, Wolf S, et al: A clinical guide to prognosis in stress diseases. *JAMA* 1952;149:1624–1628.
4. Gordon L, Mooney RL: *Mooney Problem Checklist.* New York, Psychological Corp, 1950.
5. Cassell JE: Summary of major findings of the Evans County Health Department Heart Project. *Arch Intern Med* 1971;128:887–889.
6. Kane R, Kane R: *Assessing the Elderly: A Practical Guide to Measurement.* Lexington, MA, D.C. Heath, 1981.
7. Pfeiffer E: A short portable mental status questionnaire for the assessment of organic brain deficit in elderly patients. *Am Geriatr Soc* 1975;23(10):433–441.
8. Dudley DL, Hudson LD, Smith CK: Psychological Aspects of Chronic Obstructive Lung Diseases. North Chicago, IL, Abbott Laboratories, 1973.
9. Fink DH: *Release from Nervous Tension.* New York, Simon & Schuster, 1962.
10. Davis MH, Saunders DR, Creer TL, et al: Relaxation training facilitated by biofeedback apparatus as a supplemental treatment in bronchial asthma. *J Psychosom Res* 1973;17:121–128.
11. Vachon L, Rich ES: Visceral learning in asthma. *Psychosom Med* 1976;38:122–130.
12. Brown BB: *New Mind, New Body.* New York, Harper & Row, 1974.
13. Roveti D: Electrical safety test procedures for hospitals. *Med Electronics & Data* Nov–Dec 1971;2:34–39.
14. Green E, Green A: *Beyond Biofeedback.* New York, Dell Publishing Co, 1977.
15. Berzins GF: An occupational therapy program for the chronic obstructive pulmonary disease patient. *Am J Occup Ther* 1970;24:181–186.
16. Rusk HA: Pulmonary problems, in Reha-

bilitation Medicine, ed 3. St. Louis, Missouri. CV Mosby Co, 1971.

17. Lustig F, Haas A, Castilio R: Clinical and rehabilitation regimen in patients with chronic obstructive pulmonary disease. *Arch Phys Med Rehabil* 1972;53:315–322.

18. Miller WF, Taylor HF, Pierce AK: Rehabilitation of the disabled patient with chronic bronchitis and pulmonary emphysema. *Am J Public Health* 1963;53 (suppl):18–24.

19. Gordon EE, Haas A: Energy cost during various physical activities in convalescing tuberculosis patients. *Am Rev Tuberc* 1955;71:722–731.

20. Kass I, Dyksterhuis JE: The Nebraska COPD rehabilitation project: A program to identify the factors involved in the rehabilitation of patients with chronic obstructive pulmonary disease: A multidisciplinary study of 140 patients. Final Report, Social and Rehabilitation Service, Department of Health, Education, and Welfare, Project RD 2517 M. December 1971.

21. Kass I, Dyksterhuis JE, Rubin H, et al: Correlation of psycho-physiological variables with vocational rehabilitation; outcome in chronic obstructive pulmonary disease patients. *Chest* 1975;67:433–440.

22. Haas A, Luczak A: The application of physical medicine and rehabilitation to emphysema patients. Rehabilitation Monograph XXII, Institute of Rehabilitation Medicine. New York University Medical Center, November 1963.

23. Haas A, Cardon H: Rehabilitation in chronic obstructive pulmonary disease: A five-year study of 252 male patients. *Med Clin North Am* 1969;53:593–606.

24. Daughton DM, Fix AJ, Kass I, et al: Role of intelligence test scores in predicting vocational rehabilitation success of patients with chronic obstructive pulmonary disease (COPD). *J Chron Dis* 1979;32:405–409.

25. Dudley DL, Sitzman J, Rugg M: Psychiatric aspects of patients with chronic obstructive pulmonary disease. *Adv Psychosom Med* 1985;14:64–77.

26. *Diagnostic and Statistical Manual of Mental Disorders,* ed 3. Washington, DC, The American Psychiatric Association, 1980.

27. Antipsychotic medication: A question of dosage. *J Clin Psychiatry* 1985;46(5):3–40.

28. Movement disorders and tardive dyskinesia. *J Clin Psychiatry* 1985;46(4):3–53.

29. Depression and chronic disease: Proceedings from a symposium. *J Clin Psychiatry* 1984;45(3):4–57.

30. Monograph Series: Depression and chronic disease. *J Clin Psychiatry* 1984; 2(4):3–47.

31. Update on the clinical management of affective illness. *J Clin Psychiatry* 1985; 46(10):3–56.

32. Dominquez RA, Goldstein BJ: 25 Years of benzodiazepine experience: Clinical commentary on use, abuse and withdrawal. *Hospital Formulary* 1985;20:1000–1014.

33. Richelson E: Pharmacology of neuroleptics in use in the United States. *J Clin Psychiatry* 1985;46:8–14.

34. Richelson E: Pharmacology of antidepressants in use in the United States. *J Clin Psychiatry* 1982;43:4–11, and 1983;44:4–9.

35. Lerer B: Alternative therapies for bipolar disorder. *J Clin Psychiatry* 1985; 46:309–316.

13

PULMONARY REHABILITATION

JOHN E. HODGKIN

The Council on Rehabilitation in 1942 defined rehabilitation as the restoration of the individual to the fullest medical, mental, emotional, social, and vocational potential of which he or she is capable. The rehabilitation process has found widespread acceptance for patients with musculoskeletal and neuromuscular disorders for many years. In addition, rehabilitation programs for patients with cardiovascular disease have become common in recent years. However, in spite of multiple reports that pulmonary rehabilitation programs result in benefits for patients with chronic obstructive pulmonary disease (COPD), such programs have still not achieved uniform acceptance by the medical community.[1-11]

During the mid-1970s, the Human Interaction Research Institute (HIRI) in Los Angeles, California, coordinated a study that showed many physicians were not aware of or using many proven components of care for patients with pulmonary disease.[12] The HIRI project developed a state-of-the-art paper on diagnosis and treatment of COPD. After this paper was published in the Journal of the American Medical Association in 1975,[13] hundreds of allied health professionals and physicians were invited to review the paper and make recommendations or modifications that were felt to be important. Using this input, an expanded article was published in 1979 as a book by the American College of Chest Physicians.[14] A major goal of the HIRI project was to disseminate information as widely as possible to physicians and allied health personnel regarding components of care that were felt to be beneficial to patients with respiratory impairment.

154

Attempts have been made to clarify which aspects of care are useful and to define pulmonary rehabilitation. In 1974, a committee of the American College of Chest Physicians[15] developed a definition that was later incorporated into the American Thoracic Society statement below.

As more and more pulmonary rehabilitation programs made their appearance in the late 1970s, many pulmonary physicians developed a concern that some of the programs were business ventures more intent on making money by selling and servicing respiratory therapy equipment than on providing good care for patients. Because of that concern, as well as a growing realization that pulmonary rehabilitation meant many different things to pulmonary specialists, the American Thoracic Society Scientific Assembly on Clinical Problems appointed an ad hoc committee in 1979 to try to clarify the meaning of the term. The committee not only defined pulmonary rehabilitation but also listed the recommended sequence for a pulmonary rehabilitation program and summarized the services that should be available if a facility is going to offer such a program. The recommendations developed by this committee were published in 1981 as an ATS official position statement,[16] which is reprinted here by permission of the American Thoracic Society.

PULMONARY REHABILITATION*

Introduction

The purpose of this statement is to define pulmonary rehabilitation and to describe the essential elements of a pulmonary rehabilitation program. In order to provide comprehensive pulmonary rehabilitation services, a program should be able to carry out the described components of pulmonary rehabilitation and to provide the essential services required as defined in this statement.

Definition of Pulmonary Rehabilitation

Rehabilitation was defined by the Council of Rehabilitation in 1942 as the restoration of the individual to the fullest medical, mental, emotional, social, and vocational potential of which he/she is capable. Instead of addressing solely the physical and mental aspects, rehabilitation should be tailored to maximize one's improvement and minimize the impact of an illness, or a state of progressive deterioration from optimal health, not only on the person, but also his/her family and community.

The American College of Chest Physicians' Committee on Pulmonary Rehabilitation adopted, at its annual meeting in 1974, the following definition:

"Pulmonary rehabilitation may be defined as an art of medical practice wherein an individually tailored, multidisciplinary program is formulated which through accurate diagnosis, therapy, emotional support, and education, stabilizes or reverses both the physio- and psychopathology of pulmonary diseases and

---

*This official ATS statement was adopted by the ATS Executive Committee, March 1981.

attempts to return the patient to the highest possible functional capacity allowed by his pulmonary handicap and overall life situation."

The two principal objectives of pulmonary rehabilitation are to: (1) control and alleviate as much as possible the symptoms and pathophysiologic complications of respiratory impairment, and (2) teach the patient how to achieve optimal capability for carrying out his/her activities of daily living. Depending on the needs of the specific patient, comprehensive care may include the delivery of a structured, defined "rehabilitation program" as an element of the patient's care. However, in the broadest sense, pulmonary rehabilitation means providing good, comprehensive respiratory care for patients with pulmonary disease. A facility caring for such individuals should be capable of either providing or having access to a regional medical center that is able to offer such a comprehensive care program. The components of pulmonary rehabilitation described in this statement are most useful for patients with chronic obstructive pulmonary disease (COPD), e.g., emphysema, chronic bronchitis, and asthma. However, certain aspects may be selected for patients with other pulmonary disorders.

Sequence of Pulmonary Rehabilitation

A certain sequence should be followed when outlining an appropriate treatment plan. This process involves careful evaluation of the patient, developing a treatment program that best meets the patient's needs, proper assessment of the patient's progress, and a plan for patient follow-up. A logical sequence would proceed as follows:

A. *Patient Selection.* Any patient with symptomatic COPD should be considered for pulmonary rehabilitation. Those patients with either very mild or very severe disease will not generally be placed on as intensive and comprehensive a rehabilitation program as those with moderate to moderately-severe disease.

Multiple factors affect the ultimate success of rehabilitation for any individual. These include, in addition to severity of the disease, the presence of other disabling diseases such as cancer or arthritis, age, intelligence, level of education, occupation, family support, and personal motivation.

B. *Evaluation.* A careful assessment of the patient should be performed initially. This evaluation would include:

1. *Diagnostic Workup.* Proper identification of the patient's specific respiratory ailment is important because the treatment regimen prescribed should be geared to the patient's disease process. Essential diagnostic information would include: appropriate pulmonary function studies, a chest radiograph, an electrocardiogram, and, when indicated, arterial blood gas measurements at rest and during exercise, sputum analysis and blood theophylline measurements.

2. *Behavioral Considerations.* The best rehabilitation results require personal commitment from the patient, determination and persistence. Additionally, significant psychiatric symptoms of any sort profoundly disrupt compliance. For these reasons, the patient should receive emotional screening assessments and treatment or counseling when required.

Thorough understanding of the disease and its treatment is one of the more important factors in patient motivation, cooperation, and anxiety reduction. This is particularly true in pulmonary rehabilitation during which the patient must master a large amount of knowledge. Yet learning abilities among these patients are often subtly impaired. This can be remedied in two ways: (a) Estimating the patient's learning skills and adjusting the program to the patient's ability, and (b) Requiring the patient to demonstrate new knowledge and skills before progressing further.

The patient must be reviewed in terms of the personal and environmental assets at his/her disposal. These include family and social support, potential employment skills, employment opportunities, and community resources. These all need to be evaluated and mobilized for practical help to the patient and to bolster his/her motivation.

C. *Determine Goals.* It is crucial that short and long-term goals be developed for each individual following the evaluation. The patient and his/her family need to help determine and fully understand these goals, so that they realistically approach the treatment phase.

D. *Components of Pulmonary Rehabilitation*
   1. *Physical Therapy.* Good bronchial hygiene, e.g., effective coughing, clapping, and bronchial drainage is particularly important to those patients who produce excess mucus within the airways. Pursed-lip breathing may help to slow the respiratory rate and lessen small airway collapse during periods of increased dyspnea. Relaxation techniques can be useful in anxious patients.
   2. *Exercise Conditioning.* A physical conditioning (exercise) program should be considered in any patient with exercise limitations. Selection of appropriate, safe exercise routines is enhanced by measuring workloads, gas exchange behavior, heart rate, and electrocardiogram. However, in selected patients, assessment of the functional work capacity may be possible with such techniques as determining the number of steps the individual can climb or the distance the patient can walk at a certain speed.
   3. *Respiratory Therapy.* Supplemental oxygen and aerosolization of medications such as bronchodilators and corticosteroids are useful for certain patients. In an attempt to limit the inappropriate and excess use of oxygen and respiratory therapy equipment in the home, the American Thoracic Society has developed statements regarding these treatment modalities.
   4. *Education.* If patient compliance is to be optimized, both the patient and his/her family need to understand the underlying pulmonary disorder. Those individuals outlining the treatment plan should instruct the patient and family about the purpose for medications, as well as their side effects. Proper nutrition, the use and cleaning of respiratory therapy equipment, techniques of physical therapy modalities, and details of an exercise conditioning program must all be carefully explained.
   5. *General.* The importance of smoking cessation must be emphasized. Attention should be paid to such environmental factors as temperature, humidity, inhaled irritants, and altitude. Although there is little objective data that adequate hydration liquefies airway secretions, it is agreed that dehydration should be prevented. Immunization with the influenza and pneumococcal vaccines is recommended. An appropriate use of such pharmacologic agents as beta$_2$ agonists, methylxanthines, antimicrobials, and corticosteroids is important, and their indications must be understood by the primary care physician.

E. *Assessment of Patient's Progress.* While the treatment plan is being developed, the patient's progress should be monitored. This will help both the patient and the health care team objectively evaluate the plan outlined, so that any needed changes can be initiated.

F. *Long-Term Followup.* Ongoing care will generally be the responsibility of the primary care physician. Periodic reassessment can be beneficial to the patient, as a way of objectively evaluating progress and allowing for educational reinforcement.

Services Required for Pulmonary Rehabilitation

A variety of services are provided through a pulmonary rehabilitation program. Many patients with COPD will not need these services; however, they should be available for those patients with special needs or more severe disease.

A. *Essential Services*
   1. *Initial Medical Evaluation and Care Plan.* Perform a complete history and physical examination. Obtain appropriate laboratory tests. Make the correct diagnosis. Outline a proper therapy regimen for ongoing care.
   2. *Patient Education, Evaluation, and Program Coordination.* Educate patient regarding lung anatomy and physiology, disease process, useful therapeutic modalities, and other relevant matters. Coordinate allied health personnel involved in the patient's care. Make home visits, as necessary.
   3. *Respiratory Therapy Techniques.* Educate patient concerning proper use and cleaning of respiratory therapy equipment. Administer therapy as prescribed by attending physician. Make home visits as needed to insure compliance.
   4. *Physical Therapy Techniques, Including Exercise Conditioning.* Educate patient regarding relaxation techniques, proper breathing, clapping and bronchial drainage. Measure functional work capacity and develop an exercise conditioning program. Record physiologic changes resulting from exercise training.
   5. *Daily Performance Evaluation.* Evaluate activities of daily living. Teach energy conservation (work simplification) and self-care techniques.
   6. *Social Service Evaluation.* Obtain social history and determine patient's psychosocial assets and needs. Evaluate potential for compliance as well as actual compliance. Mobilize family or other interested individuals as part of extended support system to be used following discharge from the hospital. Evaluate third-party payer problems and help in resolving such problems. Assist in making arrangements for needed community resources, including financial aid, homemaker services, and extended care facilities.
   7. *Nutritional Evaluation.* Evaluate the patient's nutritional status. Outline dietary prescription based on the patient's specific nutritional needs.

B. *Additional Services*
   1. *Psychological Evaluation.* Administer psychometric battery that includes tests designed to measure organic brain dysfunction, IQ, personality profile, psychosocial assets, impact of illness on person, his/her family, etc. Help patient and family develop coping mechanisms to control not only chronic anxiety or depression but also acute exacerbations.
   2. *Psychiatric Evaluation.* Categorize personality pattern. Make psychiatric diagnosis if one exists. Provide specific psychiatric support and/or therapy when needed. If necessary, make specific recommendations regarding optimal psychopharmacologic agents.
   3. *Vocational Evaluation.* Assess vocational rehabilitation potential for those patients with significant impairment. Includes vocational tests, interviews, on-the-job observation, as well as determining whether the subject has the work capacity to meet the oxygen requirements of his/her job. Work output can generally be sustained for an eight-hour period if one does not exceed 30–40% of his/her attained maximum oxygen consumption.

A physician knowledgeable about respiratory diseases should perform the initial complete examination and assist in outlining a proper regimen of treatment.

The specific provider for the other services may vary from program to program. A multidisciplinary team that might include a professional nurse, respiratory therapist, physical therapist, occupational therapist, dietitian, social worker, and pulmonary or cardiopulmonary technologist expert in pulmonary rehabilitation techniques is appropriate for those settings where large numbers of patients are referred and for teaching or research purposes. However, in other settings, it may be possible to provide similar services with fewer individuals if they are highly-qualified and specially-trained in evaluation and management of the patient with COPD. In selected patients, the evaluation and delivery of a comprehensive care program can be accomplished in an outpatient setting. Thus, the techniques of rehabilitation should be within the reach of all physicians, applying the principles expressed in this document.

Benefits and Limitations of Pulmonary Rehabilitation

A. *Benefits.* A comprehensive respiratory care program can result in definite benefits to the patient. There is overwhelming evidence that a comprehensive respiratory care program can result in an improved qualify of life and a significantly improved capability for carrying out his/her daily activities.

Participation in a comprehensive pulmonary rehabilitation program has repeatedly been shown to decrease the hospital days required per patient per year. Some patients may be able to return to useful employment, thus making a contribution to the work force. Patients can achieve a significant reduction in anxiety, depression, and somatic concern with an associated improvement in their own ego strength. Numerous studies have shown that the physical conditioning of patients with COPD can be substantially improved with a regular exercise training program.

Cessation of smoking can result in improved pulmonary function, reduction of cough, decreased sputum production, and lessened dyspnea. The course of COPD may be altered if the airway abnormality is detected early.

B. *Limitations.* Event though all of the above benefits have been documented, an extension of lifespan and slowing of pulmonary function deterioration have not been shown in the majority of published studies. Through the use of routine office spirometry, COPD can be detected at a much earlier stage when institution of a comprehensive respiratory care program may more effectively achieve an alteration in the patient's course.

A significant problem relates to the fact that only approximately 20–35% of the participants in smoking cessation programs quit permanently. More effort needs to be applied to the prevention of respiratory disease, rather than concentrating on treatment after significant disability has occurred.

Another major factor interfering with delivery of good care is the unevenness in our capacity to delivery community-based services. A visiting nurse association (or its equivalent) does not exist in every community, nor do socially-oriented service programs, such as Meals on Wheels, Homemaker's, etc.

Which tests are required to appropriately determine impairment/disability needs to be more clearly determined. Ideally, patients should be adequately evaluated and treated comprehensively *prior to* a final disability determination.

Conclusion

In the 17th century, Jeremy Taylor said, ''To preserve a man alive in the midst of so many diseases and hostilities, is as great a miracle as to create him.'' In the past, rehabilitation has been applied rather loosely to vaguely described various approaches to long-term management of the chronically ill patient. The time has come for us to not only define what we mean by pulmonary rehabilitation but to describe the essential services required. This comprehensive approach to patient evaluation will result in improved care for respiratory patients so that they may be restored to their most optimal potential.

This statement was prepared by an *ad hoc* committee of the Scientific Assembly on Clinical Problems. The committee members are as follows:

JOHN E. HODGKIN, *Chairman*

MICHAEL J. FARRELL

SUZANNE R. GIBSON

RICHARD E. KANNER

IRVING KASS

LAWRENCE M. LAMPTON

MARGARET NIELD

THOMAS L. PETTY

References

1. Masferrer R, O'Donohue WJ Jr., Seriff NS, et al: Home use of equipment for patients with respiratory disease [ATS statement]. *Am Rev Respir Dis* 1977;115:893–895.

2. Block AJ, Burrows B, Kanner RE, et al: Oxygen administration in the home [ATS Statement]. *Am Rev Respir Dis* 1977;115:897–899.

3. California Thoracic Society guidelines for pulmonary rehabilitation, a statement by the CTS Respiratory Care Assembly, Newsletter, Respiratory Care Assembly of California Thoracic Society, September 1979, 8(#1).

4. Daughton DM, Fix AJ, Kass I, et al: Physiological-intellectual components of rehabilitation success in patients with chronic obstructive pulmonary disease (COPD). *J Chronic Dis* 1979;32:405–409.

5. Hodgkin JE (ed): *Chronic Obstructive Pulmonary Disease. Current Concepts in Diagnosis and Comprehensive Care.* Park Ridge, Ill, American College of Chest Physicians, 1979.

6. Hodgkin JE: Pulmonary rehabilitation, in Simmons D (ed): *Current Pulmonology III.* New York, John Wiley & Sons, 1981.

7. Intermittent positive pressure breathing (IPPB). *Clin Notes Respir Dis,* Winter 1979, pp 3–6.

8. Kimbel P, Kaplan AS, Alkalay I, et al: An in-hospital program for rehabilitation of patients with chronic obstructive pulmonary disease. *Chest* 1971; 60 (suppl):6S-10S.

9. Lertzman MM, Cherniack RM: Rehabilitation of patients with chronic obstructive pulmonary disease. *Am Rev Respir Dis* 1976;114:1145–1165.

10. Moser KM, Bokinsky GE, Savage RT, et al: Physiological and functional effects of a comprehensive rehabilitation program upon patients with chronic obstructive pulmonary disease. *Arch Int Med* 1980;140:1596–1601.

11. Nield M: The effect of health teaching on the anxiety level of patients with chronic obstructive lung disease. *Nursing Res* 1971;20:537–541.

12. Petty TL (ed): *Chronic Obstructive Pulmonary Disease.* New York, Marcel Dekker, 1978.

13. Petty TL: Pulmonary rehabilitation, *Basics of RD.* New York, American Thoracic Society, 1975.

14. Pierce AK, Paez PN, Miller WF: Exercise therapy with the aid of a portable oxygen supply in patients with emphysema. *Am Rev Respir Dis* 1965; 91:653–659.

15. Skills of the Health Team Involved in Out-of-Hospital Care for Patients with COPD, a statement by the Section on Nursing, Scientific Assembly on Clinical Problems, American Thoracic Society. *ATS News* 1977;3:18.

STRUCTURE OF THE PULMONARY REHABILITATION TEAM

A physician who is knowledgeable about respiratory disease is a key part of the pulmonary rehabilitation team. By performing an initial history and physical examination, the physician can assist the team in developing an appropriate treatment program for the individual by defining the patient's disease process and determining his or her needs. A multidisciplinary team that includes a respiratory nurse, respiratory therapist, occupational therapist, physical therapist, dietician, social worker, chaplain, and psychologist or psychiatrist is particularly useful for programs to which large numbers of patients are referred and for teaching or research purposes. However, it is possible to perform a thorough assessment and deliver similar services with fewer allied health professionals if the individuals on the team are appropriately trained in the evaluation and management of COPD patients. The specific provider of essential services may vary from program to program, depending on the size of the facility and the availability of allied health professionals who are trained to assess patients with COPD. Although every patient with COPD will not need all of the services described in the ATS Statement, all of these services must be available, since there are many patients who will need them all.

Pulmonary rehabilitation is generally accomplished in the outpatient setting, particularly now that third-party payers are reluctant to pay for inpatient care for those who are not acutely ill. However, it can be very helpful for pulmonary rehabilitation team members to perform their initial evaluation and to outline an appropriate treatment program while a patient is hospitalized for an acute exacerbation in order to help insure a smooth transition from inpatient to outpatient.

BENEFITS OF PULMONARY REHABILITATION

Pulmonary rehabilitation requires the use of individually tailored treatment modalities designed to help the patient achieve and maintain the highest functional capacity possible. The components of a comprehensive respiratory rehabilitation program are listed in Table 13–1. Although each of these components of care is not discussed here, the reader is referred to other chapters in this book describing them.

A summary of benefits reported through the use of the treatment modalities described in this book are listed in Table 13–2. A reduction in respiratory symptoms as well as the reversal of anxiety and depression and an improvement in ego strength can be achieved in most patients.[17–19] All programs have reported an improved ability for most patients to carry out activities of daily living,[1–7, 20–27] enhanced exercise capacity,[28–41] and better quality of life.[1–7, 20–27] Some are able to continue or return to gainful employment.[4, 20, 42]

Table 13–1. **Components of Pulmonary Rehabilitation**

General
  Patient and family education
  Proper nutrition including weight control
  Avoidance of smoking and other inhaled irritants
  Avoidance of infection (immunization, etc.)
  Proper environment
  Adequate hydration

Medications
  Bronchodilators
  Expectorants
  Antimicrobials
  Corticosteroids
  Cromolyn sodium
  Digitalis
  Diuretics
  Psychopharmacologic agents

Respiratory Therapy Techniques
  Aerosol therapy
  Oxygen therapy
  Home use of ventilators

Physical Therapy Modalities
  Relaxation training
  Breathing retraining
  Chest percussion and postural drainage
  Deliberate coughing and expectoration

Exercise Conditioning

Occupational Therapy
  Evaluate activities of daily living
  Outline energy-conserving maneuvers

Psychosocial Rehabilitation

Vocational Rehabilitation

A reduction in the number of days of hospitalization required by patients with COPD following pulmonary rehabilitation has been reported by several groups.[27, 43–45] A study of 80 patients participating in the pulmonary rehabilitation program at Loma Linda University Medical Center (LLUMC) showed a reduction from approximately 19 days of hospitalization in the year prior to the pulmonary rehabilitation program to approximately six days of hospitalization per year in the first year following completion of the program.[43] This trend has continued for the eight years for which follow-up data have been analyzed (Fig. 13–1).[46, 47] The number of days of hospitalization required over the eight-year period for only those patients still surviving at the end of eight years was very similar to the curve reflecting data for all of the patients showing that this reduction was not simply due to the death of the sickest patients during the initial years of follow-up (leaving healthier patients toward the end of the eight-year period). This reduction in hospital days can obviously result in a significant decrease in cost by avoiding costly hospitalizations.

Table 13–2. **Demonstrated Benefits of Pulmonary Rehabilitation**

- Reduction in respiratory symptoms.
- Reversal of anxiety and depression and improved ego strength.
- Enhanced ability to carry out activities of daily living.
- Increased exercise ability.
- Better quality of life.
- Reduction in hospital days required.
- Prolongation of life in selected patients, i.e., use of continuous oxygen in patients with severe hypoxemia.

The reported decrement in forced expiratory volume in one second (FEV_1) for patients with COPD ranges from 40 to 80 ml/year[48–54] rather than the 20 to 30 ml/year decrease reported for normal individuals.[55, 56] No pulmonary rehabilitation study has shown a significant alteration in the mean rate of decrease in their COPD patients. Unfortunately, however, most reports to date have described patients who entered into pulmonary rehabilitation programs after severe impairment of pulmonary function had developed. The fact that pulmonary function may improve significantly, or even return to normal, in patients with early obstructive airway disease who stop smoking provides hope that, by applying the principles of pulmonary rehabilitation to patients much earlier in the course of their disease, it will be possible to alter the ultimate course of the disease, e.g., slow down the progression of or even improve the obstructive airway defect.[57]

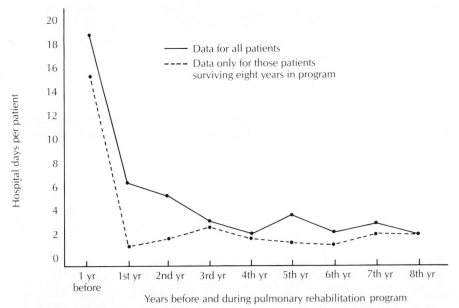

Figure 13–1. Analysis of hospital days before and during pulmonary rehabilitation program at the Loma Linda University Medical Center.

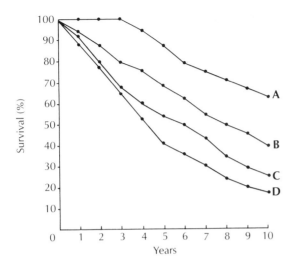

Figure 13–2. Cumulative survival rates of COPD patients. A, Hodgkin and associates.[46] B, Postma and associates.[53] C, Burrows and associates.[51] D, Petty and associates.[48]

A review of the reports of survival in COPD patients undergoing pulmonary rehabilitation shows quite a variation in survival curves (Fig. 13–2). Table 13–3 compares information relating to the patients in the four pulmonary rehabilitation study groups depicted in Figure 13–2. A description of the characteristics of the patients participating in these programs has been published elsewhere.[46, 48, 51, 53, 58] A possible reason for the improved survival curve in the LLUMC study by Hodgkin and associates is that patients entered into that pulmonary rehabilitation program earlier in the course of their disease. The study did, however, look at the cumulative survival rate for only those patients with an initial FEV_1 above 1.24 L in an attempt to compare that data with a survival curve from the Burrows study, which evaluated survival in patients with an FEV_1 above 1.24 L.[49, 59] Figure 13–3 compares those curves. The survival rate for the LLUMC patients was significantly better (P value < 0.05) for years two through seven. This could be related to the fact that the LLUMC patients went through a comprehensive pulmonary rehabilitation program with continuing follow-up by team members, including home visits. The normal cumulative survival rate for the U.S. population at 60 years

Table 13–3. **Comparison of Pulmonary Rehabilitation Study Groups**

	Hodgkin and Associates[46, 58]	Petty and Associates[48]	Postma and Associates[53]	Burrows and Associates[51]
Number	75	182	129	200
Mean age (years)	60	61	54	59
Mean FEV_1 (L)	1.55	0.94	0.61	1.04
Mean Pa_{O_2} (mmHg)	68	—	—	—
Mean Pa_{CO_2} (mmHg)	42	—	44	44
Nonsmokers (%)	23	—	36	38

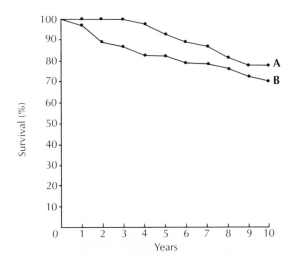

Figure 13–3. Cumulative survival rates of COPD patients with FEV$_1$ > 1.24 L. *A*, Hodgkin and associates (N = 46).[46] *B*, Burrows and associates (N = 52).[49]

of age is 91% at five years and 80% at 10 years, while the cumulative survival rate in the LLUMC study group (mean age of 60 years) was 88% at five years and 63% at 10 years.

The possibility that a comprehensive pulmonary rehabilitation program, including close follow-up, may improve survival was suggested by the cumulative survival curve for patients in the NIH/IPPB study[60] in which mortality was less for the three years of follow-up than in most previously published studies (Fig. 13–4). Patients in this study had moderate to severe COPD (mean FEV$_1$ was 36% of predicted).

It seems reasonable that, in order to achieve a significant reduction in the rate of respiratory function deterioration and a definite prolongation of life, good comprehensive care must be instituted earlier in the course of the disease rather than waiting until severe, irreversible impairment of function is present. Prolongation of life has, of course, been reported in selected patients,

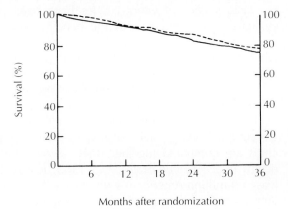

Figure 13–4. Survival of randomized patients. Dotted line represents intermittent positive-pressure–breathing patients; solid line represents compressor nebulizer patients. (From the IPPB Trial Group: Intermittent positive pressure breathing therapy of chronic obstructive pulmonary disease. *Annals of Internal Medicine*, 1983; 99:612–620, by permission.)

Months after randomization

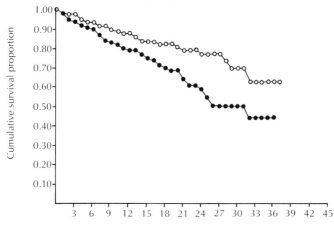

Time from randomization (months)

Figure 13–5. Overall mortality. Ordinate is fraction of patients surviving; abscissa is time from randomization or duration of treatment. Open circles represent continuous oxygen therapy group; squares represent nocturnal oxygen therapy group. Of the total group, 80 nocturnal and 87 continuous oxygen therapy patients were followed for 12 months, and 29 nocturnal and 37 continuous oxygen therapy patients were followed for 24 months. (From Nocturnal Oxygen Therapy Trial Group: Continuous or nocturnal oxygen therapy in hypoxemic chronic obstructive lung disease. *Annals of Internal Medicine* 1980; 93:391–398, by permission.)

such as those COPD patients with severe hypoxemia who use supplemental oxygen continuously (Fig. 13–5).[61]

COST-EFFECTIVENESS OF PULMONARY REHABILITATION PROGRAMS

Cost studies of various types have been performed in an attempt to evaluate in economic terms the benefits of pulmonary rehabilitation. If a rehabilitation program is to be cost-effective, increased tangible benefits, when compared to traditional treatment programs, must be identified in terms of the program's monetary worth and its health-related benefits.[62]

The Epidemiology of Respiratory Diseases Task Force Report published in 1980 states that one in five people in the United States reports some type of chronic respiratory problem, and that COPD shows the most rapid increase among the leading causes of death.[63] When emphysema and chronic bronchitis are combined together, they account for approximately 2.5% of all deaths in the United States.[63] In 1980, it was estimated that there were at least 7.9 million Americans with chronic bronchitis, 6.8 million with asthma, and 2.5 million with emphysema.[64] The number of people with emphysema is probably much higher, but respiratory diagnoses have been inconsistently reported in the past, thus making it difficult to obtain accurate figures.

In 1975, the total cost of health care related to diseases of the respiratory system was estimated to be $19.7 billion.[63] In 1979, the cost of health care, lost wages, and time away from work for people with COPD exceeded $15 billion.[64]

Health care expenditures averaged $146.30 per person in 1965, $1,067.06 per person in 1980, and $1,459 per person in 1983. As a percent of the gross national product, health care expenditures increased from 6% in 1965 to 9.4% in 1980[65] and to 10.8% in 1983. It is estimated that over $360 billion annually is now being spent on health care in the United States. Pulmonary rehabilitation programs seem justifiable if they result in less suffering and an improved quality of life. However, if such programs can also result in a reduction in the cost of medical care for the individual, this is certainly an additional bonus.

As mentioned earlier,[4, 20, 42] some individuals with COPD, through pulmonary rehabilitation, are able to maintain or return to gainful employment. This, of course, is a cost benefit to society when these individuals remain productive members of the work force. Helping patients achieve independence in their activities of daily living, including self-care, can be an economic benefit by reducing their dependence on health care providers. Indicators of such improvement following pulmonary rehabilitation programs include a reduction in the need for hospitalization, emergency room visits, doctors' office visits, extended care facility placements, and home care visits.

The reduction in hospital days achieved by the COPD patients depicted in Figure 13–1 resulted in an estimated savings in hospitalization costs for the first year following the pulmonary rehabilitation program of approximately $1,935 per patient or more than $154,000 for the 80-patient group.[43] The cost of the LLUMC pulmonary rehabilitation program from July 1981 to June 1982 amounted to $519,942 (Table 13–4).[62] The LLUMC pulmonary rehabilitation team was following approximately 1150 COPD patients in 1982; consequently, the cost per patient was about $452 per year. For an 80-patient group, this would amount to a cost of $36,160 per year. Clearly, the cost of rehabilitation, when one takes into account the savings achieved by the reduction in hospital days required following a pulmonary rehabilitation program, seems justifiable.

Table 13–4. **Cost of the Loma Linda University Medical Center Respiratory Rehabilitation Program from July 1981 to June 1982**

Total direct labor	$354,785
Indirect labor	92,244
Space	52,343
Supplies	6,591
Travel	11,452
Miscellaneous	2,527
Total	$519,942

Hudson and colleagues also reported a significant reduction in the number of hospital days required for COPD patients following a pulmonary rehabilitation program.[44] For the 64 patients for which data regarding hospitalization days were complete, there was a total of 631 days, or 10 hospital days required per patient, prior to the rehabilitation program and an average of five days per patient during the first year after the program. Two years following treatment, the average of hospital days per patient per year was still five. The savings was estimated at approximately $51,120 per year for the group of 44 patients who survived for the four years of follow-up. The cost for the year prior to the pulmonary rehabilitation program was approximately $94,730 and averaged $43,610 for each of the next four years. At the time of their study, their outpatient program cost was estimated at $30,379 per year. This included personnel costs as well as the cost of home oxygen. The expense of oxygen ($16,200 to $21,600 per year depending upon the number of patients on oxygen) added considerably to the outpatient costs. Even with the inclusion of outpatient oxygen, there was still a savings of $20,741 per year for this group of 44 survivors.

Another study reporting on the cost-effectiveness of a respiratory rehabilitation program was undertaken at Barlow Hospital in Los Angeles by Johnson and colleagues.[45] They reported on 194 patients with severe COPD (mean FEV_1 of 0.83 L), 80% of whom required supplemental oxygen in the year before entering the program. These patients averaged 39 hospital days per patient in the previous year. After the program, the hospital need had decreased by 46% to 17.8 days per patient per year. The patients who survived the second year of follow-up, when studied separately, had a reduction of 20.8 days per year or a 59% reduction. This study reported that the cost of respiratory rehabilitation at Barlow Hospital was balanced off in less than one year through cost-savings from reduced hospitalization alone.

These three studies[43-45] are of note in that they all look at the effect of respiratory rehabilitation on the number of hospital days required following the program. All studied patients with significant COPD. All found a significant reduction in the number of hospital days after the program. The socioeconomic impact on society and third-party payers is apparent. If these results could be duplicated in all health facilities that offer pulmonary rehabilitation services, millions of dollars could be saved each year.

SUMMARY

Any COPD patient with symptoms is a candidate for pulmonary rehabilitation. A careful assessment of the individual to determine the patient's precise disease process and needs is essential to outlining an appropriate treatment program. Following the sequence described in the ATS Statement on Pulmonary Rehabilitation included in this chapter provides the best potential for successfully returning the patient to the highest level of function possible. An increase in the availability of pulmonary rehabilitation programs should allow more COPD patients to participate in this process, resulting in an enhanced ability to carry out daily activities, an improved quality of life, and a reduction in the long-term costs of caring for such individuals.

REFERENCES

1. Barach AL: The treatment of pulmonary emphysema in the elderly. *J Am Geriatr Soc* 1956;4:884–887.
2. Miller WF: Rehabilitation of patients with chronic obstructive lung disease. *Med Clin North Am* 1967;51:349–361.
3. Balchum OJ: Rehabilitation in chronic obstructive pulmonary disease. *Arch Environ Health* 1968;16:614.
4. Haas A, Cardon H: Rehabilitation in chronic obstructive pulmonary disease: A five-year study of 252 male patients. *Med Clin North Am* 1969;53:593–606.
5. Cherniack RM, Handford RG, Svanhill E: Home care of chronic respiratory disease. *JAMA* 1969;208:821–824.
6. Petty TL: Ambulatory care for emphysema and chronic bronchitis. *Chest* 1970; 58: 441–448.
7. Kimbel P, Kaplan AS, Alkalay I, et al: An in-hospital program for rehabilitation of patients with chronic obstructive pulmonary disease. *Chest* 1971;60 (suppl):6S–10S.
8. Lertzman MM, Cherniack RM: Rehabilitation of patients with chronic obstructive pulmonary disease. *Am Rev Respir Dis* 1976;114:1145–1165.
9. Hodgkin JE, Gray LS, Connors GA (eds): Pulmonary Rehabilitation and Continuing Care (special issue). *Resp Care* November 1983;28:1419–1528.
10. Hodgkin JE, Zorn EG, Connors GI (eds): *Pulmonary Rehabilitation: Guidelines to Success.* Boston: Butterworths, 1984.
11. Petty TL (ed): *Chronic Obstructive Pulmonary Disease,* Ed 2. New York: Marcel Dekker, 1985.
12. Glaser EM: Strategies for facilitating knowledge utilization in the biomedical field. Final report to National Science Foundation, Grant No. DAR 73–07767 A06. Washington, DC: National Science Foundation, 1975.
13. Hodgkin JE, Balchum OJ, Kass I, et al: Chronic obstructive airway diseases: Current concepts in diagnosis and comprehensive care. *JAMA* 1975;232:1243–1260.
14. Hodgkin JE (ed): *Chronic Obstructive Pulmonary Disease: Current Concepts in Diagnosis and Comprehensive Care.* Park Ridge, IL: American College of Chest Physicians, 1979.
15. Petty TL: Pulmonary rehabilitation, in *Basics of RD.* New York, American Thoracic Society, 1975.
16. Pulmonary rehabilitation: official American Thoracic Society Position Statement. *Am Rev Respir Dis* 1981;124:663–666.
17. Dudley DI, Glaser EM, Jorgenson BN, et al: Psychosocial concomitants to rehabilitation in chronic obstructive pulmonary disease. *Chest* 1980;77:413–420, 544–551, 677–684.
18. Agle DP, Baum GI, Chester EH, et al: Multidiscipline treatment of chronic pulmonary insufficiency: Psychologic aspects of rehabilitation. *Psychosom Med* 1973; 35:41–49.
19. Fishman DB, Petty TL: Physical, symptomatic, and psychological improvements in patients receiving comprehensive care for chronic airway obstruction. *J Chronic Dis* 1971;24:775–785.
20. Kass I, Dyksterhus JE: The Nebraska COPD rehabilitation project: A program to identify the factors involved in the rehabilitation of patients with chronic obstructive pulmonary disease: A multidisciplinary study of 140 patients. Final Report, Social and Rehabilitation Service, DHEW Project No. RD-2517-m. Omaha, University of Nebraska, December 1971.
21. Daughton DM, Fix AJ, Kass I, et al: Physiological-intellectual components of rehabilitation success in patients with chronic obstructive pulmonary disease (COPD). *J Chronic Dis* 1979;32:405–409.
22. Miller WF, Taylor HF, Pierce AK: Rehabilitation of the disabled patient with chronic bronchitis and pulmonary emphysema. *Am J Public Health* 1963;53 (suppl):18–24.
23. Petty TL, Nett LM, Finigan MM, et al: A comprehensive care program for chronic airway obstruction. *Ann Intern Med* 1969;70:1109–1120.
24. Shapiro BA, Vostinak-Foley E, Hamilton BB, et al: Rehabilitation in chronic obstructive pulmonary disease: A two-year prospective study. *Respir Care* 1977; 22:1045–1057.
25. White B, Andrews JL Jr, Morgan JJ, et al:

Pulmonary rehabilitation in an ambulatory group practice setting. *Med Clin North Am* 1979;63:379–390.

26. Krumholz RA: Pulmonary outpatient rehabilitation; A four-year follow-up. *Ohio State Med J* 1973;69:680–684.

27. Moser KM: Rehabilitation of the COPD patient, in *Weekly Update: Pulmonary Medicine*. Princeton, NJ, Biomedia, 1979.

28. Pierce AK, Paez PN, Miller WF: Exercise therapy with the aid of a portable oxygen supply in patients with emphysema. *Am Rev Respir Dis* 1965;91:653–659.

29. Woolf CR, Suero JT: Alterations in lung mechanics and gas exchange following training in chronic obstructive lung disease. *Dis Chest* 1969;55:37–44.

30. Bass H, Whitcomb JF, Forman R: Exercise training: Therapy for patients with chronic obstructive pulmonary disease. *Chest* 1970;57:116–121.

31. Woolf CR: A rehabilitation program for improving exercise tolerance of patients with chronic lung disease. *Can Med Assoc J* 1972;106:1289–1292.

32. Rusk HA: Pulmonary problems, in *Rehabilitation Medicine*, ed 3. St. Louis, CV Mosby, 1971.

33. Schrijen F, Jezek V: Haemodynamic variables during repeated exercise in chronic lung disease. *Clin Sci Mol Med* 1978;55:485–490.

34. Nicholas JJ, Gilbert R, Gabe R, et al: Evaluation of an exercise therapy program for patients with chronic obstructive pulmonary disease. *Am Rev Respir Dis* 1970;102:1–9.

35. Unger KM, Moser KM, Hansen P: Selection of an exercise program for patients with chronic obstructive pulmonary disease. *Heart Lung* 1980;9:68–76.

36. Brundin A: Physical training in severe chronic obstructive lung disease. *Scand J Respir Dis* 1974;55:25–46.

37. Wasserman K, Whipp BJ: Exercise physiology in health and disease. *Am Rev Respir Dis* 1973;112:219–249.

38. Degre S, Sergysels R, Messin R, et al: Hemodynamic responses to physical training in patients with chronic lung disease. *Am Rev Respir Dis* 1974;110:395–401.

39. Alpert JS, Bass H, Szucs MM, et al: Effects of physical training on hemodynamics and pulmonary function at rest and during exercise in patients with chronic obstructive pulmonary disease. *Chest* 1974;66:647–651.

40. Shephard RJ: Exercise and chronic obstructive lung disease. *Exerc Sport Sci Rev* 1976; 4:263–296.

41. Hughes RI, Davison R: Limitations of exercise reconditioning in COLD. *Chest* 1983;83:241–249.

42. Petty TL, MacIlroy ER, Swigert MA, et al: Chronic airway obstruction, respiratory insufficiency, and gainful employment. *Arch Environ Health* 1970;21:71–78.

43. Burton GG, Gee G, Hodgkin JE, et al: Respiratory care warrants studies for cost-effectiveness. *Hospitals* 1975;49:61–71.

44. Hudson LD, Tyler ML, Petty TL: Hospitalization needs during an outpatient rehabilitation program for severe chronic airway obstruction. *Chest* 1976;70:606–610.

45. Johnson NR, Tanzi F, Balchum OJ, et al: Inpatient comprehensive pulmonary rehabilitation in severe COPD: Barlow Hospital study. *Resp Ther* 1980;May–June:15–19.

46. Bebout DE, Hodgkin JE, Zorn EG, et al: Clinical and physiological outcomes of a university-hospital pulmonary rehabilitation program. *Resp Care* 1983;28:1468–1473.

47. Hodgkin JE, Branscomb BV, Anholm JD, et al: Benefits, limitations, and the future of pulmonary rehabilitation, in Hodgkin ZE, Zorn EG, Connors GL (eds): *Pulmonary Rehabilitation: Guidelines to Success*. Boston, Butterworths, 1984.

48. Sahn SA, Nett LM, Petty TL: Ten-year follow-up of a comprehensive rehabilitation program for severe COPD. *Chest* 1980;77(suppl):311–314.

49. Burrows B, Earle RH: Course and prognosis of chronic obstructive lung disease. *N Engl J Med* 1969;280:397–404.

50. Boushy SF, Thompson HK, North LB, et al: Prognosis in chronic obstructive pulmonary disease. *Am Rev Respir Dis* 1973;108:1373–1383.

51. Diener CF, Burrows B: Further observations on the course and prognosis of chronic obstructive lung disease. *Am Rev Respir Dis* 1975;111:719–724.

52. Emergil C, Sobol BJ: Long-term course of chronic obstructive pulmonary disease: A new view of the mode of functional deterioration. *Am J Med* 1971;51:504–512.

53. Postma DS, Burema J, Gimeno F, et al: Prognosis in severe chronic obstructive pulmonary disease. *Am Rev Respir Dis* 1979;119:357–367.

54. Renzetti AD, McClement JH, Bertram DL: The Veterans Administration cooperative study of pulmonary function. III. Mortality in relation to respiratory function in chronic obstructive pulmonary disease. *Am J Med* 1966;41:115–129.

55. Ferris BG Jr, Anderson DO, Zickmantel R: Prediction values for screening tests of pulmonary function. *Am Rev Respir Dis* 1965;91:252–261.

56. Kory RC, Callahan R, Boren HG, et al: Veterans Administration–Army cooperative study of pulmonary function. I. Clinical spirometry in normal men. *Am J Med* 1961;30:243–258.

57. Buist AS, Sexton GJ, Nagy JM, et al: The effect of smoking cessation and modification on lung function. *Am Rev Respir Dis* 1976;114:115–122.

58. Sammer EA, Hodgkin JE, Zorn E, et al: Clinical and physiological response to comprehensive respiratory care. *Respir Care* 1979;24:1207.

59. Burrows B: Prognosis of the bronchial and emphysematous types, in *Proceedings of Symposium on Chronic Obstructive Pulmonary Disease 1974.* Berlin: Schattauer Verlag, 1975.

60. The IPPB Trial Group. Intermittent positive pressure breathing therapy of chronic obstructive pulmonary disease: A clinical trial. *Ann Int Med* 1983;99:612–620.

61. Nocturnal Oxygen Therapy Trial Group. Continuous or nocturnal oxygen therapy in hypoxemic chronic obstructive lung disease. *Ann Intern Med* 1980;93:391–398.

62. Dunham JL, Hodgkin JE, Nicol III J, et al: Cost effectiveness of pulmonary rehabilitation programs, in Hodgkin JE, Zorn EG, Connors GL (eds): *Pulmonary Rehabilitations: Guidelines to Success.* Boston, Butterworths, 1984.

63. Task Force Report, Chairman, Claude Lenfant, MD. Epidemiology of respiratory diseases. US Department of Health and Human Services, Public Health Service, National Institutes of Health, 1980; NIH Publication 81-2019:13–25, 156–158.

64. Report to the 1982 California Legislature on the Chronic Obstructive Lung Disease Project (Chairperson, Kenneth Moser, M.D.) State of California, Health and Welfare Agency, Department of Health Services, 1982;3–5, 20, 21.

65. US Department of Health and Human Services. Office of Health Research, Statistics, and Technology. Health: United States 1981. DHHS Publication (PHS) 82–1232.

14

IMPAIRMENT AND DISABILITY EVALUATION AND VOCATIONAL REHABILITATION

RICHARD E. KANNER

The disorders characterized by chronic limitation or obstruction to expiratory airflow (such as COPD) are, for the most part, common in occurrence and progressive in nature. Thus, they account for a large number of patients being unable to earn a living. The exact number of people disabled by these disorders cannot be determined with an accuracy because disability compensation may come from many different sources, such as Social Security Disability Insurance, Social Security Supplemental Security Income, the Veterans Administration (VA), private insurance companies, and self-insured industries. It is estimated that in 1983 and 1984 more than 16,000 individuals per year were awarded disability benefits for the first time from the Social Security Administration (SSA) through their disability insurance program as a result of having COPD.[1]

COPD is a progressive disease. Thus, afflicted individuals, once they reach the stage of total disability, have little hope of returning to work. Most patients with disabling COPD have a long history of cigarette smoking.

Although smoking cessation may cause some improvement in lung function, this benefit is usually seen in younger individuals with mild airways obstruction.[2] Thus, these people do not have a significant impairment due to COPD. Most smokers with an accelerated decline in lung function, however, find that the annual rate of decline slows and symptoms, such as a chronic productive cough, improve when they stop smoking.

The age that symptoms and abnormalities on pulmonary function testing first appear is an important clue to the rate of the progression of disease. The younger the subject when the disorder is first detected the more rapid the progression.[3] Mild abnormalities in a 60- or 70-year-old person are probably of little clinical significance. Most patients with COPD start complaining of significant limitations in their middle to late fifties, although there is a suggestion that the average age at which the first serious problems are experienced is increasing to 60 years or older. This is important with respect to impairment and disability evaluation because the older worker is less likely to learn a new occupation.

IMPAIRMENT AND DISABILITY EVALUATION

The terms "impairment" and "disability" must first be defined since they are not synonymous. Impairment is a medical term denoting a functional abnormality that persists after appropriate therapy and has little likelihood of reversibility. It may or may not be stable. With respect to respiratory disease, it would be an abnormality in either ventilation, diffusion, or perfusion of the lungs. The physician evaluates impairment and the findings are a vital part of the disability determination. More emphasis should be given to the residual function than to the impairment because the former determines what the patient is capable of doing. The subsequent disability determination procedure decides if it is realistic to retrain the patient for an occupation with energy requirements appropriate for the degree of residual function.

Disability determination is an administrative process that assesses the effect of an impairment on an individual's life and implies an inability to perform roles or tasks expected within a social environment. Many factors are considered in disability determination along with impairment. These include age, gender, educational level, and socioeconomic status and the energy, skills, and any toxic exposures associated with the patient's occupation. Depending on these other factors, two people with identical impairments can have very different disability ratings. Disability is determined by an administrative law judge or a panel or other agency. Physicians as well as nonphysicians with expertise specific for the situation may be involved.

Methodology for evaluating a patient with COPD for impairment and disability differs according to who is responsibile for awarding benefits. The SSA probably covers most claimants, but other sources of disability payments

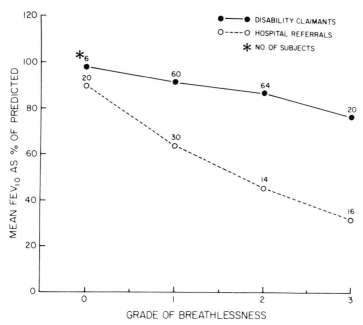

Figure 14–1. The relationship between the grade of dyspnea and FEV_1 in subjects applying for black lung benefits and in hospital patients. (From Morgan WKC: Disability or disinclination? Impairment or importuning? *Chest* 1979;75:712–715, by permission.)

include the VA and private insurance companies. SSA provides a handbook for physicians outlining the objective criteria they use to evaluate impairments.[4] In general, SSA involves benefits only for total disability. The VA guidelines are more heavily weighted to the patient's symptoms rather than objective testing and consider both partial and total disability.[5] Private insurance companies usually rely on standards set by the American Medical Association (AMA)[6] and the American Thoracic Society (ATS).[7, 7a] These organizations recommend the use of objective measurements. The AMA provides for both partial and total impairment, while the original ATS Statement[7] dealt only with total impairment. It should be pointed out that as more knowledge becomes available, the standards are being modified. The SSA is currently making revisions in their criteria, and the new ATS Statement[7a] includes partial as well as total impairment.

The use of subjective criteria to award disability benefits creates a situation where abuse of the system is possible. Claimants tend to exaggerate symptoms when applying for benefits. Several studies have shown that when compared to subjects being evaluated for medical rather than disability reasons, both groups show a fairly good relationship between dyspnea and FEV_1 measured as a percent of the predicted value (Fig. 14–1). However, claimants have a considerably greater degree of dyspnea for the same level of pulmonary function.[8–10]

Another question frequently raised in setting standards for disability is whether age should be considered. SSA guidelines provide a fixed actual value of pulmonary function as a cutoff point rather than a percent of the individual's predicted value. In this way, the older worker is not at a disadvantage, since the aging process decreases one's ability to do physical work. Thus, standards that use a percent of the older worker's predicted value would not take into account this decline in function with age. This is particularly important if the energy requirements of the job do not change as the worker grows older. The AMA and ATS believe that the percent of predicted value is more realistic because it compares the worker to his or her peers. Moreover, the question of penalizing the older worker for changes associated with aging is not a part of the physician's evaluation of impairment. The physician compares the patient to healthy people of the same age, sex, and height. It is during the disability part of the process where an administrative law judge or a panel of experts can consider the subject's age as a factor in relating the impairments noted to the energy requirements of the job and thus to the degree of disability present.

There are occupational causes of COPD, especially in disorders such as occupational asthma. Cotton dust exposure also contributes to the development of COPD. However, in most subjects with COPD, cigarette smoking is the primary etiology, with other exposures being secondary and usually minor contributors to the disorder. In one occupational lung disease, coal workers' pneumoconiosis (CWP), legislation has been enacted concerning the impairment and disability evaluation and benefits for all coal mine workers.[11] In CWP, there may be some focal emphysema, and long-term dust exposure in conditions that existed in the mines prior to the early 1970s can cause a form of chronic bronchitis termed industrial bronchitis.[9, 12] However, in the absence of the more advanced degrees of CWP, there is little functional impairment if the coal mine worker never smoked.[12] If the coal mine worker applies for benefits and meets any of the criteria for disability benefits, then the burden of proof is upon the coal mine operator to prove that the impairment is due to causes other than work in the mines.

The value of exercise testing in the determination of impairment caused by lung disease has yet to be established. In subjects with COPD, the value of the FEV_1 correlates well with exercise performance, but in one study, neither was particularly good in predicting which patient was working or unemployed.[13] Despite some enthusiasm for exercise testing, it cannot be determined at this time what physiologic measurements are the "gold standard" for determining impairment. Although exercise testing can be expensive, time-consuming and difficult to carry out, in certain subjects it can be helpful. It can diagnose previously undetected cardiac disease as an explanation for the subject's dyspnea, demonstrate poor conditioning as a factor, and estimate the relative contributions of pulmonary and cardiac disorders to the claimant's symptoms.

SSA has a handbook for physicians for use in impairment and disability evaluation.[4] The handbook specifically points out that physicians provide medical evidence for evaluation of impairment but that disability is an administrative decision. Under chronic obstructive airway disease, there is a table listing height in inches and values for the maximum voluntary ventilation (MVV) and one-second forced expiratory volume (FEV_1) for each height. In order to qualify, patients must have an MVV and FEV_1 equal to or less than the listed value for their height. These criteria may be slightly liberalized in the proposed changes in the guidelines. Patients with asthma who do not meet the criteria lised in the table can still qualify if, in spite of prescribed treatment, there are documented episodes of acute attacks occurring at least once every two months or on an average of at least six times a year, and if they demonstrate prolonged expiration with wheezing or rhonchi between attacks. The documentation should include hospital and emergency room records. This statement regarding asthma has been adopted by the AMA and ATS in their guidelines.

Previous SSA guidelines included arterial blood gas values under the heading of diffuse pulmonary fibrosis, but these values were developed under the assumption that everyone resided at sea level. The new changes state that chronic impairment of gas exchange (as assessed by arterial blood gas analysis measured during steady-state exercise) can be due to any cause, including COPD. The PO_2 is related to the PCO_2, and there are three tables: one for altitudes < 3000 feet, one for 3000 to 6000 feet, and one for > 6000 feet. Under the new proposals, a single breath or steady-state diffusing capacity measurement can also be used to measure impairment of gas exchange from any cause.

The most recent AMA Guides (1984)[6] are similar in many ways to the 1982 and 1986 ATS Statements.[7, 7a] However, the AMA partial impairment ratings included the patients' symptoms as a criterion for impairment and the degree of dyspnea. Spirometric measurements of forced vital capacity (FVC) and the FEV_1 and their ratio are compared to the prediction formulas of Crapo and coworkers[14] to arrive at a percent impairment. If the FVC is < 50% of the predicted value or the FEV_1 is < 40% of the predicted value or the FEV_1/FVC ratio is < 0.40, the impairment is considered severe. Also, a single-breath carbon monoxide diffusing capacity of < 40% of predicted, using the reference values of Crapo and Morris,[15] is considered a severe impairment. Abnormal values that do not meet these criteria fall into categories of mild and moderate impairment. Impairment can also be rated using maximal oxygen uptake ($\dot{V}O_2max$) during exercise testing. A value of $\dot{V}O_2max$ > 25 ml/(kg · min) is considered no impairment, < 15 ml/(kg · min) is a severe impairment, and values in between are rated as mild or moderate (Table 14–1).

The ATS published a statement in 1982 on impairment and disability due to respiratory disease that included an algorithm for testing claimants.[7] The initial step was spirometry followed by a single-breath carbon monoxide diffusing capacity. If these tests indicated total impairment using the cutoff values given above in the AMA guidelines, then no further testing was

Table 14–1. **Classes of Respiratory Impairment***

	Class 1 0% No Impairment	Class 2 10%–25% Mild Impairment	Class 3 30%–45% Moderate Impairment	Class 4† 50%–100% Severe Impairment
Dyspnea	The subject may or may not have dyspnea. If dyspnea is present, it is for nonrespiratory reasons or it is consistent with the circumstances of activity.	Dyspnea with fast walking on level ground or when walking up a hill; patient can keep pace with persons of same age and body build on level ground but not on hills or stairs.	Dyspnea while walking on level ground with person of the same age or walking up one flight of stairs. Patient can walk a mile at own pace without dyspnea, but cannot keep pace on level ground with others of same age and body build.	Dyspnea after walking more than 100 meters at own pace on level ground. Patient sometimes is dyspneic with less exertion or even at rest.
	or	or	or	or
Tests of ventilatory function‡ FVC FEV₁ FEV₁/FVC ratio (as percent)	Above the lower limit of normal for the predicted value as defined by the 95% confidence interval.	Below the 95% confidence interval but greater than 60% predicted for FVC, FEV₁ and FEV₁/FVC ratio.	Less than 60% predicted, but greater than 50% predicted for FVC, 40% predicted for FEV₁, and 40% actual value for FEV₁/FVC ratio.	Less than 50% predicted for FVC, 40% predicted for FEV₁, 40% actual value for FEV₁/FVC ratio, and 40% predicted for D$_{CO}$.
	or	or	or	or
V̇O₂max	Greater than 25 ml/(kg·min)	Between 20–25 ml/(kg·min)	Between 15–20 ml/(kg·min)	Less than 15 ml/(kg·min)

*Established by the American Medical Association's ad hoc committee on medical rating of physical impairment. (From *Guides to the Evaluation of Permanent Impairment,* ed 2. Chicago, American Medical Association, 1984, by permission.)
†An asthmatic patient who, despite optimum medical therapy, has had attacks of severe bronchospasm requiring emergency room or hospital care on the average of six times per year is considered to be severely impaired.
‡FVC is forced vital capacity. FEV₁ is forced expiratory volume in one second. At least one of the three tests should be abnormal to the degree described for Classes 2, 3, and 4.

necessary. Also further studies are not indicated if these measurements are within the limits of normal as defined by the prediction equations of Crapo and coworkers[14, 15] because it would be highly unlikely that such an individual would be severely impaired. Exceptions would be patients with primary pulmonary vascular disease. For those with abnormal values who do not meet the criteria for total impairment, exercise studies are recommended. A revised

ATS statement has now been published.[7a] The limits set for total impairment will be the same, and cutoff points for degrees of partial impairment have been added. There is also a category of "mild abnormality which results in no functional impairment." The revised statement also emphasizes the finding of cor pulmonale as a total impairment, regardless of arterial blood gas values, and minimizes the use of blood gas analysis in disability determination.

All guidelines for impairment evaluation require a careful medical history and physical examination. Should there be an occupational etiology for the medical impairment, then a detailed occupational history must be given, including all jobs held by the claimant and all potentially hazardous exposures. A diagnosis should be established since certain disorders (e.g., asthma) may be reversible with proper therapy while others (e.g., emphysema) have little chance of improvement. In patients with airway obstruction caused by occupational asthma, the diagnosis is important in the administrative decision regarding disability, especially if there are few abnormalities present when the claimant is away from the workplace. A careful evaluation for cor pulmonale is important because this condition is considered totally disabling by itself. In patients with COPD, the chest radiograph is of little value for impairment evaluation except when it is compatible with overinflation and/ or cor pulmonale. Even when this occurs, it adds or detracts nothing from the physiologic measurements. However, if there have been occupational exposures that could result in pneumoconiosis associated with COPD, then the radiograph becomes absolutely necessary to determine if pneumoconiosis is present. The International Labor Organization/University of Cincinnati (ILO/ UC) system of characterizing the radiograph for pneumoconiosis should be used.[16] Other laboratory studies are also useful. The volume of packed red cells (hematocrit) or hemoglobin can be helpful in looking for polycythemia resulting from hypoxemia. The electrocardiogram can help in the determination of cor pulmonale.

Exercise testing is included in the AMA and ATS guidelines. SSA includes exercise arterial blood gases but not $\dot{V}O_2$max in their revised statement. When exercise testing is performed, it should be done under standardized conditions monitoring for heart disease. A treadmill is probably preferable to a cycle ergometer because more muscle groups are used in running, but either is acceptable. Oxygen saturation should be monitored with an oximeter, and oxygen uptake is measured along with the pulse rate and blood pressure. Protocols for testing are given in the 1982 ATS Statement.[7] The use of the estimated work capacity, as described in the 1982 ATS Statement and the AMA guideines, was included to help reduce the complexity and thus the cost of the evaluation. However, this has not proven to be a reliable technique and has been omitted in the revised ATS Statement.[7a]

Arterial blood gas values are used for determining impairment. As was previously discussed, older SSA guidelines utilized these measurements primarily for patients with diffuse pulmonary fibrosis, but the new changes allow exercise blood gas values to be used for lung diseases of all types. The AMA

Guides downplay arterial blood gases, as does the 1982 ATS Statement, but the ATS Statement gives criteria for severe impairment as being a PO_2 of less than 55 mmHg while breathing room air and a PO_2 of less than 60 mmHg if any sequelae of hypoxemia are present. The current revision of the ATS Statement has removed these absolute values for the PO_2 and stresses the presence of cor pulmonale as a cause for total impairment. Arterial blood gas values require an invasive procedure, are by themselves not very sensitive or specific, and are influenced by hypo- and hyperventilation, body position, age, and altitude. The sequelae of hypoxemia, e.g., cor pulmonale or polycythemia, are a more reliable indication of impairment.

SSA still uses the MVV as a criterion, but other guidelines now omit this measurement. Experience has shown that the MVV is too effort-dependent, too fatiguing, and (since it bears a fixed relationship to the FEV_1) unnecessary. Tests of "small airways" function such as the closing volume or the maximal midexpiratory flow rate (FEF_{25-75}) are of little use in impairment evaluation. If these are the only abnormal values, then the patient does not have any limitations. Tests of small airways function would be expected to be abnormal in subjects with a decreased FEV_1.

There are special situations that cannot be completely assessed by spirometry, diffusion capacity, and exercise testing. Asthma is one such situation. The criteria for total impairment due to asthma that has been adapted by the SSA mentioned above has also been incorporated into the AMA and ATS guidelines. The proposed revisions of the ATS Statement include other aspects of airway obstruction. Asthma either aggravated or caused by occupational exposures may be asymptomatic in the pulmonary laboratory setting but can preclude the patient's returning to the workplace. This needs to be recorded in the report along with evidence demonstrating that an etiologic or aggravating substance is in the workplace that results in a significant deterioration in pulmonary function. Exercise-induced asthma is another condition, but usually this does not limit one's ability to work. However, when exercise causes significant symptoms, the subject should be tested after exercising and the established cutoff points for the FVC, FEV_1, and FEV_1/FVC ratio be used to determine the extent of the impairment.

Upper airways obstruction is another impairment that may not demonstrate severe abnormalities on routine spirometric testing but which, by increasing the work of breathing, can limit a subject's ability to work. An approach to this type of patient is presented in the revised ATS Statement. If the central airways are shown to be the site of the obstruction, then CO_2 retention would indicate the impairment is severe. A mild or moderate impairment would be present if the arterial CO_2 level is normal.

Most impairment evaluations are performed for the SSA, and their guidelines must be followed in these situations. Should the evaluating physician believe the claimant is totally impaired, even when the objective measurements would not qualify that individual for benefits, then a letter should be written explaining why further consideration should be given. An administrative law judge who rules on the claim can use the additional information and may award benefits even when the criteria are not met. The physician's letter should carefully document all the reasons why an award of benefits would be appropriate for that claimant.

Private insurance companies and self-insured industries usually allow the evaluating physician to select the methods and criteria for impairment, although they can recommend a particular set of guidelines, which is usually the AMA or ATS format. The VA has its own guidelines that are available to physicians in the VA system for impairment determination of veterans claiming benefits. A physician performing these evaluations should have copies on hand of the latest SSA guidelines, AMA guides, and the ATS Statement.

Pulmonary function testing should utilize established standardized procedure.[17] Some guidelines spell out in detail how the equipment should be calibrated and the tests performed. These requirements are similar to the ATS Snowbird Workshop recommendations.[17] Some studies, such as the single-breath carbon monoxide diffusing capacity, have yet to be standardized, but progress is being made on reaching a consensus on how to perform this study. Often the agency requesting the impairment evaluation requires the evaluating physician to submit the spirometric tracings to be certain the claimant performed in an optimum manner.

On occasion, physicians performing evaluations for impairment and disability may be requested to participate in the disability determination part of the process. This may simply be a request to assign a percent disability rating on the basis of the impairment noted and whatever other information is available. This can put physicians in an awkward position because few are knowledgeable in vocational rehabilitation. At other times, the physician's participation may be as an expert witness. In this capacity, it may be necessary to give testimony based on the impairment evaluation data to an administrative law judge, an industrial commission, or other panel or board concerned with disability determination. The testimony may be in the form of a deposition or in front of a judge or board. In these situations, the physician and lawyer must familiarize themselves with each other's jargon. When a medical term is used, it should be explained in terms understandable to nonphysicians. An example would be defining the FEV_1 as "the maximal amount of air a person can exhale in one second after inhaling the maximal amount of air possible." The abbreviation FEV_1 will have little meaning to nonmedical personnel.

Although physicians often find these settings unfamiliar, they should not be uncomfortable. Since their role is that of an expert witness, they probably know more about the subject than anyone else in the room. If the physician and lawyer work together properly, the lawyer will know what questions to ask to put the necessary information into the record. The physician should be aware that, although medical science tries to be 95% certain before accepting data as fact, the legal profession considers a "reasonable degree of certainty" to be at least 50%. As with everything else, proper preparation by both physician and lawyer is essential.

VOCATIONAL REHABILITATION

Vocational rehabilitation of patients with COPD is a difficult task at best. The disease tends to progress further and limits the patient's ability to function, even when therapy is optimal. In addition, most patients become totally impaired near the end of their working life when they are past their 55th or 60th birthday. The exceptions are the group with either occupational asthma or with asthma aggravated by nonspecific irritants. Retraining these subjects to work in environments more conducive to their well-being is a realistic goal. However, the typical subject with advanced COPD who is impaired is past age 55, and even if the cigarette habit has been broken, there is still a decline in pulmonary function, albeit at a slower rate than if smoking persists. The occasional younger subject can be retrained to perform less strenuous occupations, but if there is impairment at a relatively young age, that individual must, by definition, have a markedly accelerated rate of decline in pulmonary function.[3]

In the 1960s, it was noted that pulmonary function studies could predict who was able to work by identifying subjects with an FEV_1 of > 2 L. However, it was more difficult to relate employment to FEV_1 when the measured value was below 2 L.[13] Another study demonstrated that intelligent patients have a more favorable outcome from vocational rehabilitation, probably because such workers are often employed at jobs with lower energy requirements.[18] The success of vocational rehabilitation also has been shown to be, in part, related to the percent predicted for the FEV_1 FEV_{25-75}, and the MVV.[19]

Finally, it should be emphasized that even when there is little hope of returning the individual to gainful employment, the physician has the obligation to help the patient achieve maximal self-reliance. The patient with COPD can learn to be reasonably self-sufficient and not become a burden to the family and/or community.

References

1. Continuous Disability History Sample (unpublished) from the Division of Disability Studies, Social Security Administration.
2. Tattersfield AE: Smoking in patients with advanced lung disease. *Br Med J* 1983;286(6360):163–164.
3. Fletcher C, Peto R, Tinker C, et al: *The Natural History of Chronic Bronchitis and Emphysema.* Oxford, Oxford University Press, 1976.
4. Social Security Administration. *Disability Evaluation Under Social Security.* U.S. Dept. of Health and Human Services, SSA Publication No. 05–10089. Washington, DC, US Government Printing Office, February 1986, pp 28–34.
5. Veterans Administration. Schedule for Rating Disability. (Section 6600 for bronchitis, 6601 for bronchiectasis, 6602 for bronchial asthma, 6603 for emphysema.) September 1975.
6. The Respiratory System, in *Guides to the Evaluation of Permanent Impairment,* ed 2. Chicago, American Medical Association, 1984:85–101.
7. American Thoracic Society: Evaluation of impairment/disability secondary to respiratory disorders. *Am Rev Respir Dis* 1982;126:945–951.
7a. American Thoracic Society: Evaluation of impairment/disability secondary to respiratory disorders. *Am Rev Respir Dis,* 1986; 133:1205–1209.
8. Morgan WKC: Disability or disinclination? Impairment or importuning? *Chest* 1979;75:712–715.
9. Morgan WKC, Seaton A: Pulmonary Physiology. Its application to the determination

of respiratory impairment and disability in industrial lung disease, in Morgan WKC, Seaton A (eds): *Occupational Lung Disease,* ed 2. Philadelphia, WB Saunders, 1984, pp 18–76.

10. Cotes JE: Assessment of disablement due to impaired respiratory function. *Bull Physiopath Respir* 1975;11:210–217.

11. Department of Labor, Employment Standards Administration: Standards for determining coal miners' total disability or death due to pneumoconiosis. *Fed Reg* 45 (20CFR Part 718):13678–13712, February 29, 1980.

12. Rom WN, Kanner RE, Renzetti AD, et al: Respiratory disease in Utah coal miners. *Am Rev Respir Dis* 1981;123:372–377.

13. Gilbert R, Keighley J, Auchincloss JH Jr: Disability in patients with obstructive pulmonary disease. *Am Rev Respir Dis* 1964;90:383–394.

14. Crapo RO, Morris AH, Gardner RM: Reference spirometric values using techniques and equipment that meet ATS recommendations. *Am Rev Respir Dis* 1981;123:659–664.

15. Crapo RO, Morris AH: Standardized single breath normal values for carbon monoxide diffusing capacity. *Am Rev Respir Dis* 1981;123:185–189.

16. Guidelines for the use of ILO International Classification of Radiographs of Pneumoconioses, No. 22 (rev.). Occupational Safety and Health Series. Geneva, Switzerland, International Labour Office, 1980.

17. American Thoracic Society Statement. Snowbird workshop on standardization of spirometry. *Am Rev Respir Dis* 1979; 119:831–838.

18. Daughton DM, Fix AJ, Kass I, et al: Physiological-intellectual components of rehabilitation success in patients with chronic obstructive pulmonary disease (COPD). *J Chron Dis* 1979;32:405–409.

19. Kass I, Dyksterhuis JE, Rubin H, et al: Correlation of physiopathologic variables with vocational rehabilitation outcome in patients with chronic obstructive pulmonary disease. *Chest* 1975;67:433–440.

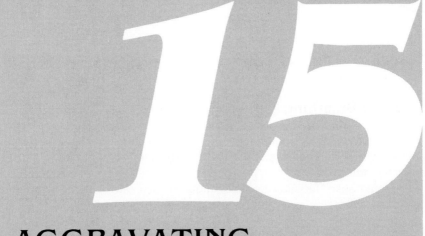

AGGRAVATING FACTORS AND COEXISTING DISORDERS

BEN V. BRANSCOMB

AGGRAVATING FACTORS

Nonspecific Dusts and Irritants

Bronchospasm is a nonspecific response to stimulation of the broncho-pulmonary irritant receptors, even in people without airways obstruction. In those with hyperreactive airways, inhalation of dusts or fumes is a major factor in the induction and perpetuation of bronchospasm. Cough and expectoration are also increased. Offending agents include primary or second-hand cigarette smoke, smoke from domestic heating, industrial sources, paint fumes, perfumes, occupational gases, dusts, and many other substances. Exacerbations of asthma and bronchitis caused by stimulation of the inhaled substances should not be misconstrued as necessarily allergic in origin.

Air pollution may increase a patient's symptoms even in communities that comply with air quality standards. Pollution levels are determined by calculating the geometric mean over a 24-hour period. Consequently, patients may be exposed for short periods to high pollution levels, particularly oxides of nitrogen and sulfur, that are sufficient to induce asthma even though the 24-hour mean satisfies the regulations. Early morning jogging in polluted environments is particularly unwise for persons with reactive or inflammatory airways disease.

Deep Breathing

Stimulation of the pulmonary stretch receptors may induce asthma in persons with highly reactive airways. Bronchospasm is sometimes induced by deep breathing during exercise, during episodes of hyperventilation, and during pulmonary function testing. Animated loud talking and laughing can also cause wheezing.

Exercise-Induced Asthma

Typically, exercise-induced asthma begins about five minutes after the onset of exercise. It may be prevented by cromolyn or prior use of adrenergic bronchodilators. The phenomenon disappears after several repeated bouts of exercise, presumably because of depletion of the responsible mediators. Inhaling very cold air, particularly through the mouth, also may induce asthma. The mechanism has been shown to be related to cooling of the airways secondary to evaporation of water into the cold desaturated inhaled air. Swimming is an excellent form of exercise in persons with exercise-induced asthma since it combines warm temperatures with high humidity.

Hyperventilation

Episodes of hyperventilation may be misinterpreted as asthma. Hyperventilation may also induce bronchospasm and regularly accompanies acute asthma. Hyperventilation is established by arterial blood gas findings. Bronchospasm is confirmed by positive physical findings and by simple tests demonstrating a fall of FEV_1 or peak flow below baseline values or by improvement in the values after treatment. Hyperventilation episodes related to fear, anxiety, or other psychological mechanisms should be addressed by reassurance, counseling, bag breathing or other forms of rebreathing, and exercise training.

Anxiety

It is doubtful that psychological mechanisms are ever the sole cause of asthma. Anxiety, stress, and emotionally laden interpersonal encounters frequently induce attacks of asthma in children and sometimes in adults. Furthermore, psychosocial and financial circumstances vastly complicate compliance and other aspects of management. Consequently, a holistic approach is important in all patients and essential in the management of more difficult subjects. The patient's coping style should be specifically addressed. Sometimes social services, psychologic, or psychiatric consultations are required. A discussion of the four more commonly encountered personality types follows:

The Low Panic-Fear, High Denial Patient[1] tends to accept his symptoms stoically and to deny the need for a consistent regimen. He particularly rejects recommendations concerning smoking, exercise, and other nonpharmacologic treatment. His approach is highly intellectualized. He feels emotions represent weaknesses and so minimizes symptoms and withholds information. He may profess understanding which, in fact, he does not have.[2] The nature of the disease, the risks and particularly the benefits of treatment should clearly but unassertively be presented to such a patient. A low-control style on the part of the physician may be appropriate; the patient may need to feel that the doctor is his consultant and that he is electing to follow the management program based on facts provided by the doctor. He should be seen often enough to reinforce the treatment regimen and to preserve the physician's role. In the face of his independence and denial, the need for treatment can be emphasized by allowing him to listen to his own chest with a stethoscope and by frequent simple office or home pulmonary function tests.

The High Panic-Fear, Low Denial Patient tends to be extremely dependent, emotionally labile, demanding, helpless, and anxious. He exaggerates and misinterprets symptoms and has poor coping ability. He tends to give up easily and to discontinue treatment because he is insecure about following advice. Nevertheless, he feels it is the doctor's responsibility to cure the disease. This patient often uses over-the-counter medications, drugs prescribed by numerous previous physicians, or medications obtained from friends. He may resort to bizarre diets, megavitamins, or irregular practitioners and may exaggerate the role of allergy.

These patients require much reassurance and education. The fact that most symptoms can be controlled with relatively simple medications if they are consistently applied should be emphasized. Physicians often switch drugs too frequently or overmedicate these patients. The physician should specifically assess the role of dependency in these patients. Initially, in order to control the acute manifestations of the disorder and to establish an effective relationship, a somewhat autocratic, firm, yet sympathetic role is appropriate. The physician must avoid vacillation or the appearance of frustration. Providing the patient with drug samples may be interpreted as lack of a confident therapeutic plan. When confidence is established and the symptoms improve, the physician's high-control style should be modified: The patient should be taught to make management decisions. Teaching the patient the use of a peak flow meter at home may be helpful. The dependency relationship should ultimately be reduced and management responsibility returned to the patient as much as possible. However, since the locus of control in high fear, low denial patients tends to be external, they may require considerable guidance.

The Alexithymic Patient. Another type of patient, representing 34% of hospitalized asthmatics in one study,[1] can be characterized as alexithymic. This patient tends to be out of touch with his feelings. He does not plan, communicates superficial feelings only, volunteers little, and answers questions in a flat, indecisive manner. Physicians tend to undertreat such patients because they are boring and noncomplaining. Frequently, they are very suggestible. Obtaining the history and assessment of symptoms requires diligence and skill in alexithymic patients. Recommendations must be clearly presented and supported by written instructions.

The Resistive Patient is particularly frustrating. He has frequently changed physicians. Medicines that initially seemed beneficial are frequently rejected because of dubious reactions and intolerances. Precise subjective symptoms are difficult to elicit, but the patient describes his misery vividly and in unnecessary detail. Frequently, he quotes specific dates, physicians' names, and pseudoscientific explanations, often in incorrect medical terminology. He is often whining and complaining, assumes no reponsibility for his problems, and has a ready reason to reject each medication suggested.

One must avoid playing the resistive patient's game, which consists of forcing one to grope for recommendations that can then be rejected. Insofar as possible, he should be brought into the care process by turning his questions back on himself. He should be made to articulate a goal that could be accomplished if his symptoms were controlled. The likelihood that he can accomplish this goal if he accepts treatment should be emphasized. When he tends to reject treatment, he should be led back to the reality of potential improvement.

Chronic Aspiration and Esophageal Reflux

Esophageal reflux may initiate reflex bronchospasm. Chronic aspiration of gastric acid also results in bronchial irritation and bronchospasm. The events occur primarily during sleep and are suggested by nocturnal cough and nocturnal asthma. Gastroesophageal symptoms, sore throat, and chronic hoarseness may suggest these mechanisms are present. Chronic laryngitis, bronchiectasis, recurrent pneumonia, and hemoptysis may be seen. Contrast radiography, esophageal motility and pH studies, measurement of cardiac sphincter tone and gastric emptying time, and endoscopy may be required. Since aminophylline relaxes the cardiac sphincter, it may be inadvisable for patients with bronchospasm secondary to reflux or aspiration. Avoidance of food and fluids for two to three hours before bedtime and through the night is important. Metoclopramide hydrochloride may help reduce reflux by increasing sphincter tone at the lower end of the esophagus and by increasing gastric motility and gastric emptying.

Infection

Acute upper and lower respiratory infections are often associated with exacerbations of asthma and chronic bronchitis. It is commonly difficult to determine whether infection exists in patients with chronic obstructive disease since they cough regularly and produce mucus when they are not infected. Body temperature and leukocyte count should be measured, although these are frequently normal when infection is present. A change in the color and viscosity of the sputum is helpful, but the sputum should be smeared and stained, since uninfected sputum may become dark when it has been retained for a long period of time. Because of these problems, it is sometimes desirable to treat the patient with antibiotics on a trial basis. Influenza and other viral infections are sometimes followed by intractable asthma that persists for weeks or months.

Sinusitis

Chronic paranasal sinusitis should be suspected in persons with sinus pain, narrow nasal passages, or postnasal drip. Vasoconstrictors should be used systematically but limited to about seven or 10 days. Topical ones are more effective than systemic ones if properly used. If antibiotics effective for gram-positive organisms prove unsuccessful, drugs should be selected by the results of culture. Antibiotic treatment should be continued for at least 10 days. Long-standing sinusitis sometimes requires treatment for four to six weeks. Radiographs of the maxilla should be obtained in chronic maxillary sinusitis that fails to respond to treatment in order to rule out periapical abscess. Allergic rhinitis may occur independently or concurrently with bacterial sinusitis and should be treated. Inhalation of topical corticosteroids through the nose may be very helpful in reducing nasal congestion and postnasal drainage. Surgery is sometimes required when chronic upper airway disorders complicate COPD.

Aspirin and Nonsteroidal Anti-Inflammatory Drugs

Aspirin and nonsteroidal anti-inflammatory drugs induce asthma in some persons with reactive airways. The mechanism is pharmacologic, not allergic. The syndrome of asthma, nasal polyps, and aspirin sensitivity is well recognized. Bronchospasm can also be induced in occasional subjects by ingestion of a food coloring dye, tartrazine yellow, and also by consumption of sodium metabisulfite or related antioxidants that are used on meat and vegetables and by commercial salad bars to preserve the appearance of freshness. Many patients are unaware of exposure to these substances. Aspirin and nonsteroidal anti-inflammatory drugs are contained in a wide variety of over-the-counter preparations. Furthermore, patients who are exposed to any of these substances on a regular basis fail to make the association between the offending agent and bronchospasm. Drugs that block the beta receptor sites, such as propranolol, may also precipitate bronchospasm.

Occupational and Environmental Exposure

Bronchospasm can be induced by immediate or delayed hypersensitivity, by exposure to nonspecific irritants or temperature changes, and by direct pharmacologic means. All of these circumstances occur in the occupational setting.[3, 4] Establishing the occupational relationship is usually difficult, particularly when the offending agent results in delayed hypersensitivity or when it is a nonspecific irritant. In these circumstances, increased symptoms in asthmatic or bronchitic patients may occur hours after they have left the worksite and may persist throughout the weekend when they are away from the job. Exposure to offending inhalants may also be related to home activities and hobbies. More than one adverse environmental factor may coexist. These factors are difficult to investigate, particularly when there is a long interval between the exposure and the symptomatic response. Informal challenge testing to an occupational or other environmental exposure is complicated by the inability to control all of the variables plus many emotional and financial issues. The principal categories of environmental respiratory hazards for the person with asthma or bronchitis are:

1. Extremes of cold and heat are encountered by such persons as foundry workers, those who work outside, and those who are required to enter refrigerated compartments.

2. Inert dust can stimulate irritant bronchopulmonary receptors resulting in bronchospasm. Inhaled dust may also overload the mucociliary escalator in bronchitic patients resulting in increased cough and secretions.

3. Many jobs and home activities are associated with exposure to irritating particles and gases. Oxides of nitrogen and sulfur, ammonia, solvents, chlorine, and cigarette smoke are examples.

4. Inhaled allergens include not only pollen and antigens from domestic animals and mites but also industrial pollutants, such as toluene diisocyanate, polyurethane from plastic foam manufacture, and platinum salts; coffee bean dust; and the wheat weevil (baking).

5. Pharmacologically active substances causing bronchospasm are seen in several occupations. Byssinosis is thought to be mediated by polypeptides from the cotton bract.

Noncompliance

Although they may profess compliance, about one third of the patients fail to follow the pharmacologic and particularly nonpharmacologic recommendations.[5] This problem should be addressed specifically in all patients. The fact that some medications may occasionally be omitted should be acknowledged and discussed in a nonjudgmental way. The patient should acknowledge any problems with the regimen to the physician. Adherence to the program should be documented as objectively as possible: theophylline levels, the number of inhaler refills, carboxyhemoglobin levels to verify smoking, and patient diaries are useful. Patients may not only omit prescribed medications but may use over-the-counter drugs or previous prescriptions that have been discontinued. The following strategies[2] are sometimes helpful in dealing with noncompliance:

The Blind Capsule. Patients with misconceptions concerning drugs and high panic-fear patients who are afraid to relinquish management decisions to the physician often accept the following approach: Patients are led through a discussion in which they acknowledge the possibility that suggestion and psychosomatic factors may influence their assessment of the benefits of medications and that they will ultimately need to make their own decisions concerning medication. Patients are invited to accept a blind capsule every six hours into which all of their medications have been placed without their knowledge of the drugs or doses. This is done with the understanding that they are not receiving a placebo and that they will eventually be informed of the contents of the capsule or allowed to look at the medical record. They are asked to record their symptoms and any side effects before being told what drugs they are taking. Most patients are sophisticated enough about psychosomatic medicine to accept this system. This program is particularly useful when the patient has erroneous convictions about the side effects of drugs or when it is desirable to increase or decrease sharply the dose of steroids in a fearful patient. The system is discontinued when the appropriate medications have been identified.

The Patient Diary. Especially useful in patients with high denial, the diary records patient activities, symptoms, medications, and side effects. This record should be reviewed with the patient in a sympathetic and nonpejorative way.

Nonpharmaceutical Prescriptions. All recommendations, not just those related to drug therapy, should be written out. This emphasizes the importance of the nonpharmacologic aspects of care.

Frequent Follow-up. The frequency with which the therapeutic regimen is reinforced has been repeatedly demonstrated as a major factor in compliance. This can be accomplished efficiently by assigning to an office nurse or other assistant the responsibility of acting as an intermediary for certain patients. The assistant collects information, is accessible to the patient by phone, and serves as a patient educator.

Scheduled Telephone Visits. The patient is taught what signs and symptoms to monitor and is told to expect a telephone call from the doctor scheduled at a specific time one or two weeks after an office visit. The call should be made during the time the physician normally sees outpatients. The conversation proceeds just as though the patient were in the office.

The Recorded Conference. Remembering instruction is often difficult for patients, particularly at the time of discharge from the hospital. A tape recording can be made during the discharge conference, which is then given to the patient to play at home.

The Patient Contract. Compliance has been shown to improve when the patient is given a written contract stating the goals of treatment, time to achieve them, and the obligations of both patient and physician.[6]

COEXISTING DISORDERS

Cardiovascular Disease

Approximately 50% of patients with COPD over the age of 50 have ischemic heart disease, hypertension, rhythm disturbances, or heart failure.[7] Left ventricular failure may be difficult to diagnose in the presence of COPD but should be suspected when there is a reduction in exercise tolerance unexplained by worsening of the underlying pulmonary disease. Nocturnal dyspnea secondary to lung disease must be differentiated from paroxysmal nocturnal dyspnea of cardiac origin. If the dyspnea is quickly relieved by bronchodilator inhalation or by expectoration of a large amount of retained sputum allowing the patient to go back to sleep rapidly, airways obstruction is probably the cause. Such accumulation of retained sputum usually occurs late at night. In contrast, nocturnal dyspnea resulting from pulmonary edema generally occurs shortly after onset of sleep. A ventricular gallop rhythm at the apex or in the epigastrium suggests left ventricular failure; however, cardiac sounds may be difficult to hear in COPD patients with an increased AP diameter of the chest.

Resting and exercise arterial blood gas studies and a stress electrocardiogram should be obtained. In addition, the patient should be observed during an informal, noninvasive, maximal exercise test. At the termination of exercise, tachycardia, sweating, low pulse volume, and peripheral vasoconstriction frequently reflect inadequate oxygen delivery to the tissues. These findings suggest left ventricular failure, provided the hemoglobin concentration is normal and the exercise arterial saturation is above 90%. Furthermore, patients with insufficient cardiac output typically complain of generalized weakness and fatigue.

Air hunger and labored breathing are the complaints when the mechanical work of breathing is the limiting factor. Prompt relief of exercise-induced dyspnea by bronchodilators also suggests that airways obstruction is the major cause. Patients with heart failure generally require a longer time to recover from activity. Abrupt gain of several pounds in body weight is helpful in detecting fluid retention and suggests heart failure. Cardiac function can be further quantitated by measuring the left ventricular ejection fraction by two-dimensional echocardiography or by gated ventriculography. Exercise gas-exchange studies are sometimes helpful in differentiating between cardiac and pulmonary limits and exercise capacity. When exercise is limited by a cardiovascular problem, the anaerobic threshold is reached at a lower level of work than is normal. However, many patients with pulmonary insufficiency are limited by dyspnea secondary either to increased work of breathing or by deconditioning before an exercise level is reached at which cardiac function can be properly assessed.

Occasionally, when patients with COPD develop left ventricular failure and pulmonary congestion, they experience a paradoxical improvement in expiratory flow rates, improvement in carbon monoxide diffusing capacity, and intensification of breath sounds. These changes reflect a restoration of the elastic recoil of the lung by the mechanical effects of vascular congestion.[8–10] The FVC is usually reduced.

Right ventricular failure secondary to pulmonary hypertension in COPD is suggested by the presence of neck vein distention during both phases of respiration, hepatomegaly, and pedal edema. A right ventricular gallop may be heard along the left sternal margin or in the epigastrium. Right ventricular failure is also suggested by unexplained reduction in exercise tolerance, increased dyspnea, weight gain, and increased cough. It is more common in older patients, those with severe chronic pulmonary impairment, those with left ventricular disease, and those with hypoxemia. Right ventricular failure is exceedingly common in persons with chronic hypercapnia, secondary polycythemia, or profound desaturation during sleep.

In order to control left ventricular failure, it may be necessary to limit an otherwise desirable exercise program. In contrast, moderately severe right ventricular failure is often tolerated well for years, compatible with a lifestyle that includes reasonable amounts of exercise. The principal treatment of right ventricular failure consists of diuretics, measures to improve alveolar ventilation, and supplemental oxygen. Increasing the oxygen tension in poorly ventilated areas of the lung lowers pulmonary artery pressure by diminishing hypoxic vasoconstriction. Oxygen therapy may also diminish myocardial work in hypoxic persons by lowering cardiac output. Diuretics must be used cautiously to prevent excessive reduction in venous return with consequent reduction in cardiac output. Mild to moderate ankle edema is common in well-managed patients. Serum potassium should be monitored and supplemented in patients receiving diuretics. Potassium-conserving diuretics, such as triamterene, are often helpful. Sodium restriction is desirable but may intensify nutritional problems that so frequently occur in patients with severe obstructive disease. If an acceptable level of chronic right ventricular failure can be maintained with diuretics and other measures, concessions to sodium restriction may be required in the interest of improved nutrition.

The risk of arrhythmias is increased with age, hypertension, coronary disease, hypoxemia, xanthines, and adrenergic drugs. Stress electrocardiography should be performed in patients with these risk factors, particularly when an exercise program is contemplated. Beta$_2$ agonists should be used rather than less selective adrenergic drugs. Systematic administration by aerosol produces greater benefits with less cardiovascular side effects than the same medication administered by subcutaneous injection or by mouth. The patient should be cautioned against excessive use of inhalers. Xanthines increase myocardial oxygen consumption out of proportion to increased coronary perfusion.[11] Plasma theophylline levels should be carefully checked because the metabolism of xanthines is usually delayed when heart failure is present. A plasma theophylline level of 8–12 µg/ml is usually acceptable in arrhythmia-prone patients. The initial intravenous theophylline dose in acutely ill arrhythmia-prone patients is about 0.5 mg/kg/hr. The arterial oxygen tension should be scrupulously monitored.

Hypertensive patients experience many of the problems discussed above. Improved left ventricular function resulting from treatment of hypertension may result in improved gas exchange. Excessive diuresis with resultant hypovolemia must be avoided since it may worsen both gas exchange and cardiac output. Nonselective beta-blocking agents, such as propranolol, may induce bronchospasm. This risk is reduced somewhat when the more cardioselective beta-blocking agents are used, e.g., metoprolol and atenolol. Nifedipine and diltiazem are acceptable as well as prazosin, methyldopa, and clonidine. However, psychological depression is often produced by the centrally acting antihypertensives, especially at higher doses. This often limits their use in COPD patients in whom depression is a common problem. The direct-acting vasodilators minoxidil and hydralazine are not contraindicated but may produce postural hypotension and reflex tachycardia.

Pregnancy

Cough and expectoration are uncomfortable and ineffective during pregnancy. Airways obstruction intensifies the difficulties. Vigorous treatment of chronic pulmonary problems should be instituted early in pregnancy. Smoking should be strongly discouraged. The pregnant patient can be supported by pillows or rolled-up blankets in a position so that postural drainage and careful, deliberate coughing may effectively remove bronchopulmonary secretions.

Asthmatic women are almost equally divided among those whose asthma improves, worsens, or remains about the same during pregnancy. The course of asthma can generally be predicted by the events during a previous pregnancy and by the diligence with which the asthma is treated. In women whose asthma has been well controlled, delivery is usually unassociated with respiratory problems.

The respiratory adaptations during pregnancy[12, 13] are as follows:
- Tidal volume, minute ventilation: Increased.
- Oxygen consumption, alveolar ventilation: Increased.
- VC, TLC, respiratory rate, FEV_1: Unchanged.
- FRC, ERV, RV: Decreased.
- Pa_{O_2}: Increased (107 in first trimester, 103 in last trimester).
- Pa_{CO_2}: Decreased (27 in first trimester, 32 in last trimester).
- Arterial pH: 7.40 to 7.47.
- HCO_3^-: Decreased to 18 to 21 mEq/L.
- Perception of increased resistive load: Increased in 65% of patients.
- Closing volume: Near FRC.

Several considerations are suggested by these data. A carbon dioxide tension above 35 is inappropriately high and may represent ventilatory failure. Both acidosis and alkalosis can develop rapidly because of the small buffering capacity secondary to the low serum bicarbonate. A Pa_{O_2} below 70 indicates hypoxemia in the mother and must be vigorously treated to prevent fetal hypoxemia. Because the closing volume is near the FRC, small changes in airway diameter result in $\dot{V}/\dot{Q}$ mismatching and hypoxemia. The increased tidal volume, increased minute ventilation, and the mechanical effect of the pregnancy on diaphragm function all tend to render the patient vulnerable to ventilatory fatigue.

In general, drugs should be avoided during the first trimester. Tetracyclines induce malformation and discoloration of the fetus's teeth. Iodides are contraindicated because they cause fetal goiter. Methylxanthines can be used but require frequent monitoring because the serum levels often fluctuate. Epinephrine is reported to increase fetal malformation when used during the first four months and may also reduce uterine perfusion. More selective beta$_2$ agonists have less effect on uterine circulation and should be used by the inhaled route to minimize systemic effects. Steroids should be avoided during the first trimester, if possible. Nevertheless, their use is preferable to uncontrolled asthma, provided that systematic beta$_2$ agonists by aerosol plus methylxanthines have failed and that the steroid risks are clearly understood.[14] Beclomethasone or other inhaled steroids have negligible systemic effects and are often beneficial, although neither has been approved in pregnancy because of the absence of human studies.

Prostaglandin $F_{2\alpha}$ is a smooth muscle constrictor that has been used to induce therapeutic abortions. It is a potent bronchoconstrictor and therefore is contraindicated in patients with reactive airways disease.[15]

Diabetes Mellitus

Steroids attenuate the responsiveness of insulin receptors and increase gluconeogenesis. Consequently, diabetes becomes hard to manage when corticosteroids must be given. Closer monitoring and higher insulin doses are needed in such patients. A reduction in the steroid dose may result in hypoglycemia, unless the insulin dose is reduced concomitantly. Diabetes secondary to steroid therapy is characterized by extreme insulin sensitivity. Smaller than usual insulin doses should be used in steroid-induced hypoglycemia. Bronchopulmonary infections are also more frequent and more difficult to manage in diabetic patients.

Thyroid Disease

Propranolol and other beta-blocking agents used in hyperthyroidism should be avoided because they may induce bronchospasm. Adrenergic drugs are thought to intensify the symptoms of hyperthyroidism. Since hypothyroidism is associated with poor theophylline clearance, smaller doses are necessary.

The Older Patient

Bronchitis and emphysema are typically diagnosed initially in older persons. Asthma also begins after the age of 50 in about one sixth of all asthmatics. In contrast to childhood asthma, in which the ratio of males to females is approximately 2 to 1, adult-onset asthma is more commonly seen in women than men. Most of the patients present with a combination of cough, expectoration, and wheezing. This form of COPD may appropriately be labeled "chronic asthmatic bronchitis."[16] Adult asthmatics frequently are difficult to manage and often dependent on steroids for symptomatic control. Osteoporosis with painful vertebral compression fracture is a devastating complication of prolonged steroid therapy. Unfortunately, this problem is often seen in postmenopausal women who are particularly at risk of osteoporosis. Corticosteroids should be used in the lowest possible dose and either intermittently or on alternate days, if possible.[17, 18] Inhaled corticosteroids[19, 20] and full use of other drug and nondrug therapeutic modalities should minimize osteoporosis and other steroid complications in older patients. Chronic deconditioning, obesity, and concomitant diseases are frequent in older patients.

Gastrointestinal Disorders

Intolerance to methylxanthines sometimes limits the use of this class of drugs to very small doses. However, serum levels as low as 8 µg/ml may produce significant benefit. Methylxanthines relax the cardiac sphincter and therefore may increase the symptoms of esophageal reflux. Gastrectomy predisposes to tuberculosis, particularly if steroids are used.[21] Corticosteroids may lead to the development of peptic ulcer, but this is not a frequent occurrence and, therefore, not an absolute contraindication when unremitting bronchospasm cannot be managed successfully by other means. Antacids or H_2 blockers should be administered to persons suspected of having ulcer disease. The stool guaiac should be monitored occasionally.

Impaired hepatic function results in delayed theophylline clearance. Serum theophylline levels must be followed carefully and smaller doses used.[22] When COPD is associated with cirrhosis, spironolactone or triamterene may be the preferred diuretic. Serum potassium must be monitored when these potassium-conserving diuretics are employed.

Obesity

Ventilation in obese persons is more rapid and tidal volume is smaller than in those of normal weight. This results in an increased ratio of dead space to tidal volume. Minute ventilation must be consequently increased to supply metabolic needs. The rapid shallow breathing pattern results in greater airways resistance and is the opposite of the slow deep breathing sought in the management of COPD. The work of breathing is increased in obese persons, many of whom experience obstructive sleep apnea, obesity and hypoventilation (pickwickian syndrome), or both.[23, 24]

Cough is less effective in obese persons, and adequate postural drainage is difficult to achieve. Spontaneous or prescribed physical activity is difficult. Smaller doses of medication should be prescribed than those estimated by tables or formulas based on body weight because such formulas usually overlook the impact of extreme obesity on metabolic activity and the volume in which the drug is diluted. Dosages of medication should be used conservatively in obese persons.

References

1. Dirks JF, Schraa JC: Patient mislabeling of symptoms and rehospitalization in asthma. *J Asthma* 1983;20:43–44.
2. Branscomb BV: The difficult asthmatic. *Clinics in Chest Medicine* 1984;5:695–713.
3. Middleton T, Reed CE: *Allergy: Principles and Practice.* St. Louis, CV Mosby Co, 1978.
4. Moira CY: Occupational assessment of asthma. *Chest* 1982;82 (suppl):20–24.
5. Eraker SA, Kirscht JP, Becker MH: Understanding and improving patient compliance. *Ann Intern Med* 1984;100:258–268.
6. Quill TE: Partnerships in patient care: A contractual approach. *Ann Intern Med* 1983;98:228–234.
7. Reynolds RJ, Buford JG, George RB: Treating asthma and COPD in patients with heart disease. *J Respir Dis* 1982;3:41–51.
8. Sharp JT, Griffith GT, Gunnell IL, et al: Ventilatory mechanics in pulmonary edema in man. *J Clin Invest,* 1958;37:111–117.
9. Sharp, JT, Griffith GT, Gunnell IL, et al: The effects of therapy on pulmonary mechanics in human pulmonary edema. *J Clin Invest* 1961;40:665–672.
10. Cook, CD, Mead J, Schreiner GL, et al:

Pulmonary mechanics during induced pulmonary edema in anesthetized dogs. *J Appl Physiol* 1959;14:177–186.

11. Foltz EL, Ruben A, Steiger WA, et al: The effects of intravenous aminophylline upon the coronary blood-oxygen exchange. *Circulation* 1950;2:215–224.

12. Schatz M, Patterson R, Zeitz S, et al: Corticosteroid therapy for the pregnant asthmatic patient. *JAMA* 1975;233:804–807.

13. Turner ES, Greenberger PA, Patterson R: Management of the pregnant asthmatic patient. *Ann Intern Med* 1980;93:905–918.

14. Mintz S: Pregnancy and asthma, in Weiss EB, Segal MS (eds): *Bronchial Asthma: Mechanisms and Therapeutics*. Boston, Little, Brown & Co, 1976.

15. Mathe AA, Hedqvist P, Holmgren A, et al: Bronchial hyperreactivity to prostaglandin F2 and histamine in patients with asthma. *Br Med J* 1973;1:193–196.

16. Dodge RR, Burrows B: The prevalence and incidence of asthma and asthma-like symptoms in a general population sample. *Am Rev Respir Dis* 1980;122:567–575.

17. Melby JC: Drug Spotlight program: Systemic corticosteroid therapy: Pharmacology and endocrinologic considerations. *Ann Intern Med* 1974;81:505–512.

18. Fanci AS, Dale DC, Balow JE: Glucocorticosteroid therapy: Mechanisms of action and clinical considerations (NIH Conference). *Ann Intern Med* 1976;84:304–325.

19. Kass I, Nair SV, Patil KD: Beclomethasone dipropionate aerosol in the treatment of steroid-dependent asthmatic patients. An assessment of 18 months of therapy. *Chest,* 1977;71:703–707.

20. Hodgkin JE, Guth RH, Nelson JC: Inhalation of triamcinolone acetonide via IPPB or compressor pump therapy. *Chest* 1976;70:428–429.

21. Preventive therapy of tuberculous infection: Official ATS statement. *Am Rev Respir Dis* 1974;110:371–374.

22. Piafsky KM, Ogilvie RI: Dosage of theophylline in bronchial asthma. *N Engl J Med* 1975;292:1218–1222.

23. Gastaut H, Tassinari CA, Duron B: Polygraphic study of the episodic diurnal and nocturnal (hypnic and respiratory) manifestations of the pickwickian syndrome. *Brain Res* 1966;2:167–186.

24. Sackner M, Landa J, Forest T, et al: Periodic sleep: Chronic sleep deprivation related to intermittent upper airway obstruction and central nervous system disturbance. *Chest* 1975;67:264–271.

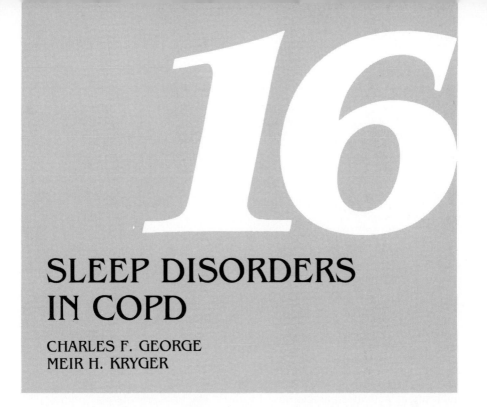

SLEEP DISORDERS IN COPD

CHARLES F. GEORGE
MEIR H. KRYGER

The average person spends seven to eight hours every night asleep, which adds up to a third of his or her lifetime. The physiology of this considerable period of time was completely ignored for many years. In the past 25 years, there has been an explosion of information on the changes in homeostasis during sleep, and with the advent of ear oximetry and polysomnography, changes in respiration have been increasingly quantitated in various disease states. The interactions of sleep and respiration in the patient with chronic obstructive pulmonary disease (COPD) is the subject of this chapter, which deals primarily with nocturnal hypoxemia, its mechanisms, extent, and consequences in the typical COPD patient.

PHYSIOLOGY OF SLEEP

Sleep is not a homogeneous state. It has been divided into various stages based on neurophysiologic findings. The presence or absence of eye movements measured by an electro-oculogram divides sleep into rapid eye movement (REM) or non–rapid eye movement (NREM) sleep. NREM sleep is subdivided into four stages; Stages 1 and 2 indicate lighter sleep, and Stages 3 and 4 refer to deep sleep or slow-wave sleep (SWS). REM sleep has not been formally subdivided, but there are two distinct phases: (1) periods of

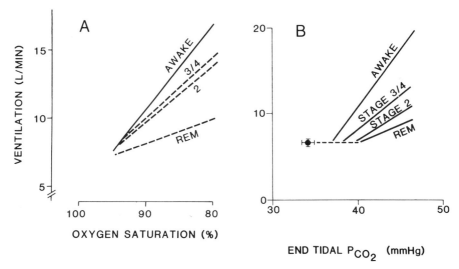

Figure 16–1. Hypoxic (*A*) and hypercapnic (*B*) ventilatory responses in normal sleep. (From Douglas NJ: Control of ventilation during sleep, in Kryger MH (ed): *Clinics in Chest Medicine* 1985;6(4):563–575, by permission.)

intermittent activity characterized by rapid eye movements and myoclonic twitches called phasic REM (PREM) and (2) an underlying background of activity characterized by muscle atonia and desynchronized electroencephalogram (EEG) called tonic REM (TREM).[1]

Studies in healthy individuals reveal that chemical drives to breathe are reduced during sleep compared with wakefulness and that the reduction is sleep-stage specific.[2–8] Patients with COPD do not tolerate face masks and other upper airway instrumentation required to assess the hypoxic and hypercapnic ventilatory responses during sleep, so there is no data. However, one can assume that the COPD patient experiences the same sleep-stage specific reduction in chemical drives. For healthy individuals, this attenuation in chemical drive permits a minor degree of hypoxia and/or hypercapnia, both of which have little clinical importance. For the COPD patient, however, who often has diminished chemical drives while awake, further reduction of these drives with the sleep stage has the potential of producing severe hypoxemia and hypercapnia.

Figure 16–1 demonstrates curves for the hypoxic and hypercapnic ventilatory responses in healthy individuals. For a given SaO_2 or end tidal Pco_2, there is a stepwise reduction in the ventilation with the sleep stage (i.e., marked attenuation in REM). It can also be appreciated that, for a given degree of hypoxia, changing sleep stage or awakening would produce a substantial increase in ventilation. This awakening or arousal in response to hypoxia is a potentially useful protective mechanism. Unfortunately, hypoxia is an unreliable arousal stimulus. Healthy individuals subjected to oxygen saturations of about 70% arouse or awaken only about 50% of the time.[2, 5, 7]

Thus, hypoxic patients may have no protective arousal or ventilatory response.

There are other normal physiologic changes during sleep that may be disadvantageous to patients with COPD. Animal data reveal that arousal in response to airway irritation is impaired during sleep,[9, 10] and it is likely that this response is also diminished in the COPD patient. In addition, airway resistance increases during sleep, and the usual compensatory increase to such resistance is reduced consequent to sleep.[11, 12] Muscle tone decreases as a function of the sleep state (i.e., less in deep sleep than light). During REM, there is almost complete muscle atonia, with the exception of the primary respiratory muscles. Accessory muscles, such as the scalenes and sternomastoid, lose their tone with REM onset.[13] When this loss of tone affects muscles of the upper airway and tongue, the potential for upper airway obstruction and apnea exists.[14] Finally, although not documented conclusively, COPD patients are likely to have reduced mucociliary clearance with sleep.[15]

SLEEP HYPOXEMIA

As a result of changes in mechanics, chemical drives, and other reflexes during sleep, the COPD patient develops hypoxemia. This sleep hypoxemia has been well characterized in an early report using spot tests of blood gases, which revealed that the PaO_2 in patients with a mean awake Pa_{O_2} of 62 mmHg fell to about 57 mmHg in NREM sleep and to about 50 mmHg in REM sleep.[16] Qualitatively similar results have been obtained in several studies reporting continuous oxygen saturation measurements. In one study of hypoxic patients, the mean awake saturation of 84.6% dropped 1.7% in Stage 1 sleep, 3.1% in Stage 2, 1.4% in slow wave sleep, and 7.7% in REM sleep.[17] Other reports have confirmed severe hypoxemia in REM and have shown hypoxemia in slow wave sleep to be more severe than in Stages 1 or 2.[18] Undoubtedly, this is due to differences in patient selection. Thus, in patients with hypoxemia while awake, there occurs a small drop in saturation when the patient enters NREM sleep and a further, often larger, fall in saturation as the patient goes into REM sleep.

The early studies with intermittent arterial blood gas sampling were able to appreciate the differences in magnitude but could not give any information on the dynamic changes of sleep hypoxemia. It is now known from studies with continuous measurement of SaO_2 by oximetry that severe sleep hypoxemia in COPD is episodic. The number of episodes reported differs from one study to another because of patient selection and the definition used for an episode of sleep hypoxemia. When hypoxemic episodes are sustained (i.e., exceeding one minute in duration with a drop in saturation > 10%), it was found that patients with severe daytime hypoxemia had a mean of three to four such episodes per night while those with less severe daytime hypoxemia had an average of about one episode per night.[19] In a large group of patients with a mean awake saturation of 84.6% ($\pm 1.6\%$ standard error of the mean

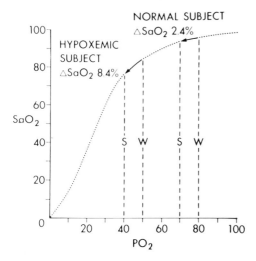

Figure 16–2. The oxygen-hemoglobin dissociation curve. Despite identical drops in P_{O_2}, there is a much greater fall in SaO_2 for the hypoxemic subject who starts on the steep part of the curve. (From Kryger MA (ed): Pathophysiology of Respiration New York, John Wiley & Sons, 1981, p 118.)

or SEM), 25% of their time asleep was spent below a saturation of 80%, 13% of the time asleep below 75%, 5% of the time asleep below 70%, and 2% of the time alseep below 65%.[17] Thus, some patients may spend a great deal of time desaturated. Patients may also have short hypoxemic dips lasting only 20 or 30 seconds.

There seem to be two factors that determine the degree of nocturnal desaturation. The first of these is the degree of hypoxemia while awake. Catterall and colleagues studied 20 patients with COPD, and the maximal

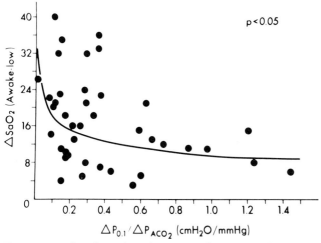

Figure 16–3. The relationship of maximum sleep oxygen desaturation and hypercapnic drive to breathe assessed with $P_{.1}$ in COPD patients. Note that patients with high drive had little desaturation and that those with large desaturation had drives in the lower range. (From Fleetham JA, Meyon B, West P: Chemical control of ventilation and sleep arterial oxygen desaturation in patients with COPD. *American Review of Respiratory Disease* 1980;122:583–589, by permission.)

drop in SaO_2 ranged from 5% to 47% with a mean of 19.7% for those with awake hypercapnia and more severe hypoxemia. For those patients with normocapnia and minimal hypoxemia while awake, the mean was 9.3%.[20] Fleetham and coworkers studied 24 hypoxemic COPD patients and found a mean drop in SaO_2 of 17.5%.[17] This variability can be accounted for in part by the starting point on the oxygen-hemoglobin dissociation curve (Fig. 16–2). Thus, although the change in saturation is different, the calculated fall in Po_2 is about the same in both studies.

Although nocturnal hypoxemia is related to awake oxygenation, there is substantial variability in the sleep SaO_2 for a given awake SaO_2. The second factor in determining the magnitude of the decrease in oxygen saturation appears to be related to $Paco_2$.[21–23] That is, large drops in sleep SaO_2 are uncommon in patients without hypercapnia or in those with a brisk ventilatory response to carbon dioxide. In other words, those with carbon dioxide retention have a decreased hypercapnic ventilatory response and are more likely to exhibit large falls in oxygen saturation with sleep (Fig. 16–3). Thus, carbon dioxide sensitivity may protect against severe sleep hypoxemia in COPD.

PHYSIOLOGY OF SLEEP HYPOXEMIA

There are several factors contributing to the sleep hypoxemia in COPD patients including hypoventilation, changes in functional residual capacity (FRC) and ventilation perfusion mismatching, and changes in breathing pattern. None of these are mutually exclusive.

Hypoventilation

Changes in alveolar ventilation can be measured directly or inferred from changes in Pco_2 during sleep. As mentioned above, patients with COPD do not tolerate the face mask and apparatus required to accurately quantitate ventilation during sleep; therefore, indirect measures such as magnetometers, respiratory inductance plethysmography (RIP), or impedance plethysmography must be used. Despite various claims, these devices are not completely reliable. At the very best, they are within $\pm 10\%$ of the spirometrically measured tidal volumes and require tedious calibration to account for position changes during sleep.[24] Nonetheless, within a given body position and/or sleep stage, relative changes in ventilation can be appreciated. Hudgel and coworkers reported on a group of severe COPD patients and, using an inductance vest, found a decrease in ventilation and tidal volume in NREM compared to wakefulness with a further reduction in REM sleep.[25] Johnson and Remmers studied the accessory respiratory muscles and concluded that, during REM, loss of inspiratory activity of ribcage muscles causes chest-wall distortion (as measured by RIP changes in rib-cage and abdominal excursion) and hypoventilation in severe COPD patients.[13]

The $Paco_2$ increases during sleep in COPD, as shown by Pierce and colleagues who found a 6.6 mmHg rise in Pco_2.[26] Koo and associates using spot tests of blood gases reported that the greatest increase in Pco_2 during sleep was 8.3 (± 4.4) mmHg compared to wakefulness with the Pco_2 increasing by 4 to 5 mmHg during NREM and another 4 to 5 mmHg during REM sleep.[16] Coccagna and Lugaresi found $Paco_2$ increased 3 to 5 mmHg in NREM sleep and about 8 mmHg in REM.[27] Catteral and coworkers found a 4.2 mmHg rise in Pco_2 in sleeping COPD patients who had hypoxemia while awake.[20] Measuring transcutaneous Pco_2 in a group of severe COPD patients, Goldstein and colleagues found only minor elevations of Pco_2 (maximum 6 mmHg) during sleep regardless of whether the patient breathed air or oxygen.[28] Thus, the weight of the evidence using either indirect measures of ventilation or changes in Pco_2 suggests that hypoventilation does occur in COPD during sleep but the magnitude is variable.

Ventilation-Perfusion Mismatching

A decrease in FRC during sleep could result in worsening ventilation perfusion imbalance in the COPD patient and contribute to the hypoxemia observed during sleep. Using uncalibrated magnetometers, Muller and associates showed a decrease in the end expiratory lung volume during REM in healthy subjects and in young patients with cystic fibrosis.[29] Findings consistent with intercostal muscle and diaphragm hypotonia were also measured with surface electromyography during REM in this and other studies.[30] These findings suggest that FRC decreased. Hudgel and colleagues demonstrated a decrease in end expiratory lung volume during REM in patients with COPD.[25] They have also measured FRC during sleep in healthy individuals using a helium dilution method and confirmed a small decrease in FRC.[31] Thus, a change in FRC with sleep is likely, and this change is maximal during REM.

Findlay and co-workers have shown that the most important determinant of hypoxemia for healthy individuals deliberately holding their breath is the initial lung volume.[32] For a given breath-hold time, the lower the starting lung volume the greater the oxygen desaturation. The extrapolation for COPD patients is that the lower the FRC the more likely they are to develop hypoxemia.

Previously quoted studies have shown a larger fall in arterial Po_2 than rise in Pco_2 during sleep. It has therefore been suggested that the worsening gas exchange is due to worsening ventilation-perfusion matching, i.e., an increase in units with low ventilation-perfusion ratios.[16] Such suggestions are based on the assumption of steady-state conditions, so that oxygen uptake, carbon dioxide output, ventilation, cardiac output, and gas concentrations in mixed venous blood and inspired gas are all constant. Under those conditions, a change in ventilation with an increase in alveolar and arterial carbon dioxide produces a decrease of similar magnitude in PaO_2. Not all requirements for steady-state analysis are present in sleep. Indeed, during non–steady-state conditions, an acute reduction in ventilation (as in breath-holding) causes decreases in PaO_2 that are much larger than changes in PCO_2. Because of the very large body stores of carbon dioxide, sudden hypoventilation results in a slow rise in $PaCO_2$.

Cardiac output has been measured by two groups in REM and NREM sleep. Catterall and associates[20] and Fletcher and Levin[33] found no significant difference in the mean cardiac output on NREM compared with REM. However, there was considerable variation, and some patients obviously had an increase in their cardiac output. These authors found a significant fall in directly measured arterial venous oxygen content differences, suggesting that cardiac output did increase in REM sleep. From similar measurements including blood respiratory exchange ratio values, Fletcher and colleagues suggested that the shunt fraction increased during REM sleep.[34] However, their calculations depended on the assumption of steady-state gas exchange, which is unlikely with the transient period of disturbed ventilation during REM sleep. Thus, episodes of hypoxia without comparable carbon dioxide retention are due to transient hypoventilation as much as due to changes in ventilation-perfusion matching. Until methods are developed to quantitate accurately the shunt component (and alveolar ventilation) continuously during non–steady-state conditions of REM sleep, the relative contribution of each of these mechanisms will remain unknown.

Breathing Patterns

While hypoventilation alters ventilation-perfusion matching and contributes to a lower FRC, none of these changes occur in isolation, and they are influenced further by the pattern of breathing. There are difficulties with assessing the impact of breathing pattern on the degree of sleep hypoxemia. This is a result of differences in patient selection among investigators and also imprecise terminology. Guilleminault and associates reported that obstructive sleep apnea was responsible for most of the hypoxemia in 21 of the 26 patients with COPD whom they studied. It is important to note that these patients were very obese and selected on the basis of excessive daytime sleepiness. As such, they were not representative of the typical COPD patient. None had an FEV_1 of less than 1 L and 12 of the 26 had an $FEV_1 > 2$ L![35]

Both obstructive sleep apnea and COPD are common disorders, so it is not unexpected that both might occur in the same individual. This has been seen in other studies but not to the same degree as Guilleminault and associates reported, because their patients were being evaluated for COPD. Douglas and Coworkers report one out of 10 patients had both obstructive sleep apnea and COPD.[19] One of the patients reported by Wynne had episodes of obstructive apnea.[36] Of the 10 patients reported by Arand and colleagues, one had obstructive sleep apnea, while three had partial upper airway obstruction manifested as snoring.[37] These three had large swings in intrathoracic pressure and changes in SaO_2, sleep state, and heart rate similar to those seen in classic sleep apnea. Those patients had significant episodes of desaturation that were short and repetitive and that were seen in all sleep stages. This clearly differentiates them from the usual patient with COPD in whom prolonged, severe desaturation occurs primarily in REM sleep.

It is worthwhile and important to reassess patients with both disorders, after treatment of the obstructive apnea, since treatment of the sleep apnea may not be sufficient to abolish nocturnal hypoxemia. Fletcher and Brown have studied 11 patients with both obstructive sleep apnea (OSA) and moderate COPD (FEV_1 55% of predicted value). Before treatment, the nocturnal oxygen profile was of a typical OSA patient with frequent desaturations in both NREM and REM. Following tracheostomy, the obstructive apneas were abolished and the oxygen profile resembled that of a typical COPD patient with desaturations predominantly in REM.[38]

There are changes in breathing patterns during REM when hypoxemia is most obvious. However, the definitions of apnea, hypopnea, and periodic breathing are not standardized among investigators and often cause some confusion about the breathing pattern contribution to sleep hypoxemia.[39] Hypopnea is variously defined as a decrease in oronasal airflow or respiratory effort (rib-cage and/or chest-wall motion). Some have included oxygen desaturation of > 4% as a necessary condition for defining hypopnea, thus biasing results towards the association of breathing patterns and hypoxemia.[40] It is clearly preferable, therefore, to define hypopnea in terms of volume and timing.

There is limited information on the pattern of breathing in patients with COPD during REM sleep. Skatrud and Dempsey[40] reported hypopnea in three patients during REM. Their definition of hypopnea included oxygen desaturation. They found a reduced contribution of the rib cage to tidal volume that was 48% while awake and fell to 34% and 19% during tonic and phasic REM, respectively. They felt these changes reflected loss of tone in the intercostal and accessory respiratory muscles as part of the general loss of muscle tone in REM. Johnson and Remmers extended this and have shown conclusively that, with the onset of REM sleep, there is almost complete loss of EMG activity in the anterior scalene and sternomastoid muscles.[13]

The authors of this chapter have found differences in oxygenation in phasic and tonic REM in patients with COPD (oxygenation is lower during phasic than tonic REM).[41] In association with the phasic REM episode, there was a change in breathing pattern more than 75% of the time. This was most often with a sudden decrease in amplitude and increase in frequency with the onset of the phasic REM and a subsequent return to baseline values over the extended episode of phasic REM.[42] In addition, Catterall and associates found hypopnea (defined as at least 50% reduction in rib-cage motion for 10 seconds or longer) during 75% of all hypoxemic episodes during REM.[20] While there was no obvious breathing pattern irregularity in the other 25% of REM hypoxemic episodes, abnormalities in abdominal motion may account for the hypoxia. Their group found that the incidence of abnormal breathing patterns in COPD was not different from that of healthy subjects. These results were similar to those reported in chronic mountain sickness patients, in whom there was a detectable breathing pattern abnormality 25% of the night compared to 22.6% in controls. Yet, only the chronic mountain sickness patients desaturated significantly in sleep.[43] Thus, some patients become hypoxic when they develop the breathing pattern dysrhythmias of sleep seen in healthy individuals.

In summary, some normal irregularities occur in the breathing pattern during sleep along with changes in FRC and changes in the rib-cage and abdominal components of breathing. COPD patients have similar changes, but if they are hypoxemic during wakefulness, i.e., on the steep part of the oxygen-hemoglobin dissociation curve (Fig. 16–2), then these irregularities serve to produce marked decreases in SaO_2. Hypoxemia persists because of chemical drives blunted by disease and further attenuated by the sleep state. COPD patients become hypoxemic most severely during REM when drives are lowest and changes in the breathing pattern are most common.

CONSEQUENCES OF SLEEP HYPOXEMIA IN COPD

Cardiac Complications

Several years ago, Smolensky and colleagues reported that patients with COPD were most likely to die in the middle of the night.[44] Nocturnal cardiac arrhythmias or myocardial ischemia could be the explanation for this. Depending on the study reported, the incidence of arrhythmias in hypoxic COPD patients ranges from 30% to 100%. However, these are not a homogeneous group of patients and were often studied when they were acutely ill at a time when the incidence of arrhythmias is undoubtedly increased.[45–47]

Flick and Block found that cardiac arrhythmias occur more frequently at night in patients with COPD.[48] There are many factors that could contribute to arrhythmias such as medications (methylxanthines, beta adrenergic agents), degree of hypoxia, sleep stage, and the presence or absence of heart disease. Two studies have looked at the effect of nocturnal hypoxemia on ventricular ectopic activity. Tirlapur and Mir studied 12 patients, nine of whom had carbon dioxide retention.[49] All patients had transient hypoxemia defined as a fall in saturation > 10% that lasted for more than one minute. During these episodes, there was an increased rate of atrial and ventricular ectopic activity as well as some changes in the S-T segment in a few patients. These changes were largely alleviated with oxygen therapy. The difficulty with this study is that information is given on oxygen saturation and ventricular ectopy at hourly intervals and at those times when the oxygen saturation was low. However, the variability in ventricular ectopy at other times during the night is not known. A study by Shepard and associates reports on the relationship of ventricular ectopy to nocturnal oxygen desaturation in patients with moderate obstructive lung disease (FEV_1 42% of predicted value).[50] There was no significant relationship between ventricular ectopy and oxygen saturation, except in those patients who desaturated below 80%. However, their study did not address the effect of blood theophylline level, and although they did not look at specific sleep stages in NREM, there was no significant difference between the rates of ectopy in REM versus NREM sleep.

The authors of this chapter studied 16 patients with severe COPD (mean FEV_1 21% of predicted value) in an attempt to examine the effects of oxygen saturation, level of theophylline, and/or sleep stage on ventricular ectopy.[51] While the rates of ventricular ectopy varied between patients, there was no consistent difference between sleep stages. In addition, the level of arterial oxygenation, expressed as a mean for the stage, bore no relationship to the ventricular ectopy. When periods of ventricular ectopy were obvious (e.g., runs of bigeminy, trigeminy, couplets, or evidence of ventricular tachycardia), the oxygenation at the time of those arrhythmias was not significantly lower than the preceding period with no arrhythmia. The effect of blood theophylline level was studied in eight of the 16 patients, and although theophylline increased both the mean heart rates for each sleep stage and the oxygen saturation percent, the effect of theophylline on ventricular ectopy was variable. In those patients who initially had a very low level of ventricular ectopy, there was no clear pattern of change in arrhythmias. However, in those patients who had a high rate of ventricular ectopy, increasing their theophylline levels significantly increased the frequency of ventricular ectopy in each sleep stage. Overall, there is little correlation between sleep stage and instantaneous dips in oxygenation on rates of ventricular ectopic activity, and increasing theophylline levels has a variable effect on simple or complex arrhythmias.

In general, COPD patients have a resting tachycardia that is maintained during sleep. The tachycardia may be related to sustained hypoxemia since nocturnal oxygen therapy reduces the heart rate.[52] It is unclear whether heart rate in COPD changes with sleep stage per se or whether the heart rate changes with hypoxemic episodes. Arand and coworkers reported a slight reduction in heart rate during desaturations in COPD patients.[37]

Other ECG abnormalities have been observed in COPD patients including partial right bundle branch block, S-T segment depression, and lengthening of the Q-T interval. These abnormalities are probably related to SaO_2 saturation levels since oxygen therapy reverses several of them.[49] In general, patients with severe hypoxemia had much more improvement with oxygen than those with less hypoxemia. Thus, sustained sleep hypoxemia probably has a deleterious effect on the myocardium and conducting system.

Pulmonary Hypertension

During sleep, transient hypoxemia is associated with transient increases in pulmonary artery pressure, and since oxygen saturation is lowest during REM, it is not surprising that pulmonary artery pressure is highest then. Coccagna and Lugaresi[27] found that pulmonary artery pressure rose on average by 1.29 mmHg for each 1% fall in arterial saturation, which is very similar to that reported by Boysen and colleagues.[53] Because pulmonary artery pressure increases in response to changes in arterial PCO_2 and pH, these may also contribute to the changes in pulmonary artery pressure during REM sleep. However, the transient changes in SaO_2 and pulmonary artery pressure reported by Boysen and colleagues were probably too short in duration to have been associated with significant elevations in PCO_2. In addition, Coccagna and Lugaresi reported that the changes in pulmonary artery pressure in specific sleep stages correlated much better with PaO_2 than with PCO_2 or pH. The fact that oxygen therapy markedly reduces episodic pulmonary hypertension during sleep lends further support to the primary importance of oxygenation rather than carbon dioxide or pH in influencing the pulmonary artery pressure.

Repeated episodes of transient pulmonary hypertension during sleep have been suggested as promoting sustained pulmonary hypertension.[52] There is no direct evidence for this in humans. In one large series, mean pulmonary artery pressure was better related to mean nocturnal SaO_2, which was in turn closely related to awake SaO_2 than to the degree of desaturation during hypoxemic episodes.[22] However, a recent study by Fletcher and Levin demonstrated that chronic oxygen therapy improved nighttime oxygenation and minimized episodes of sleep hypoxemia in REM.[33] This was associated with a reduction in pulmonary artery pressure and pulmonary vascular resistance with no significant change in cardiac output. When these patients were taken off oxygen, their pulmonary artery pressure and pulmonary vascular resistance values were similar to those before the oxygen was administered. These results are compatible with the hypothesis that oxygen therapy causes regression of hypoxia-induced increase in vascular smooth muscle tension, which renders the pulmonary artery pressure very sensitive to further hypoxia.

Sleep Quality

Sleep quality refers to the amount of total sleep and how that sleep is distributed through the night. Unfortunately, there is no large single series that compares sleep quality in COPD patients and in similarly instrumented age- and sex-matched healthy individuals. Therefore, comparisons of sleep quality are made from data acquired by different laboratories, usually under different conditions. Accepting this limitation, sleep quality appears to be poor in patients with severe COPD.

Nocturnal sleep time is reduced in COPD patients, being only four to five hours per night. They also sleep less efficiently, with about one third of the night in bed spent not sleeping. This may be due to the fact that they often nap during the day, but this is only speculation. However, when compared with healthy individuals, the distribution of sleep stage expressed as percent of total sleep time is not statistically different.[17] This result stems from the large scatter in the normal sleeping population. Data from COPD patients can be found to cluster at one end of the normal distribution and, as such, are clearly different from the normal population. COPD patients have a reduced amount of REM sleep, an increased amount of light sleep, many arousals, a shortened duration of uninterrupted sleep, and very frequent sleep stage changes.

The cause of disturbed sleep is not clear. Fleetham and coworkers found that 40% of arousals were associated with dips in SaO_2.[17] However, increasing oxygenation by oxygen administration did not improve sleep or reduce arousal frequencies. Arousals were still associated with small dips in SaO_2. These decreases were minor so that arousals occurred at much higher levels of SaO_2, suggesting that arousals were not caused by hypoxemia per se but by associated phenomena, possibly hypercapnia or acidemia. This is consistent with the notion that hypoxemia is an unreliable arousal stimulus. Calverley and colleagues showed that the greater the number of hypoxemia episodes in a group of patients with severe hypoxemia while awake, the less perturbed the sleep.[18] In their study, a hypoxemic episode was defined as exceeding a minute with at least a 10% drop in SaO_2. They did not report arousal frequency. These investigators suggested that unstable sleep may be protective, preventing prolonged hypoxemia. In the same report, some measures of sleep quality in five out of six very hypoxemic patients were improved with oxygen administration, suggesting that hypoxemia may have disturbed their sleep originally. These results differ from those of Fleetham and coworkers but may be due to the more severe hypoxemia present in the patients of Calverley and colleagues. Sleep quality may differ with the degree of hypoxemia; the major arousal stimulant or factor disturbing sleep may be carbon dioxide in moderate hypoxemia, so arousal frequency would not be expected to decrease with oxygen therapy. On the other hand, with very severe hypoxemia and carbon dioxide retention during wakefulness, the hypoxemia may be an important arousal stimulus, so oxygen therapy might improve sleep.

Other factors may disturb sleep. Nocturnal cough is one such possibility. Power and associates have recently studied nocturnal cough in patients with chronic bronchitis and emphysema.[54] In 10 patients, there was a mean of 14.6 ($\pm$4.5 SEM) bouts of coughing per patient per night. Of these coughing bouts, 85% occurred during electroencephalographically confirmed wakefulness, and coughs during true sleep were rare—only one patient coughed during REM sleep and none during Stage 3 and Stage 4 sleep. Cough was only once followed by arousal, and there was no correlation between cough and either apneas or hypoxemia during sleep. It remains unclear whether such coughing impairs sleep quality.

Medications used to treat COPD such as methylxanthines may contribute to abnormal sleep. The authors have found that theophylline decreases the amount of REM sleep and increases light sleep (specifically Stage 2 sleep) but does not significantly change the total sleep time in patients with COPD.[42] Fleetham and colleagues report similar decreases in REM sleep but also found the total sleep time was decreased.[55]

Neuropsychiatric Impairment

Neuropsychiatric impairment might theoretically result from the very severe nocturnal hypoxia frequently observed in severe COPD. Although little clinical evidence supports this hypothesis, there is ample evidence that patients with severe COPD demonstrate neuropsychiatric abnormalities that are inversely related to the awake arterial oxygenation.[56] In one study, CNS abnormalities related better to daytime rather than to sleep oxygenation.[22] Continuous, rather than nocturnal, oxygen therapy has been shown to improve neuropsychiatric abnormalities.[57, 58] This suggests that sustained, rather than episodic (nocturnal), hypoxemia is more important in the development of these abnormalities.

TREATMENT OF SLEEP HYPOXEMIA IN COPD

Oxygen Therapy

There is no doubt that sleep hypoxemia can be prevented by nocturnal oxygen therapy, which has been shown in several studies. Tirlapur and Mir[49] administered 24% oxygen to 12 COPD patients—a dose that virtually abolished hypoxemic dips in patients with little daytime hypoxemia. In patients with more severe daytime hypoxemia, this oxygen dose ameliorated but did not prevent arterial oxygen saturations of $< 85\%$ during sleep in five out of seven patients. Douglas and associates administered oxygen at 2 L/min via nasal prongs to hypoxemic patients and found the lowest saturations of the night to be greatly increased.[19] The same group later administered oxygen at 2 L/min to six very hypoxic patients (mean awake oxygen saturation of 81%), which increased mean sleep SaO_2 from 53% to 90% (the lowest increased from 33% to 76%). Low flow oxygen significantly improves nocturnal hypoxemia but does not abolish it completely.

Better results can be obtained when oxygen dosage is individualized.[56] Patients were given a nocturnal oxygen flow of 1 L more than the lowest oxygen flow rate that increased resting awake arterial PO_2 to 65 mmHg. Using this guideline, mean sleep saturation was increased over 90% with the average lowest saturation of the night being $> 85\%$.

There were initial concerns that nocturnal oxygen therapy might produce severe carbon dioxide retention in COPD patients. However, these fears are unfounded because subsequent studies show very little increase in Pco_2 through the night in stable patients.[19, 24, 59, 60] Thus, nocturnal oxygen therapy is tolerated very well by COPD patients.

The effects of nocturnal oxygen administration on sleep quality have been systematically examined by two groups and reviewed above.[17, 18] The differences in results are probably related to the types of patients. In the study that showed improvement, all patients were hypercapnic, while in the other, which showed no improvement, the patients were not hypercapnic. The former group was apparently treated only with inhaled beta$_2$ sympathomimetic agents, while the latter was treated in addition with methylxanthines, which impair sleep quality.

Two trials have shown that long-term oxygen therapy in hypoxemic COPD patients can prolong life,[61] but at present, it is impossible to assess the therapeutic value of oxygen administered exclusively during sleep. The British MRC trial gave patients oxygen for at least 15 hours per day, including the hours of sleep.[61] Here, there was a better survival than with no therapy at all. In similar patients, the Nocturnal Oxygen Therapy Trial showed that mortality was lower when oxygen was administered for approximately 20 hours a day than when nocturnal oxygen therapy was given for 12 hours a day.[56] Although sleep oxygenation was worse during the daytime, correction of just the sleep hypoxemia produced less benefit than continuous oxygen therapy. Therefore, patients with COPD who are hypoxemic while awake, i.e., Pao_2 of 55 mmHg or less, should be treated with continuous oxygen. In these patients, specific sleep studies are not needed to make this decision since COPD patients with the most severe nocturnal hypoxemia are already hypoxemic while awake. There may be patients who are hypoxemic during sleep but not during wakefulness. If severe episodic nocturnal hypoxemia exists and obstructive sleep apnea can be ruled out, then nocturnal oxygen therapy should be prescribed, although there are no studies yet showing benefit from this approach.

DRUG THERAPY OF SLEEP HYPOXEMIA

There are several respiratory stimulant agents available that may ameliorate sleep hypoxemia in COPD, but there are no long-term clinical trials. Skatrud and colleagues evaluated medroxyprogesterone acetate (MPA) in five sleeping hypercapnic COPD patients who were selected because they had previously been shown to increase their awake ventilation in response to MPA.[62] MPA increased nocturnal ventilation and reduced $Paco_2$. Sleep Sao_2 also improved, with the greatest changes occurring in REM sleep. It is important to note, however, that this sleep stage was studied in only three patients. Dolly and Block assessed the effect of MPA in 19 patients with moderate COPD in a randomized double-blind trial.[63] MPA in awake patients was associated with an increased mean PaO_2, reduced $PaCO_2$, and increased pH. Although there was no significant change in the number of episodes of sleep apnea, hypopnea, desaturation, or lowest saturation during sleep, MPA marginally decreased the number of minutes of total sleep time when oxygen saturation was less than 90%. Most of these patients did not have significant carbon dioxide retention during the day, and only five had a carbon dioxide level > 45 mmHg, which may account for differences between investigators. In chronic mountain sickness, a disorder afflicting high-altitude residents who demonstrate waking hypoxemia and hypoventilation with worsening hypoxemia during sleep, MPA has been shown to increase ventilation and improve sleep oxygenation and has been an effective form of chronic therapy.[43] Thus, it is not known at present what the value of MPA in sleep hypoxemia in patients with COPD may be. MPA may have a beneficial effect in selected patients with daytime carbon dioxide retention who can voluntarily reduce their carbon dioxide level, but the numbers are too small to comment with certainty.

A carbonic anhydrase inhibitor, acetazolamide, has been evaluated in five sleeping hypercapnic COPD patients.[40] In three, there was a reduction of the sleep PCO_2 to normal, but arterial PO_2 had a mean increase of 9 mmHg in all five of these carefully selected patients. There are no other studies with acetazolamide for improving sleep hypoxemia in COPD.

Almitrine stimulates peripheral chemoreceptors, specifically the carotid body, and thus increases ventilatory response to hypoxia in humans. It has been shown to increase ventilation in COPD patients during the waking state.[64] Connaughton and coworkers have recently studied the effects of almitrine using a double-blind placebo-control crossover study in 9 patients with severe irreversible airways obstruction (FEV_1 < 1 L), daytime hypoxemia (PaO_2 < 60 mmHg), and hypercapnia ($PaCO_2$ > 45 mmHg).[65] They found that almitrine improved arterial blood gas tensions while awake and also improved nocturnal oxygen saturation with the mean rising from 83% ($\pm$ 4%) to 89% ($\pm$ 3%), and the lowest SaO_2 during sleep increased from 65% to 77%. Also, the time spent below 80% was reduced from 135 to 46 min. They concluded that almitrine improved arterial gas tensions when awake and reduced the frequency and severity of nocturnal hypoxemia without impairing sleep quality, and that the improvement in nocturnal oxygen saturation was related to a higher position on the oxygen-hemoglobin dissociation curve when awake. In the resting state, almitrine increases pulmonary artery pressure when studied in patients with hypoxia and hypercapnia caused by chronic bronchitis and emphysema.[66] The effects of orally administered almitrine on the pulmonary vascular response during sleep in humans is unknown. Any increase in oxygen saturation may be offset by potential increases in pulmonary vascular resistance, and so the usefulness of this drug awaits further studies.

References

1. Moruzzi G: Active processes in the brain stem during sleep. *Harvey Lect* 58: 233–297, 1963.

2. Berthon-Jones M, Sullivan CE: Ventilatory and arousal responses to hypoxia in sleeping humans. *Am Rev Respir Dis* 1982; 125:632–639.

3. Berthon-Jones M, Sullivan CE: Ventilation and arousal responses to hypercapnia in normal sleeping humans. *J Appl Physiol* 1984; 57:59–67.

4. Bradley CA, Fleetham JA, Anthonisen NR: Ventilatory control in patients with hypoxemia due to obstructive lung disease. *Am Rev Respir Dis* 1979; 120:20–21.

5. Douglas NJ, White DP, Weil JV, et al: Hypoxic ventilatory response decreases during sleep in man. *Am Rev Respir Dis* 1982; 125:286–289.

6. Douglas NJ, White DP, Weil JV, et al: Hypercapnic ventilatory response in sleeping adults. *Am Rev Respir Dis* 1982; 126:758–762.

7. Gothe B, Goldman MD, Cherniack NS, et al: Effect of progressive hypoxia on breathing during sleep. *Am Rev Respir Dis* 1982;126:97–102.

8. Reed DJ, Kellogg RH: Changes in respiratory responses to CO_2 during natural sleep at sea level and at altitude. *J Appl Physiol* 1958;13:325–330.

9. Sullivan CE, Kozar LF, Murphy E, et al: Arousal, ventilatory and airway responses to bronchopulmonary stimulation in sleeping dogs. *J Appl Physiol* 1979;47:17–25.

10. Sullivan CE, Murphy E, Kozar LF, et al: Waking and ventilatory responses to laryngeal stimulation in sleeping dogs. *J Appl Physiol* 1978;45:681–689.

11. Iber C, Bersenbrugge A, Skatrud JB, et al: Ventilatory adaptations to resistive loading during wakefulness and non-REM sleep. *J Appl Physiol* 1982;52:607–614.

12. Wilson PA, Skatrud JB, Dempsey JA: Effects of slow wave sleep on ventilatory compensation to inspiratory elastic loading. *Respir Physiol* 1984; 55:103–120.

13. Johnson MW, Remmers JE: Accessory muscle activity during sleep in chronic obstructive pulmonary disease. *J Appl Physiol* 1984;57:1011–1017.

14. Remmers JE, Anch AM, Degroot NJ: Respiratory disturbances during sleep. *Clin Chest Medicine* 1980;1:57.

15. Bateman JRM, Pavia D, Clarke SW: The retention of lung secretions during the night in normal subjects. *Clin Sci* 1978; 55:523–527.

16. Koo KW, Sax DS, Snider GL: Arterial blood gases and pH during sleep in obstructive lung disease. *Am J Med* 1975; 58:663–670.

17. Fleetham J, West P, Mezon B, et al: Sleep, arousals and oxygen desaturation in chronic obstructive pulmonary disease. *Am Rev Respir Dis* 1982;126:429.

18. Calverley PMA, Brezinova V, Douglas NJ, et al: The effect of oxygenation on sleep quality in chronic bronchitis and emphysema. *Am Rev Respir Dis* 1982;126: 206–210.

19. Douglas NJ, Calverley PM, Leggett RJ, et al: Transient hypoxemia during sleep in chronic bronchitis and emphysema. *Lancet* 1979;1:1–4.

20. Catterall JR, Douglas NJ, Calverley PMA, et al: Transient hypoxemia during sleep in COPD is not a sleep apnea syndrome. *Am Rev Respir Dis* 1983;128:24–29.

21. Conway WA, Kryger MH, Timms RM, et al: Hypercarbia predicts nocturnal desaturation in COPD. *Am Rev Respir Dis* 1982;125:100.

22. Conway WA, Kryger M, Timms RM, et al: Clinical significance of sleep desaturation in COPD. *Chest* 1982;82:237.

23. Fleetham JA, Mezon B, West P, et al: Chemical control of ventilation and sleep arterial oxygen desaturation in patients with COPD. *Am Rev Respir Dis* 1980; 122:583–589.

24. Gonzalez H, Haller B, Watson HL, et al: Accuracy of respiratory inductive plethysmograph over wide range of rib cage and abdominal compartmental contributions to tidal volume in normal subjects and in patients with chronic obstructive pulmonary disease. *Am Rev Respir Dis* 1984; 130:171–174.

25. Hudgel DW, Martin RJ, Capehart M, et al: Contribution of hypoventilation to sleep oxygen desaturation in chronic obstructive pulmonary disease. *J Appl Physiol* 1983; 55:669–677.

26. Pierce AK, Jarrett CE, Werkle G, et al: Respiratory function during sleep in patients with chronic obstructive lung disease. *J Clin Invest* 1966;45:631–636.

27. Coccagna G, Lugaresi E: Arterial blood gases and pulmonary and systemic arterial pressure during sleep in chronic obstructive lung disease. *Sleep* 1978;1:117–124.

28. Goldstein RS, Ramcharan V, Bowes G, et al: Effect of supplemental nocturnal oxygen on gas exchange in patients with severe obstructive lung disease. *N Engl J Med* 1984;310:425–429.

29. Muller NL, Francis PW, Gurwitz D, et al:

Mechanism of hemoglobin desaturation during rapid eye movement sleep in normal subjects and in patients with cystic fibrosis. *Am Rev Respir Dis* 1980; 121:463–469.

30. Tusiewicz K, Moldofsky H, Bryan AC, et al: Mechanics of the rib cage and diaphragm during sleep. *J Appl Physiol* 1977;43:600–602.

31. Hudgel DW, Devadatta P: Decrease in functional residual capacity during sleep in normal humans. *J Appl Physiol* 1984;57:1319–1322.

32. Findlay LJ, Ries AL, Tisi GM, et al: Hypoxemia during apnea in normal subjects: Mechanisms and impact of lung volume. *J Appl Physiol* 1983;55:1777–1783.

33. Fletcher EC, Levin DC: Cardiopulmonary hemodynamics during sleep in subjects with chronic obstructive pulmonary disease. The effect of short and long term oxygen. *Chest* 1984;85:6–14.

34. Fletcher EC, Gray BA, Levin DC: Nonapneic mechanisms of arterial oxygen desaturation during rapid eye movement sleep. *J Appl Physiol* 1983;54:632–639, 1983.

35. Guilleminault C, Cummiskey J, Motta J: Chronic obstructive airflow disease and sleep studies. *Am Rev Respir Dis* 1980;122:397–406.

36. Wynne JW, Block AJ, Hemenway J, et al: Disordered breathing and oxygen desaturation during sleep in patients with chronic obstructive lung disease. *Am J Med* 1979;66:573–579.

37. Arand DL, McGinty DJ, Littner MR: Respiratory patterns associated with hemoglobin desaturation during sleep in chronic obstructive pulmonary disease. *Chest* 1981;80:183–190.

38. Fletcher EC, Brown DL: Nocturnal oxyhemoglobin desaturation following tracheostomy for obstructive sleep apnea. *Am J Med* 1985;79:35–42.

39. George CF, Kryger MH: When is an apnea not an apnea? editorial. *Am Rev Respir Dis* 1985;131:485–486.

40. Skatrud JB, Dempsey JA: Relative effectiveness of acetazolamide versus medroxyprogesterone acetate in correction of chronic carbon dioxide retention. *Am Rev Respir Dis* 1983;127:405–412.

41. George CF, West P, Lertzman M, et al: Oxygenation in phasic and tonic REM in patients with chronic obstructive pulmonary disease. *Am Rev Respir Dis* 1985;131 (suppl):302.

42. George CF, West P, Kryger MH: Personal communication.

43. Kryger MH, Glas R, Jackson D, et al: Impaired oxygenation during sleep in excessive polycythemia of high altitude. *Sleep* 1978;1:3–17.

44. Smolensky M, Halberg F, Sargent F: Chronobiology of the life sequence, in Itoh S, Ogata K, Yoshimura H (eds): *Advances in Climatic Physiology.* Tokyo, Igaku Shoin Ltd, 1972, pp 281–318.

45. Corazza LJ, Pastor BH: Cardiac arrhythmias in chronic cor pulmonale. *N Engl J Med* 1958;259:862–865.

46. Holford FD, Mithoefer JC: Cardiac arrhythmias in hospitalized patients with chronic obstructive pulmonary disease. *Am Rev Respir Dis* 1973; 108:879–885.

47. Hudson LD, Kurt TL, Petty TL, et al: Arrhythmias associated with acute respiratory failure in patients with chronic airways obstruction. *Chest* 1973;63:661–665.

48. Flick MR, Block AJ: Nocturnal vs. diurnal cardiac arrhythmias in patients with chronic obstructive pulmonary disease. *Chest* 1979;75:8–11.

49. Tirlapur VG, Mir MA: Nocturnal hypoxemia and associated electrocardiographic changes in patients with chronic obstructive airways disease. *N Engl J Med* 1982;306:125–130.

50. Shepard JW Jr, Garrison MW, Grither DA, et al: Relationship of ventricular ectopy to nocturnal oxygen desaturation in patients with chronic obstructive pulmonary disease. *Am J Med* 1985;78:28–34.

51. George CF, West P, Kryger MH: Personal communication.

52. Block AJ: Dangerous sleep oxygen therapy for nocturnal hypoxemia. *N Engl J Med* 1982;306:166–167.

53. Boysen PG, Block AJ, Wynne JW, et al: Nocturnal pulmonary hypertension in patients with chronic obstructive pulmonary disease. *Chest* 1979;76:536–542.

54. Power JT, Stewart IC, Connaughton JJ, et al: Nocturnal cough in patients with chronic bronchitis and emphysema. *Am Rev Respir Dis* 1984;130:999–1001.

55. Fleetham JA, Fera T, Edgell G, et al: The effect of theophylline therapy on sleep disorders in COPD patients. *Am Rev Respir Dis* 1983 127(suppl):85.

56. Nocturnal Oxygen Therapy Trial Group. Continuous or nocturnal oxygen therapy in hypoxemic obstructive lung disease. *Ann Intern Med* 1980;93:391–398.

57. Brezinova V, Calverley PMA, Flenley DC: The effect of long-term oxygen therapy on the EEG in patients with chronic stable ventilatory failure. *Bull Eur Physiopath Resp* 1979;15:603.

58. Heaton RK, Grant I, McSweeny AJ, et al: Psychological effects of continuous and

nocturnal oxygen therapy in hypoxemic chronic obstructive pulmonary disease. *Arch Intern Med* 1983;143:1941.

59. Kearley RW, Wynne JW, Block, AJ, et al: Effects of low flow oxygen on sleep disordered breathing in patients with COPD. *Chest* 1980;78:682–685.

60. Leitch AG, Clancy LJ, Leggett RJE, et al: Arterial blood gas tensions, hydrogen ions and electroencephalogram during sleep in patients with chronic ventilatory failure. *Thorax* 1976;31:730–735.

61. Report of the Medical Research Council Working Party. Long-term domociliary oxygen therapy in chronic hypoxic cor pulmonale complicating chronic bronchitis and emphysema. *Lancet* 1981;1:681–685.

62. Skatrud JB, Dempsey JA, Iber C, et al: Correction of CO_2 retention during sleep in patients with chronic obstructive pulmonary diseases. *Am Rev Respir Dis* 1981;124:260–268.

63. Dolly FR, Block AJ: Medroxyprogesterone acetate and COPD. Effect on breathing and oxygenation in sleeping and awake patients. *Chest,* 1983;84:394–398.

64. Powles ACP, Tuxen DV, Mahood CB, et al: The effect of intravenously administered almitrine, a peripheral chemoreceptor agonist, on patients with chronic airflow obstruction. *Am Rev Respir Dis* 1983;127:284–289.

65. Connaughton JJ, Douglas NJ, Morgan AD, et al: Almitrine improves oxygenation when both awake and asleep in patients with hypoxia and carbon dioxide retention caused by chronic bronchitis and emphysema. *Am Rev Respir Dis* 1985;132:206–210.

66. MacNee W, Connaughton JJ, Hayhurst MD, et al: The effects of almitrine on pulmonary arterial pressure and right ventricular performance in chronic bronchitis and emphysema. *Respiration* 1984;46:157–158.

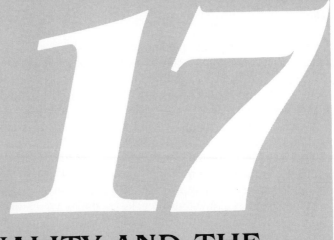

SEXUALITY AND THE COPD PATIENT

PAUL A. SELECKY

Comprehensive care of the patient with chronic obstructive pulmonary disease (COPD) is a complex process that should address all of the patient's needs. The primary focus of care is generally directed at the respiratory function of the patient and includes prescribing appropriate medications and attempting to improve bronchial hygiene.

As with any patient with a chronic disease, the needs of the total patient must be taken into consideration. For the modern health care provider, this includes understanding how the disease affects the patient's sexuality and helping to solve any problems that may arise as a result of an impairment. In order to fulfill that charge, it is important to have an understanding of the broad concept of sexuality as well as the effects of both the aging process and lung disease on this integral part of the patient's life.

SEX VERSUS SEXUALITY

For many, a discussion of a patient's sexual nature immediately brings to mind specific functions, principally the ability to participate in intercourse. It is more productive for the health care provider to focus on a broader concept that considers the total person. The term "sexuality" conveys this message and conjures up a complex process involving body, mind, and soul, i.e., the patient's personality and value system as well as his or her bodily functions.

The term "sex" has many meanings, e.g., gender, role, emotion, or physical pleasure that, depending upon one's frame of reference at the moment, may lead to miscommunication and confusion. It most commonly brings to mind physical functions and actions, usually genital. Genitality is an integral part of our sexuality, but it is a narrow focus.

Intimacy is another ingredient of our sexuality and an important human need and function. It implies closeness, warmth, and affection. It implies a relationship that is special, personal, and sometimes very private. Moreover, intimacy can take many forms of physical expression from the loving glance and tender touches to the physical intimacy of sexual intercourse.

Our sexuality, therefore, speaks to the power and meaning of being sexual, being a man or woman, being masculine and feminine. It is also a relational term implying interaction with others on all levels of our human function. In brief, sexuality has been wisely described as something you are, not just something you do.

SEXUALITY IN LATER LIFE

Modern marketing and entertainment practices have drawn our thinking of sexuality into a narrow physical focus. As a result, a discussion of sex and sexuality is often limited to the young and beautiful and excludes the elderly. Images of an elderly couple may bring to mind feelings of warmth and closeness generally associated with grandparents, but the physical aspects of their sexuality are often ignored or avoided and may conjure up feelings of awkwardness and humor. We hear ill-conceived references to the "dirty old man" and the "funny-looking old lady." The health care provider must identify and attempt to change such attitudes.

Patients with COPD are most often in their sixties or older. Younger patients with asthma generally do not need professional support or treatment regarding their sexuality.

Clinical experience with many COPD patients has revealed that the difficulties they may have with sexuality are often linked to the normal aging process. Everyone expects and tolerates the skin wrinkles, the loss of hair, the slowing of pace and energy associated with aging, but only in recent years has the popular press begun to address the effect of aging on sexuality.

Care for the older patient with COPD should be based on the thesis that sexuality lasts a lifetime. There should be no regimented expectations about the sexual performance or attitudes of the elderly. The significance that sexuality plays in later life should simply be considered an extension of past experiences in addition to the normal aging process, health changes, and sometimes the lack of a partner.[1] As a senior citizen might comment, "Elderly people stop having sex for about the same reason they stop riding a bicycle—they think it may look ridiculous, they're too tired, or they don't have a bicycle."[2]

The effect of the aging process on sexual function is often just a slowing of physical activity with little change in attitude. People who are sexually active as younger persons can be expected to be less active as they get older, whereas people who are relatively less active as younger persons may become inactive in later life.

Studies at the Duke University Center for the Study of Aging and Human Development revealed a decrease in the frequency of sexual intercourse in later life, but noted that over 75% of men and 33% of women in the seventh decade of life were sexually active, having intercourse at least once a month.[3] These statistics do not necessarily reflect a decrease in sexual interest because they are partly influenced by the loss of a spouse, which impacts more commonly on the female.[3, 4] The increasing frequency of second marriages later in life and changing attitudes are likely to alter these statistics, but sometimes create new problems. A poignant example is illustrated in the following letter to columnist Abigail van Buren:

DEAR ABBY: This is the second marriage for both of us, and I haven't the courage to face my family and friends and admit that it was a mistake. I feel like I'm just a cook, housekeeper and sex partner whenever my husband is in the mood. I'm starved for some real affection. All he wants is a five-minute sex affair with no hugging, kissing or sweet words. When we first met he was passionate, and insisted on going all the way on our second date. I should have known he wasn't a real lover—that all he wanted was sex.

I am 74 and he is 80, and we've been married for five years . . . . We appear to be an ideal couple. If we were to divorce, our children would be shocked and our pastor would be surprised . . . . I just know that I would be so much happier if I didn't have to keep putting up a front. What should I do?

                                                                    MADE A MISTAKE

DEAR MADE: "All the world's a stage," and this is no dress rehearsal, so don't worry about what your friends, family or pastor will say. Tell your husband where he has disappointed you. If he wants a chance to win you by changing his ways, give him a limited probation period. And if he doesn't shape up—ship him out. Life is too short.

                                                      (*Los Angeles Times*, 9/22/83)

LUNG DISEASE AND SEXUALITY

In addition to the aging process, the symptoms of progressive COPD can have an impact on sexual function, but the data is controversial. A study by Fox and Light of male COPD patients at the Long Beach VA Hospital revealed no correlation between sexual activity and FEV_1.[5] Over half of those men labeled as having severe respiratory impairment still described themselves as sexually active. As expected, there was some correlation between their exercise tolerance and the amount of sexual activity, but no correlation was noted between lung function and the incidence of specific sexual dysfunctions, i.e., impotence, premature ejaculation, or decreased desire.

On the other hand, a study by Fletcher and Martin of a slightly younger group of patients at the Oklahoma City VA Medical Center suggested that sexual dysfunction worsened as lung disease worsened.[6] They also noted an association between impotence and pulmonary impairment. Semple and colleagues have suggested that this may be related to an observed decrease in the serum testosterone level compared with an age-matched control group.[17] A correlation between testosterone level and the degree of hypoxemia was also noted.

Regardless of the effect of physiologic dysfunction on sexual performance, the health care provider can readily understand the impact of the chronicity of the disease process on the patient's sexuality. Characteristically, the disability of COPD often makes patients feel depressed and have poor self-esteem. They tire easily, notice decreased energy, and generally fear that any physical activity may aggravate their dyspnea.

The male patient in particular may feel his manliness threatened. He is often no longer the breadwinner and has difficulty performing routine household activities such as carrying groceries and doing chores. This feeling is then aggravated by the unwelcomed difficulty in achieving and maintaining erections. This may be the result of the natural aging process, but it further compounds his fear of failure as a sexual partner.

The female patient with COPD often senses a loss of her femininity. She perceives her chronic cough and sputum production as being unattractive, and she suffers further embarrassment by episodes of urinary incontinence during coughing. This loss of self-esteem causes her to become discouraged and depressed. She begins to use less makeup, and she is often too tired to groom herself, which can result in a self-perpetuating downhill cycle.

Some may also be struggling with the "empty-nest syndrome" if their children have moved away or are busy raising families of their own. This may further accentuate feelings of being useless and unneeded. As one can see, these circumstances provide a fertile field for the attention and skills of the health care provider.

SEXUAL PROBLEMS

Dr. Mary Calderone defined a sexual problem as "the malfunction of part of an individual's organism or life in such a way as to cause his sexual life to appear to him unrewarding or inadequate, or to be potentially harmful

Table 17–1. **Types of Sexual Dysfunctions**

1. Inhibited sexual desire.
2. Inhibited sexual arousal, e.g., impotence in men and decreased lubrication or vasocongestion in women.
3. Inhibited orgasm.
4. Other problems, e.g., premature or retarded ejaculation in men and dyspareunia or vaginismus in women.

to another individual and therefore to himself."[8] This broad approach to the understanding and treatment of sexual problems or dysfunction is particularly suited to those who minister to the needs of the COPD patient. Most of us are not trained or experienced in the treatment of sexual dysfunctions, but all can orient our skills to provide general support and direction for many of the general sexual problems in this patient population. Specific sexual dysfunctions can be identified, but these are often best treated by referring the patient to the appropriate specialist. Some of the more common dysfunctions are listed in Table 17–1.

ROLE OF THE HEALTH CARE PROVIDER

There are many settings in which the health care provider can help COPD patients with problems concerning their sexuality. The physician has ready access during the many meetings with the patient, both in the office and in the hospital. The pulmonary nurse specialist, respiratory therapist, physical therapist, and social worker often have personal interactions with the COPD patient as a part of the respiratory care program and can be a ready ear and source of information. This is particularly productive in a formal pulmonary rehabilitation program, where sexuality can be addressed in an organized fashion. Ideally, any interaction with patients and their families or significant others may provide an opportunity for discussing sexuality.

Many of us do not see ourselves in the role of sex counselor or advisor, feeling that our training and experience is limited or nonexistent. Dr. Jack S. Annon has described a model for sexual counseling that may ease our anxieties.[9] He recommends providing sexual information and advice in a progressive fashion according to the needs of the patient and the ability of the health care provider. It is a four-step process described as the PLISSIT model (Table 17–2). Dr. Howard Kravetz has aptly applied it to the COPD patient[10] and has developed accompanying patient education materials.[11, 12]

Table 17–2. **PLISSIT Model of Sexual Counseling**

1. P = Permission-Giving
2. LI = Limited Information
3. SS = Specific Suggestions
4. IT = Intensive Therapy

Table 17–3. **Permission-Giving (P)**

1. Introduce the subject of sexuality.
2. Convey acceptance by your body language and words.
3. Use open-ended questions.
4. Avoid medical terms and slang words.
5. Avoid labeling patients' attitudes and behavior.
6. Be a good listener.

Step 1: Permission-Giving

This is an important first step in helping patients with problems or fears concerning their sexuality. It creates an opportunity for communication, giving permission to patients to have sexual feelings and thoughts, sexual fantasies, and to regain or strengthen their masculinity and femininity. Further, it gives patients permission to talk about sex if they want to. Clinical tips are listed in Table 17–3.

It may help to introduce the subject of sexuality when interacting with the patient. This can be accomplished by routinely including questions on sexual activities and feelings while taking the patient's history. The physician can do this during the patient evaluation. Some basic principles of taking a sexual history are listed in Table 17–4.[13]

The pulmonary nurse specialist or respiratory therapist can introduce the subject during the admission interview for the pulmonary rehabilitation program. Information about sexuality can also be included in the patient questionnaire, which perhaps should be filled out by both the patient and spouse, either together or separately. Some rehabilitation programs include sexuality in the list of patient education lectures. The topic can also be presented to a patient support group, e.g., Better Breathers Club.

Regardless of the method, we should convey acceptance of the patient's attitudes and practices by what we say and do. We should try to be relaxed and comfortable and perhaps matter-of-fact when addressing sexuality with the patient. It is important to examine our own attitudes first in order to avoid passing judgment on the patient through our nonverbal and occasionally verbal messages. This often requires a conscious effort, including paying attention to our body language.

Table 17–4. **Basic Principles of Taking a Sexual History**

1. Be comfortable and at ease.
2. Establish empathy with the patient.
3. Your values should not affect the interview.
4. Interview skills improve with knowledge.
5. Use precise and tactful questions.
6. Approach emotionally charged subjects gradually.
7. Progress from learning to attitudes to behavior.
8. If necessary, state that a sexual behavior is common.

In other words, it's not only what you say but also the look on your face that tells the patient how you feel. Strive to create an atmosphere that says "sex can be spoken here." You might attempt open-ended questions, avoiding those that can be answered by a simple yes or no, e.g., "How does your breathing affect your lovemaking?" or "What questions do you have concerning the effect of your pulmonary problem on your sexual activity?"

In your responses to the patient, avoid complicated medical terms. Minimize the use of words such as "coitus," "libido," and "impotence." Choose everyday words that you feel comfortable with, such as "making love," "sexual desire," "difficulty having an erection," or words that the patient uses. Try to use positive-sounding words and avoid slang. Above all, don't make offhand teasing remarks such as "You're too old," or "What a way to go." They are not humorous and will likely cut off communication.

At the very least, work at being a good listener. Maintain eye contact, nod in approval, and be a mirror to the patient's feelings. Assume that the patient is anxious and attempt to put him or her at ease. Insuring the confidentiality of your discussion can be a big help. Be sure that others are not within earshot, and don't speak too loudly. Choose a time when you can approach the patient alone or with only the spouse present. Be professional but also interested and approachable.

The general process of permission-giving may be enhanced by providing the patient the opportunity to review educational materials concerning sexuality. A number of them are available from private and public organizations, as well as other sources.[11, 12, 14, 15]

Not every COPD patient feels the need or inclination to discuss sexuality with a health professional. We must remember that many of our patients' attitudes stem from those of another generation that may not have discussed this subject openly. It may be difficult for them to discuss such intimate matters with anyone, let alone a relative stranger, especially if he or she is single and of the opposite sex. Moreover, the patient's interest and concern may be nil. We must avoid being overzealous.

Step 2: Limited Information

Once the opportunity for discussion has been created, the patient may decide to pursue the subject further. This may be what the interviewer fears most if he or she is unprepared to answer the patient's questions. As in many

Table 17–5. **Limited Information (LI)**

1. Describe sexuality as involving the total person.
2. Explain the expected changes of aging.
3. Dispel fears and myths.
4. Indicate that the physiologic stress of lovemaking is limited.
5. Review the possible effects of medications.
6. Encourage discussion with the partner or spouse.

Table 17–6. **Effects of Aging on the Sexual Response**

Men
1. Erections may be slower to achieve and may require more stimulation.
2. Erections may not be as firm.
3. Time to ejaculate may be longer.
4. Amount or force of ejaculation may be less.
5. Refractory time to next ejaculation may be longer.

Women
1. Vagina may decrease in length or width.
2. Vagina may become less elastic.
3. Onset of vaginal lubrication may be slower.
4. Amount of vaginal lubrication may be less.
5. Uterine spasms may occur during intercourse.

aspects of health care, it is advisable to be prepared at least on a limited basis (Table 17–5).

Attempt to broaden the patient's focus. Emphasize that sexuality is more than just a genital function and is part of the total person, involving body, mind, and soul. Explain that sexuality is also how a person thinks and feels, not just what he or she does. Take time to understand and accept the patient's attitudes and beliefs as well. Avoid comments such as "That's silly," or "Don't feel that way." Try not to impress your own attitudes on the patient.

Involve the patient's partner as much as possible (with the patient's permission). He or she is also probably facing the aging process, has fears and anxieties, may feel depressed, and has lost self-esteem. In addition, the partner may be afraid of hurting the patient's feelings or, worse, aggravating breathing problems by what he or she says or does. Both may be focusing attention only on their genital function and often can be helped by developing a broader understanding of their relationship. You might point out that a sexual relationship has been aptly defined as one that includes a partner who gives and receives pleasure and that it is more than orgasm, has many expressions, is not dependent on physical ability, and involves the total person.[16]

Included in the list of items of limited information is to describe the normal and expected effect of aging on the sexual response of both men and women (Table 17–6).[17, 18] This often aids in easing patients' concerns that they are too old or that there is something wrong with them. They also should be led to understand that the physiologic stress of sexual intercourse is not severe for most patients. They should be told to expect some shortness of breath, some increase in heart rate, and some degree of fatigue but that these responses are unlikely to be overwhelming. Those with severe lung impairment should perhaps be more cautious. Patients who have coexisting ischemic heart disease may fear that sexual intercourse can lead to death from a heart attack and may be reassured by the knowledge that this is rare.[19]

Patients often have questions about the effect of medications on their sexual function. The male suffering from impotence may be particularly

Table 17–7. **Possible Effects of Medications on Sexual Performance**

1. Sympathomimetics: urinary retention.
2. Theophyllines: no direct effect.
3. Corticosteroids: no direct effect.
4. Antihypertensives: decreased libido and impotence.
5. Sedatives: decreased libido and impotence.
6. Cimetidine: decreased libido and impotence.
7. Digoxin: decreased libido and impotence.
8. Antibotics: vaginal thrush.

interested in knowing whether any medications prescribed for his lung disease are aggravating his sexual problem. As a general rule, the majority of pulmonary medications have little effect on sexual performance. Categories of drugs often used by COPD patients are listed in Table 17–7. More complete lists can be found in the referenced texts.[20, 21]

Step 3: Specific Suggestions

Once you have begun discussing the general impact of aging and lung disease on sexuality, patients may begin to ask specific questions about their sexual function. On the other hand, we also must accept and understand patients who have decided to be sexually inactive. Many widows or widowers and divorced persons choose to remain celibate, and we must respect their decisions. Well-meaning suggestions that the patient consider seeking a sexual partner may be offensive. An alternative might be to point out that older people have a variety of sexual beliefs and practices, indicating that the patient has a choice and that it is largely a personal decision.

For those who are sexually active, specific suggestions might be offered to ease their dyspnea and any other respiratory discomfort that they may experience during sexual activity (Table 17–8). A detailed sexual history may be needed to make your suggestions more meaningful.

Many solutions involve just a common-sense approach. The interviewer might help patients arrive at their own solutions by asking apropriate questions, such as "What do you think might ease some of the shortness of breath you have during lovemaking?" The answers might motivate patients to be sure

Table 17–8. **Specific Suggestions (SS) for Lovemaking**

1. Create a conducive atmosphere.
2. Avoid times when fatigued or upset.
3. Choose the "best breathing time."
4. Avoid alcohol or a heavy meal prior to lovemaking.
5. Use bronchodilators and oxygen in a timely fashion.
6. Start slowly and gradually work up.
7. Sexual intercourse and climax are not necessary goals.
8. Consider sexual pleasuring exercises.
9. Choose less strenuous body positions.
10. Use your imagination.

they are rested and not already dyspneic before participating in lovemaking. You might point out the benefits of daytime sexual activity, choosing a time when their breathing is the best. This might be in the middle of the day, timed according to the effects of medications and breathing treatments. Working spouses might respond to the suggestion by arranging an occasional visit home at lunchtime or during the early afternoon for lovemaking. For those patients dependent on supplemental oxygen during physical activity, wearing the oxygen cannula with appropriate adjustments in the oxygen flow rate may be helpful during lovemaking.

The patient should be cautioned about attempting sexual intercourse after a heavy meal, which may bring on fatigue and somnolence. In addition, some patients experience increased dyspnea with a full stomach. Alcohol should be avoided as well, especially by men who have difficulty achieving and maintaining an erection.

Patients should be advised to broaden their understanding of lovemaking and to avoid what psychologist Mary Ann Sviland calls the "touchdown mentality," indicating that it is not necessary to "score" every time.[22] Sexual intercourse and climax should not necessarily be the goal. Quality, not quantity, should be stressed. Many couples enjoy just being close, cuddling, and sharing intimate caresses—sometimes proceeding to intercourse, sometimes not.

The couple might also benefit from suggestions of less strenuous positions for sexual intercourse[23] or that the spouse be the active partner. Others might be interested in learning specific sexual pleasuring exercises (caresses).[24] It is important to realize that this is a personal and private part of the patient's life, and the interviewer must proceed slowly and cautiously. The specific suggestions or SS component of this counseling model might also be called *sensitive suggestions*.

Step 4: Intensive Therapy

Some patients with COPD have sexual problems that may improve with specific therapy. The majority of problems that confront the respiratory care practitioner can be resolved with the above steps, but he or she should be familiar with possible solutions for specific dysfunctions and be prepared to refer those patients for appropriate therapy. These might take several forms, as identified in Table 17–9.[25, 26] Discerning the nature of the patient's problem and making an appropriate referral require some professional skill, which the

Table 17–9. **Intensive Therapy (IT)**

1. Marriage counseling.
2. Urologic or gynecologic evaluation.
3. Psychiatric counseling.
4. Sex therapy.

respiratory care practitioner may want to develop with appropriate training and education. It is wise to identify resources in the community for the diagnosis and treatment of these disorders.

SUMMARY

Those of us who care for patients with COPD should examine our interest, ability, and willingness to address the subject of sexuality with our patients. Once we have accepted this responsibility, it is important to review and increase our knowledge about normal and abnormal sexual functioning. More importantly, our own attitudes about sexuality and sexual behavior should be evaluated and understood, as they are likely to affect our patients.

Our focus should be broad, approaching the patient as a total person—not just sex but sexuality, not just genital function but feelings and attitudes.

We might best approach the patient's needs in a step-wise fashion. At the very least, we should provide the opportunity for the patient to discuss the subject or to remain silent. If the patient is receptive, we can explain the expected effects of aging and the change in lung function on lovemaking and make suggestions if there is a problem. We should help patients in their decision making by being supportive, providing encouragement, and making appropriate suggestions and referrals to meet their needs.

References

1. Pfeiffer E: Sexual behavior in old age, in Busse EW, Pfeiffer E (eds): Behavior and Adaptation in Late Life, ed. 2. Boston, Little, Brown & Co, 1977, pp 130–141.
2. Comfort A: Sexuality and aging. SIECUS Rep 1976;4(6):1–9.
3. Pfeiffer E, Verwoerdt A, Davis GC: Sexual behavior in middle life. Amer J Psych 1972;128:1262–1267.
4. Pfeiffer E: Sexuality in the aging individual. J Amer Ger Soc 1974;22:481–484.
5. Fox LS, Light R: Physiological correlates of sexual performance capacity in the male pulmonary patient. Symposium on Sexual Counseling in the Patient with Chronic Lung Disease. Annual Meeting, American Thoracic Society, Los Angeles, May 18, 1982.
6. Fletcher EC, Martin RJ: Sexual dysfunction and erectile impotence in chronic obstructive pulmonary disease. Chest 1982; 81:413–421.
7. Semple PD, Brown TM, Beastall GH, et al: Sexual dysfunction and erectile impotence in chronic obstructive pulmonary disease, letter. Chest 1983;83:587–588.
8. Calderone MS: Sexual problems in medical practice. J Amer Med Wom Assoc 1968; 23:140–146.
9. Annon JS: Brief Therapy, in The Behavioral Treatment of Sexual Problems. Honolulu, Enabling Systems, 1974.
10. Kravetz HM, Weiss M, Meadows R: Sexual Counseling for the Male Pulmonary Patient (slide-tape program). Prescott, AZ, Howard M Kravetz, MD, 1980.
11. Kravetz HM: A Visit with Harry (slide-tape program). Prescott, AZ, Howard M Kravetz, MD, 1981.
12. Kravetz HM: A Visit with Helen (slide-tape program). Prescott, AZ, Howard M Kravetz, MD, 1982.
13. Lief HI, Berman EM: Sexual interviewing throughout the patient's cycle, in Lief HI (ed): Sexual Problems in Medical Practice. Monroe, WI, American Medical Association, 1981, pp 119–129.
14. Butler RN, Lewis MI: Love and Sex after Sixty: A Guide for Men and Women for Their Later Years. New York, Perennial, 1976.
15. Lobsenz NM: Sex After Sixty-Five. (Public Affairs Pamphlet #519) Public Affairs Committee, Inc, 381 Park Avenue South, New York, NY 10016, 1975.
16. Tibballs SC: Sexual counselling in COPD. Symposium on Sexual Counselling in the Patient with Chronic Lung Disease. An-

nual Meeting, American Thoracic Society, Los Angeles, May 18, 1982.

17. Croft LH: *Sexuality in Later Life: A Counseling Guide for Physicians*. Boston, John Wright, 1982, pp 47–64.

18. Kolodny RC, Masters WH, Johnson VE: *Textbook of Sexual Medicine*. Boston, Little, Brown & Co, 1979, pp 103–116.

19. Papadopoulos C, Beaumont C, Shelley SI: Myocardial infarction and sexual activity of the female patient. *Arch Intern Med* 1983;143:1528–1530.

20. Buffum J, Smith DE, Moser C, et al: Drugs and sexual function, in Lief HI (ed): *Sexual Problems in Medical Practice*. Monroe, WI, American Medical Association, 1981, pp 211–242.

21. Kolodny RC, Masters WH, Johnson VE: *Textbook of Sexual Medicine*. Boston, Little, Brown & Co, 1979, pp 321–352.

22. Sviland MAP: Helping elderly couples attain sexual liberation and growth. *SIECUS Rep* 1976;4(6):3–4.

23. Della Bella L: Sexuality and the pulmonary patient, in Hodgkin JE, Zorn EG, Connors GL (eds): *Pulmonary Rehabilitation*. Boston, Butterworth, 1984, pp 239–262.

24. Hartman WE, Fithian MA: Treatment of Sexual Dysfunction: A Bio-Psycho-Social Approach. Long Beach, CA, Center for Marital and Sexual Studies, 1972.

25. Levay AN, Sharpe L: Sexual dysfunction: Diagnosis and treatment, in Lief HI (ed): *Sexual Problems in Medical Practice*. Monroe, WI, American Medical Association, 1981, pp 141–158.

26. Kolodny RC, Masters WH, Johnson VE: *Textbook of Sexual Medicine*. Boston, Little, Brown & Co, 1979, pp 587–600.

18

PREOPERATIVE EVALUATION AND PERIOPERATIVE CARE

WILLIAM F. MILLER

Patients with chronic obstructive pulmonary disease (COPD) may require surgical treatment but, because of their lung disease, are usually at increased risk for cardiorespiratory complications that may result in not only increased morbidity but increased mortality as well. Careful evaluation alerts the physician to the presence and severity of various risk factors and provides the opportunity to initiate measures to reduce the risk of serious problems or, at least, to help the patient cope with the problems that may arise.

Risk is a function of many variables that involve the patient, the operation, the surgeon, the anesthesiologist, and the postoperative care staff. Many aspects of these matters have been reviewed recently.[1]

This subject is presented here in three parts. First, the physiologic consequences of the anesthetic-surgical procedure. Secondly, the current status of preoperative evaluation of risk factors. Finally, the pertinent aspects of perioperative care.

RESPIRATION DURING ANESTHESIA

Anesthesia for surgical procedures and endotracheal intubation for control of the airway are more than 100 years old, and pulmonary complications

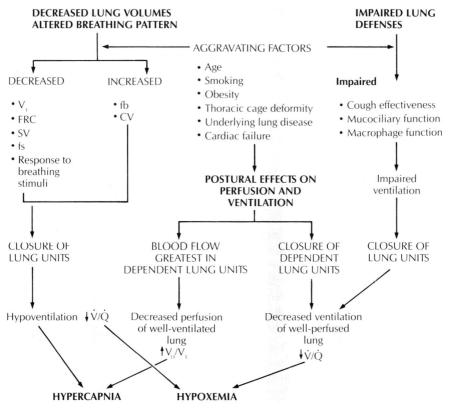

Figure 18–1. Simplified inter-relationships of anesthesia and perioperative complications. Tidal volume (V_T), functional residual capacity (FRC), sigh volume (SV), sigh frequency (fs), breathing frequency (fb), closing volume (CV), wasted ventilation fraction (V_D/V_T), and ventilation-perfusion ratio ($\dot{V}/\dot{Q}$).

have been known all this time. Although mechanical ventilation during surgery was introduced 86 years ago, it wasn't until about 40 years ago that physiologic assessment of the respiratory consequences of the conditions associated with general anesthesia and surgery began to receive attention. The historical aspects of anesthesia and surgery are reviewed elsewhere.[2] The effects of anesthesia have been reviewed specifically in terms of current physiologic concepts.[3] There is no evidence that anesthesia per se causes significant perioperative complications. The practical straightforward interrelationships are summarized in Figure 18–1. There are three primary effects: (1) decreased lung volumes and altered breathing pattern, (2) impaired lung defenses, and (3) postural effects on ventilation and perfusion.

The studies on the effects of posture per se have been reviewed by Tyler.[1] The decrease in volume and increase in perfusion of dependent segments are emphasized.

The fact that pulmonary functional changes were associated with the intraoperative period, even in normal subjects, was recognized as early as 1908 by W. Pasteur. Churchill and McNeil in 1927 as well as Beecher in

1933 made limited functional assessment of intraoperative changes. Further definition of functional changes had to await the development of improved functional methods.

Studies by Wu and colleagues in 1956 were the first to show comprehensive changes under general anesthesia including: a progressive decrease in compliance, a variable increase in resistance, and an increase in breathing frequency and minute ventilation with a decrease in tidal volume.[4] These changes were accompanied by a decrease in Pa_{O_2} and an increase in Pa_{CO_2} secondary to changes in distribution of ventilation and closure of lung units associated with lung volume changes.

These studies were followed by the specific lung volume measurements in humans by Anscombe in 1958 and the studies of Mead and Collier in 1959 on dogs, wherein the role of deep breathing and lung expansion was clearly demonstrated to reverse many of the effects of posture and anesthesia. This was subsequently confirmed in humans by Ferris and Pollard in 1960.[5] Further blood gas studies were not reported until 10 years later by Diament and Palmer. The many reports of postoperative complications following abdominal and thoracic surgery serve to substantiate the great importance of the integrity of the pulmonary system during this period.

Decisions concerning anesthetic-surgical risk should be based on all available information with respect to the risk-benefit ratio. Risk factors have been discussed at length by Tisi in a recent review.[6]

Those risk factors related to the patient include: (1) most importantly, the presence of lung or thoracic cage disease, especially the presence of active airways disease; (2) the presence of heart disease, especially coronary artery disease or heart failure; (3) severe obesity, especially with concomitant physical deconditioning or muscle weakness; (4) advanced age, i.e., over 70 years of age with concomitant physical deconditioning or muscle weakness; (5) habitual tobacco smoking; and (6) the poorly defined, but very important, factor of general mental and physical status. General physical conditioning and muscle strength are likely to be associated with a good cough, early mobility, and ambulation. Mental status has received some attention but not nearly enough. Experienced physicians are aware of the fact that the outgoing, mentally tough patient with a positive outlook does better under most kinds of stress. Methods of evaluation are not well established or widely available for clinical practice.

The presence of any of the problems listed above would justify pulmonary function assessment because any of them might affect the integrity of ventilatory function. This would be especially true if the patient were to undergo a prolonged intra-abdominal or thoracic operation.

PREOPERATIVE EVALUATION

A careful history and physical examination is mandatory and yields clues with respect to many of the elements discussed above. Additional points that

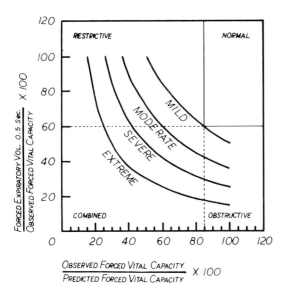

Figure 18–2. Quadrant system for grading ventilatory defects. (From Miller WF, Wu N, Johnson RL Jr: Convenient method of evaluating pulmonary ventilatory function with a single breath test. *Anesthesiology* 1956;17:480–493, by permission.)

should receive attention include: (1) any systemic disease that could lead to problems during and after the high stress period of anesthesia and surgery; (2) a current or recent (less than six weeks) acute illness, especially pulmonary infection; and (3) major life changes in the past year and, even more importantly, the patient's physical and mental reaction to them. This includes any previous episodes of general anesthesia or surgical procedures.

The value of pulmonary function tests for assessing operative risk first received major impetus from the studies of Ed Gaensler, a Boston thoracic surgeon. In 1955, Gaensler and associates found that half of their patients undergoing pneumonectomy, who had maximal breathing capacities (later identified as maximal voluntary ventilation or MVV) of < 50% of predicted and forced vital capacities (FVC) of < 70% of predicted, died following the procedure.[7] In spite of the lack of specificity of this test (since 50% of the patients lived), the possible role of pulmonary function tests received considerable attention. There was no discussion of the relation of functional changes to morbidity.

The next year, the author and colleagues introduced a quadrant system based on the observed forced expiratory volume at 0.5 seconds ($FEV_{0.5}$), the observed forced vital capacity (FVC), and the predicted forced vital capacity (PVC) for grading ventilatory defects (Fig. 18–2). We studied 24 subjects prior to general anesthesia and abdominal surgery in an attempt to identify the high ventilatory risk patient. The quadrant system was widely adopted and sometimes adapted inappropriately to our data. In the original study, patients who sustained significant postoperative pulmonary complications, in spite of aggressive pulmonary care, constituted a group of patients considered at increased risk. This was based on the ratio of $FEV_{0.5}$ to PVC values, which ranged between 0.15 and 0.25 and showed evidence of carbon dioxide retention. This level of change was considered indicative of severe ventilatory risk. Patients with more impaired functions were not subjected to elective surgery for multiple reasons, but not because of the ventilatory impairment alone. Unfortunately, the term "prohibitive" was used to describe their risk. We no longer think this term is appropriate and suggest "extreme ventilatory risk" instead. The identification of this level of impairment is intended to warn the anesthesiologist and surgeon that special attention must be paid to the patient's respiratory system, especially when tracheal intubation and general anesthesia are used. The patient probably should return to the recovery room with the endotracheal tube in place and on ventilatory assistance until it is determined that his or her ventilatory status is adequate.

Several authors have tried to modify this system by substituting the more widely used FEV_1. The author and colleagues found the $FEV_{0.5}$ a better predictor, probably because, as part of the early expiratory flow from total lung capacity, it relates better to the effectiveness of the cough mechanism. Our data for FEV_1 do not entirely agree with those of other authors with respect to definition of risk for reasons that are not apparent. Table 18–1 is our definition of degree of risk for FEV_1 compared to $FEV_{0.5}$ based on the relationship of FEV_1 to $FEV_{0.5}$.

In a study of the operative risk in patients undergoing thoracic surgery, Mittman in 1961 found that patients who were < 40 years of age had normal electrocardiograms and who had maximal breathing capacity > 50% of predicted, exhibited a mortality rate of no more than 5%; whereas those with abnormal electrocardiograms and maximal breathing capacity < 50% of predicted had a mortality rate of 71%.

In 1962, Stein and colleagues recommended a multiple function approach to assess perioperative risk, based on FVC, FEV_1, forced expiratory flow between 200 ml and 1200 ml of the forced vital capacity ($FEF_{200-1200}$), single breath nitrogen index, RV/TLC, and Pa_{CO_2} estimated by a rebreathing test. Only 3% of the patients who had normal values for all these measurements had a pulmonary complication postoperatively. On the other hand, 70% of those with one or more abnormal functions had significant pulmonary complications. This scheme, like others, lacked specificity. Moreover, the $FEF_{200-1200}$ cannot be used to evaluate the same mechanical factors of venti-

Table 18–1. **Definition of Degree of Risk**

Degree of Risk	$FEV_{0.5}$/PVC*	FEV_1/PVC†
Normal	≥ 0.50	≥ 0.64
Mild	0.35 to < 0.50	0.45 to < 0.64
Moderate	0.25 to < 0.35	0.30 to < 0.45
Severe	0.15 to < 0.25	0.20 to < 0.30
Extreme	< 0.15	< 0.20

*Observed $FEV_{0.5}$/predicted FVC
†Observed FEV_1/predicted FVC

lation in all subjects because fixed volume parameters have different significance in persons of different lung volumes owing to morphometric determinants. The first quarter forced expiratory flow ($FEF_{0-25\%}$) is the preferred test. For instance, a patient with restrictive disease and no air flow disturbance has an FVC of 1200 ml (60% of predicted); the early expiratory flow as indicated by $FEF_{0-25\%}$ is 3.4 L/sec (100% of predicted), whereas the $FEF_{200-1200}$ is 0.5 L/sec, which is very abnormal. Similarly, small normal persons have abnormally low $FEF_{200-1200}$ values with normal $FEF_{0-25\%}$ values. Thus, $FEF_{200-1200}$ values must be interpreted very cautiously because, even if there were adequate reference standards, this test would assess different mechanical factors in different patients.

In 1973, Lockwood proposed an even more elaborate system of evaluation based on multiple functions. Statistical limits were evolved for functions that would divide patients into four categories of risk for postoperative complications. The limits defining his low-risk and the very high-risk categories are listed in Table 18–2. Patients who exceed the limits of low risk in all three Group I functions or three of the five Group II functions are considered average. On the other hand, patients who exceed the limits of the very high-risk category for all three Group I functions or three of the five Group II functions are at significantly above-average risk.

Lockwood emphasized that this system alone could not determine who was fit for thoracic operations and that other physiologic assessment as well as clinical evaluation is ultimately necessary to determine this, which could be said for any single test. Furthermore, when values are proposed to define limits, absolute milliliter values should not be used. Measures should be expressed as a percentage of a predicted reference level specific for age, sex, and size. Values lower than those listed in the low-risk column could be 100% of predicted for small older women, and some of these values could be as low as 50% of predicted for large younger men. These data cannot be

Table 18–2. **Anesthetic-Surgical Risk Assessment Limits for Patients Undergoing Resectional Lung Procedures***

Function	Low-Risk Limit	Very High-Risk Limit
GROUP I		
FVC (L)	< 3.33	< 1.70
FEV_1 (L)	< 2.23	< 1.20
MVV (L/min)	< 77.5	< 35% FVC
GROUP II		
MVV (L/min)	< 77.5	< 28.0
RV (L)	> 1.54	< 3.30
TLC (L)	> 5.08	> 7.90
RV/TLC (%)	> 30.0	> 47.0
N_2 mixing time (sec)	>108.0	>265.0

*From the data of Lockwood P: The principles of predicting the risk of post-thoracotomy-function related complications in bronchial carcinoma. *Respiration* 1973;30:329–344, by permission.

Table 18–3. **Anesthetic-Surgical Risk Assessment***

Function	Low Risk	Moderate Risk	High Risk
Pa_{CO_2} (mmHg)	45–49	50–55	> 55
Pa_{O_2} (mmHg)	61–70	50–60	< 50
$FEF_{200-1200}$ (L/sec)	1.67–3.33	0.83–1.66	< 0.83
MVV (% predicted)	51–75	33–50	< 33
FEV_1 (L)	0.5–1.0	0.3–0.49	< 0.3
FVC (L)	1.0–1.5	0.6–0.9	< 0.6

*Adapted from Ayers LN, Whipp BJ, Ziment I: Preoperative evaluation, in *A Guide to Interpretation of Pulmonary Function Tests*, New York, Roerig Pfizer Pharmaceuticals, 1975.

related to reference levels without a definition of the restricted population from which they were obtained.

In 1969, Gerson reported a study of 61 patients who were candidates to have lung resection for bronchogenic carcinoma and found that of the conventional forced spirometric tests, the peak flow (FEF_{max}), and the FEV_1/FVC ratio were the most useful indices of mortality and morbidity. The $FEF_{0.5}$ was not measured, but the FEF_{max}, a component of $FEV_{0.5}$, also relates well to the effectiveness of cough. However, as a measure, the FEF_{max} is very effort-dependent and more variable.

In 1971, Boushy and associates investigated a multifactorial analytic approach for 142 patients with bronchogenic carcinoma. They found that changes in FEV_1, $FEF_{25-75\%}$, RV, FRC, and MVV all correlated with increased risk. In 40% of the patients over 60 years of age, an FEV_1 of < 2.0 L was accompanied by increased mortality. Again, no measure of early expiratory flow was made, and the limitations of absolute values should be remembered.

The effects of tobacco smoking were recognized as early as 1939 when Morton demonstrated in a three-year study of 1267 adult cases that the risk of complications in smokers is six times that of nonsmokers. Moreover, the complications in smokers were noted to be associated with more serious constitutional disturbances.

Ayers and coworkers summarized the literature and presented a multiple-function basis for classifying risk as low, moderate, or high (Table 18–3). It is impossible to reconcile these values, which appear to be low, with Lockwood's, which seem high (see Table 18–2). As previously pointed out, the limitations of the $FEF_{200-1200}$ does not measure the same mechanical properties of persons at the extremes of morphometric characteristics and age.

Gracey and associates, in a study of 157 patients with COPD, report difficulty in determining which patients would develop pulmonary complications among those who did not require mechanical ventilation. However, the group that requires mechanical ventilation postoperatively could be predicted on the basis of the type of operation and $FEF_{25-75\%}$ and MVV values of < 50% of predicted. A sputum volume > 60 ml also indicated increased risk. Their study and the earlier one by Veith and Rocco emphasize the importance of preoperative airway clearance in relation to risk of postoperative pulmonary complications.

Arterial blood gas studies are valuable in assessing the probable need for supplemental oxygen or mechanical ventilation but are of little value for determining risk. When the ventilatory indicators such as FEF_{max}, $FEV_{0.5}$, FEV_1, and $FEF_{25-75\%}$ are severely impaired, gas exchange is usually, but not necessarily, significantly impaired. Even though the author knows of no systematic evaluation, an expired air analysis that indicates a very high wasted ventilation fraction ($VD/VT \geq 0.6$, with CO_2 retention) should be significantly related to increased operative risk in patients undergoing procedures known to impair ventilation and circulation the most.

Resectional lung surgery brought with it the need to assess regional lung function and to assess the risk of postoperative respiratory failure. Cardiac catheterization studies (in which the artery to the lung to be resected is occluded by an inflatable balloon on a catheter) have suggested that a poor prognosis for pneumonectomy can be predicted when the mean resting pulmonary artery pressure (PAP) exceeds 25 mmHg. Further, if the PAP exceeds 35 mmHg or the Pa_{O_2} falls below 45 mmHg during exercise with the balloon occluded, the prognosis for successful pneumonectomy was very poor. Unfortunately, these techniques have not been systematically compared to other less invasive techniques.

Bronchospirometry was originally used to estimate the effect of pneumonectomy on breathing capacity. Rogers and colleagues proposed extension of the principle of split-function assessment to a method using radioactive ^{133}Xe as a more convenient and less invasive approach. The details of these techniques have been discussed in a recent state-of-the-art review by Wagner.[9] In essence, the method involves measurement of FVC, FEV_1, or MVV preoperatively, then the postoperative function values are estimated by multiplying the fraction of ventilation or perfusion estimated from the radioisotope scans to represent the remaining lung postresection.[10] Arborelius has described a special formula for estimating postoperative function from this method. However, the accuracy of such estimates hardly justifies the complexity of the method.

Recent studies suggest that, as the remaining function falls below 40% of normal (approximately 800 ml for FEV_1 in adult males), the prognosis for successful resection becomes increasingly poor, and when the estimated remaining function falls below 25% of normal, the prognosis was found to be grave.

Risk defined by these methods places emphasis on pulmonary problems. Reichel described in 1972 a noninvasive approach using exercise to assess both cardiac and pulmonary function. Patients who were able to complete a 12-minute graded treadmill walk, starting at 2.0 miles per hour (mph) and increasing to 3.0 mph at a 7.5% grade, tolerated pneumonectomy without complication.

Cardiac risk can be evaluated by the nine-point multifactorial cardiac risk index of Goldman and associates (Table 18–4). "Risk points" are used to classify cardiac risk on a scale of I to IV as follows: I = Mild (0 to 5 points);

Table 18–4. **Nine-Point Multifactorial Cardiac Risk Index***

Factors in Order of Discriminatory Value	Risk Points (see text)
1. S_3 gallop or jugular vein distention	11
2. Myocardial infarction in past 6 months	10
3. Abnormal rhythm or PACs on ECG	7
4. More than 5 PVC/min on ECG	7
5. Age over 70 years	5
6. Emergency operation	4
7. Significant aortic valve stenosis	3
8. Surgery (intrathoracic or intraperitoneal)	3
9. Poor general medical condition†	3

*Adapted from Goldman L, Caldera DL, Nussbaum SR, et al: Multifactorial index of cardiac risk in noncardiac surgical procedures. *New England Journal of Medicine* 1977;297:845–850.

†$Pa_{O_2} < 60$ mmHg, $Pa_{CO_2} > 50$ mmHg, $K^+ < 3.0$, $HCO_3^- < 20$ mEq, BUN > 50, creatinine > 3.0, and SGOT elevated for bedridden patient.

II = moderate (6 to 12 points); III = severe (13 to 25 points); IV = extreme (26 or more points).

Bronchospirometry studies by Bergan in 1952 revealed that when a person is moved from the supine to lateral position, the functional residual capacity (FRC) increases because of the increase in the volume of the up lung. The increase is greatest in a normal lung and is invariably proportional to the impairment of the ventilation-perfusion ratio in the respective lung. Another approach to assessing the impact of unilateral disease was the lateral position test. DeMeester and coworkers in 1974 found the test statistically inferior to radionuclide ventilation-perfusion scans, and Jay and colleagues in 1980 demonstrated further that the variability in this test limits its usefulness.

PERIOPERATIVE CARE

Those patients with active pulmonary problems that impair functional capacity or pulmonary clearance must be considered candidates for preoperative treatment whenever possible. The nature and duration of treatment vary with the problems presented by the patient and the time available.

Dripps and Deming in 1946 reported a very impressive experience with 1240 patients undergoing intra-abdominal surgery. Preoperative therapy reduced the incidence of postoperative atelectasis and pneumonia from 11% in the untreated group to 4% in the treated group.

The author and associates in 1957 re-emphasized the use of preoperative functional evaluation and respiratory therapy in patients with obstructive airways, detailing what are essentially the current approaches in principle; only the technology has changed. Bartlett and coworkers in 1973 discussed treatment with emphasis on deep-breathing maneuvers with incentive devices.

To the author's knowledge, the only current prospective study demonstrating the value of preoperative preparation was done in 1979 by Gracey and associates.[8] This study was very limited in its scope, since only 48-hour preoperative therapy was used consisting of aerosol isoproterenol (a very short-acting bronchodilator) four times a day supplemented by 200 mg of oral aminophylline four times a day. A small amount of guaifenesin (15 ml) was given three times a day along with three quarts of fluids per day. The latter is helpful if the patient is dehydrated or likely to become dehydrated during the intraoperative period, but there is no evidence that this has any effect on secretions that have already accumulated and inspissated in the airways. Nevertheless, significant reduction in postoperative complications was demonstrated—19% in the treated group compared with 40% in previously untreated groups, even though this brief period of treatment did not significantly change ventilatory function.

There has been no systematically controlled study evaluating the various specific modalities widely used for the perioperative therapy. The measures that have been described are directed at airway clearance and attempts to improve pulmonary function. The methods involve vigorous bronchodilator and bronchial hygiene therapy including, wherever possible, respiratory physical therapy with deep breathing, chest percussion, and postural bronchial drainage as well as exercise.

The main concerns are the presence of one or more of the following problems: (1) unstable or hyperreactive airways disease, especially if frequent use of glucocorticosteroids is necessary, (2) productive or nonproductive persistent cough, (3) evidence of active infection with abundant purulent sputum, (4) history of heavy cigarette smoking or air pollution exposure, and (5) subacute or chronic physical deconditioning or weakness.

The methods available for improvement of airway clearance with pharmacologic and respiratory therapy have been detailed in Chapters 7 and 8 of this book and by Miller and Geumei.[11] Patients who are moderate or greater risks should be given the maximum period reasonably available for treatment to achieve optimal control of the factors listed above and, wherever possible, reduction of the risk factors, including abstinence from smoking. When surgery is an emergency, therapy should be instituted immediately with appropriate bronchodilator therapy, especially with emphasis on aerosol agents and glucocorticosteroids, if the patient has been on steroids in the past. Usually, 40–50 mg of prednisolone every six to 12 hours for 24 to 48 hours is quite adequate. Ventilation and lung volume is protected as much as possible. Arterial blood gases are monitored to determine the need for supplemental oxygen and mechanical ventilatory assistance.

When time is available, vigorous effort should be made to maximize the patient's state of physical conditioning, especially if the patient is a moderate to severe risk and likely to be on the ventilator postoperatively.

INTRAOPERATIVE CARE

Maintenance of adequate humidification and avoidance of excessive use of anticholinergic agents are sometimes necessary to prevent the inspissation of airway secretions. Adequate deep airway suctioning can be facilitated by instillation of small amounts (2–5 ml at a time) of saline as needed.

The presence of purulent secretions should prompt a culture of an aspirated specimen for culture and the institution of an appropriate antibiotic, which could be selected on the basis of the sputum smear and the Gram stain.

The prophylactic parenteral administration of a gastric histamine H-2 antagonist and metoclopramide to enhance gastric emptying and increased lower esophageal sphincter tone has been found effective in decreasing risk of gastroesophageal reflux and aspiration. This is especially important in those patients who have an increased incidence of this problem that is aggravated by the bronchodilator and glucocorticosteroids.

The importance of maintaining lung volume inflation during the intra-operative period has been well substantiated not only in minimizing the physiologic impairment resulting from anesthesia and the operative procedure but also in reducing postoperative atelectasis and respiratory gas exchange impairment.[4, 5] If patients are unable to maintain adequate gas exchange as reflected by arterial blood gas assessment, then mechanical ventilation should be instituted and sustained into the postoperative period. This step should probably be instituted immediately in extreme-risk patients with marginal maximal inspiratory pressure of < 30 cm H_2O, especially if increased work of breathing during the intraoperative period can be anticipated, as in obese persons or patients with fever. Also, early supported ventilation is indicated when ventilatory drive is inadequate because of sedation or problems of cerebral circulatory insufficiency.

In the high-risk patient, especially with known airways instability, regular aerosol bronchodilator of a short-acting agent, such as isoproterenol or isoetharine, should be delivered every one to three hours during the intra-operative period via metered-dose inhalers, one to four inhalations via an in-line or side-arm delivery into the patient's breathing circuit. This should be given with ventilatory assistance so that a deep breath can be initiated and an inspiratory hold of 10 seconds is possible. During prolonged procedures with high gas flow anesthetic techniques, supplemental humidifaction via an in-line nebulizer or vaporizor is desirable to prevent drying of secretions in the patient known to produce > 60 ml. of sputum per day.

POSTOPERATIVE PERIOD

The key to a successful postoperative period free of serious complications is the maintenance of adequate lung expansion, uniformly adequate alveolar ventilation, and good clearance of the airways. These conditions can be monitored by assessment of arterial blood gases and ventilatory capacity indexes such as: maximum inspiratory pressure, FVC, and $FEV_{0.5}$ or FEV_1. Careful auscultation of the chest and evaluating a chest x-ray film in full inspiration (a tube-to-cassette distance of six feet) helps to localize problems.

When patients can be aroused early in the postoperative period and can effectively cooperate with deep breathing and airway clearance, they should be extubated, mobilized, and a program of deep breathing and airway care instituted. The respiratory therapy procedures should be as intense as necessary, depending on the severity of the problems the patient presents. Bland mist therapy should be considered for patients with obstructive disease postextubation. Heated mist is effective and better tolerated than unheated mist by patients with hyperirritable airways.

Regular aerosol bronchodilator therapy can be given unassisted when the patient is able and willing to take deep inhalations. When the patient cannot or will not take deep breaths, ventilatory assistance is appropriate. However, arbitrary reimbursement policies based on generalizations rather than selective physiologic criteria often determine the therapy used.

In small women, the incidence of postextubation laryngeal spasm and edema is quite frequent. We have found that a prophylactic aerosol of racemic epinephrine, 0.5 cc in 4 cc saline, and 1 cc (10 mg) triamcinolone acetonide repeated once in three to four hours has virtually eliminated this problem. Institution of helium oxygen as a gas to administer the above aerosol is extremely effective in preventing re-intubation of patients with laryngeal spasm and edema.

Patients who are being monitored with many tubes and wires are often kept immobilized on their backs, in which case basal segment atelectasis is almost inevitable. The treatment for this easily correctable problem is adequate patient mobilization with deep breathing.

A very common problem in patients with severe obstructive disease that creates major difficulties is tachypnea and airtrapping. Coughing, pain, anxiety, and uncontrolled deep breathing may precipitate such episodes. Inappropriate and improperly used ventilatory assistance can precipitate or aggravate airtrapping, which can lead to marked impairment of gas exchange due to exaggerated ventilation-perfusion imbalance, pulmonary hypertension, and decreased cardiac output resulting from alveolar overdistension. Such episodes are often not recognized as being primary, and thus, control of breathing is not involved as essential management. This can be a major factor interfering with ventilator withdrawal.

When patients cannot be extubated promptly because of inadequate gas exchange or inadequate ventilatory capacity, mechanical ventilation must be continued until the patient can achieve a level of gas exchange compatible with either preoperative values or anticipated postoperative ventilatory capacity. If a patient is known to have a preoperative, stable optimum Pa_{CO_2} of ≥ 50 mmHg, it is not reasonable to maintain the Pa_{CO_2} below that level on the ventilator. Similarly, if patients maintain a Pa_{O_2} on room air of 50 mmHg under stable optimal conditions preoperatively, they cannot be expected to do any better postoperatively. Thus, if the patient can achieve ventilatory capacity criteria of maximum inspiratory pressure ≥ 20 cm H_2O, FVC ≥ 15 mg/kg, and $FEV_1 \geq 10$ ml/kg or $FEV_{0.5} \geq 7$ ml/kg, extubation and removal from mechanical ventilation can proceed. The exception would be the patient who had preoperative stable optimal values that were no better or less than those indicated by these criteria. In this situation, the patient could not be expected to achieve such a goal, and the maximum inspiratory pressure and FVC with evidence of clinical stability would be relied upon as a basis for discontinuing intubation and mechanical ventilation.

When postoperative mechanical ventilation is indicated, a spontaneous breathing circuit should be provided with a so-called intermittent mandatory ventilation system (IMV) to avoid the risk of aggravated airtrapping that occurs if COPD patients are allowed to cycle the ventilator at will. The arguments that IMV systems increase the work of breathing apply only if the systems are set up improperly. The contention that IMV systems are more expensive is unjustifiable.

Most definitely, patients with COPD should not be ventilated to Pa_{CO_2} levels below their usual clinically stable level because this only makes the withdrawal from mechanical ventilatory assistance more difficult, if not impossible. When ventilator withdrawal is attempted, breathing control and avoidance of airtrapping are critical to success.

References

1. Proceedings of Vail Conference on Perioperative Care, Respir Care, 1984;(5, 6).
2. Knapp RB: The Gift of Surgery to Mankind. A History of Modern Anesthesiology. Springfield, IL, Charles C Thomas, 1983.
3. Gelb AW, Southorn P, Rehder K: Effect of general anesthesia on respiratory function. Lung 1981;159:187–198.
4. Wu N, Miller WF, Luhn NR: Studies of breathing in anesthesia, Anesthesiology 1956;17:696–707.
5. Ferris BG Jr, Pollard DS: Effect of deep and quiet breathing on pulmonary compliance in man, J Clin Invest 1960;39: 143–149.
6. Tisi Gennaro M: Preoperative evaluation of pulmonary function. State of the Art. Am Rev Respir Dis 1979;119:293–310.
7. Gaensler EA, Cugell DW, Lindgren I, et al.: The role of pulmonary insufficiency in mortality and invalidism following surgery

for pulmonary tuberculosis, J Thorac Surg 1955;29:163–187.
8. Gracey DR, Divertie MB, Didier EP: Preoperative pulmonary preparation of patients with chronic obstructive pulmonary disease. Chest 1979;76:123–129.
9. Wagner HN Jr: The use of radioisotope techniques for the evaluation of patients with pulmonary disease. Am Rev Respir Dis 1976;113:203–218.
10. Boysen PG, Block AJ, Olsen GN, et al: Prospective evaluation for pneumonectomy using the ^{99m}Technetium quantitative perfusion lung scan. Chest 1977;72:422–425.
11. Miller WF, Geumei AM: Respiratory and Pharmacologic Therapy in COPD. In Petty TL: Chronic Obstructive Pulmonary Disease, Lung Biology in Health and Disease, ed 2. New York, Marcel Dekker, 1985, pp 205–338.

19

AMBULATORY AND HOME CARE FOR INDIVIDUALS WITH COPD

GERARD J. CRINER
BARRY J. MAKE

The management of chronic obstructive pulmonary disease (COPD) remains a challenge for both patients with this disorder and physicians caring for them. Although patients with mild or easily reversible airflow obstruction may respond favorably to bronchodilator therapy alone, those patients with moderate or severe disease present difficult management problems. Each member of the health care team must realize that this disorder is chronic, may have a limited response to currently available therapeutic interventions, and may demonstrate a clinical course frequented by disabling exacerbations. The only chance of preventing COPD or limiting its devastating course once the disorder is established, is to discontinue cigarette consumption. Once COPD exists, various modalities can be implemented on an outpatient basis to achieve three main goals:

1. Decrease airflow obstruction
2. Reduce morbidity and prevent mortality
3. Improve the patient's functional capabilities.

Although advanced COPD has effects on various organ systems, its major consequence is to impair ventilatory pump and gas exchange functions of the

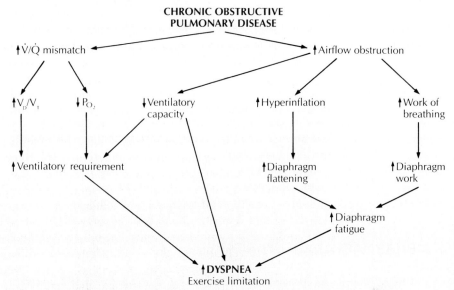

Figure 19–1. Mechanism of dyspnea in COPD. (Modified from Belman MK, Wasserman K: Exercise training and testing in patients with chronic obstructive pulmonary disease. *Basics of RD* 1981;2(10):1, by permission.)

respiratory system (Fig. 19–1). The mechanical disadvantage placed upon the muscles of inspiration by hyperinflation and the increased work of breathing caused by reduced airway caliber leads to respiratory muscle (pump) dysfunction. Loss of elastic recoil, airways disease, and destruction of pulmonary parenchyma can account for the adverse effects of emphysema on gas exchange. Despite the temptation to conveniently separate the respiratory system into ventilatory pump and gas exchange components, dysfunction of either component adversely affects the other unit. For example, an increase in airways resistance not only affects gas exchange by altering ventilation-perfusion relationships but also requires increased respiratory muscle force to ventilate through narrowed airways. These physiologic effects of COPD on the patient must be considered in developing any therapeutic plan.

A treatment plan should be multifaceted and include active patient involvement in four major aspects:

1. Discontinuation of cigarette consumption should be of paramount importance to both the patient and the physician.

2. Pharmacologic therapy should be employed to treat any reversible airflow obstruction and also to improve respiratory muscle performance.

3. The presence of frequent complications of COPD, such as pulmonary infections, cor pulmonale, hypoxemia, mental and sexual dysfunction, and respiratory failure, should be elevated and treated expeditiously when present.

4. Pulmonary rehabilitation programs that promote patient education, specific exercise conditioning, respiratory muscle training, and vocational counseling should be implemented.

This chapter explores the therapeutic modalities useful to COPD patients in the outpatient setting and also describes new therapies that may become important tools in the near future.

SMOKING CESSATION

A review of smoking cessation methods is included in Chapter 5. Educational efforts concerning smoking prevention targeted at children are probably more productive than smoking cessation techniques directed to adults. Although the latter proclaims an initial high success rate, long-term maintenance of smoking cessation succeeds in only 20% to 25% of adult patients.

PHARMACOLOGIC THERAPY

The hallmark of pharmacologic therapy for treating the reversible airways component of COPD has been the use of methylxanthines, beta adrenergic agonists and corticosteroids. Recent attention has also been directed toward examining the effects of anticholinergic agents and calcium channel blockers on airflow obstruction in these patients. For a complete discussion of pharmacologic therapy see Chapter 7. The following is an attempt to provide rational guidelines for these medications in ambulatory patients.

Theophylline

Although theophylline has been used extensively as a bronchodilator for years, the mediation of its effects remains unclear. For many years, the proposed action was through phosphodiesterase inhibition, but it is now recognized that this effect is minimal at the theophylline levels used in clinical practice.[1] Recent studies have proposed several different mechanisms for theophylline's actions including stimulation of catecholamine release,[2] inhibition of prostaglandin action,[3] translocation of intracellular calcium,[4] stimulation of the medullary respiratory center,[5] and adenosine receptor antagonism.[6] The latter action is considered by many to be theophylline's most important effect, but controversy also surrounds this proposed mechanism.[7] Whatever its mode of action at the biochemical level, theophylline is widely used as a bronchodilator of moderate potency. In addition to its efficacy as a bronchodilator, theophylline has other actions in patients with chronic airflow obstruction. These other effects include the lowering of pulmonary artery pressure,[8] reversal and delay in the onset of inspiratory muscle fatigue,[9, 10] increasing of mucociliary clearance,[11] and accentuating of the ventilatory response to hypoxemia.[12]

Table 19–1. **Conditions Affecting Theophylline Metabolism**

Increased Metabolism	Decreased Metabolism
Cigarette smoking	Liver dysfunction
Marijuana smoking	Heart failure
Children, adolescents	COPD
Corticosteroids	Cimetidine
High-protein diet	Erythromycin, clindamycin
Phenytoin	Infants (< 6 months)
Benzodiazepines	Old age
Barbiturates	
Alcohol	
Obesity	
Allopurinol	

Limitations to the use of theophylline include the drug's narrow therapeutic index, interaction with other drugs, and its metabolism that varies with the patient's age and medical condition (Table 19–1).[13–35]

When the decision has been made to institute theophylline therapy, rapid therapeutic levels can be achieved in the ambulatory setting with oral solutions or uncoated tablets.[36] Less rapidly achieved therapeutic theophylline levels can be accomplished over several days by using coated tablets or long-acting preparations. Recommended initial maintenance dosage for adults is approximately 400 mg/day; initiating therapy slowly decreases the incidence of unwanted caffeine-like side effects.[37] After three to five days, if symptoms of airflow obstruction persist, theophylline dose may be increased to 600 mg/day. Subsequently, if needed to control symptoms, a second increase in dose may be made to 800 mg/day. Above doses of 800 mg/day, determinations of serum theophylline levels are recommended to maintain levels in the range of 10 to 20 μg/ml. Serum levels of theophylline can now be easily and rapidly obtained on whole blood or saliva in the outpatient setting by immunoassay.[38] When obtaining serum theophylline levels to guide drug administration, attention must be paid to product formulation and the timing of serum level determination and drug ingestion. When using sustained-release tablets three to four half-lives are needed for the drug to reach a steady-state level. In certain patients, peak and trough levels rather than just a single serum theophylline level may be needed to adequately define dosing interval. For example, in those individuals whose symptoms are not easily controlled, peak and trough blood levels should be obtained six and 10 to 12 hours, respectively, after ingesting twice-a-day sustained-release tablets.[36]

For chronic oral theophylline administration, several sustained-release preparations are being marketed for single or twice daily dosing. Although these agents have the potential to provide more stable blood levels and increase patient compliance, those individuals with rapid metabolism of theophylline may have wide fluctuations in serum theophylline levels with longer dosing intervals. Additionally, current preparations vary widely in their ability to achieve slow absorption and thus permit dosing once or twice a

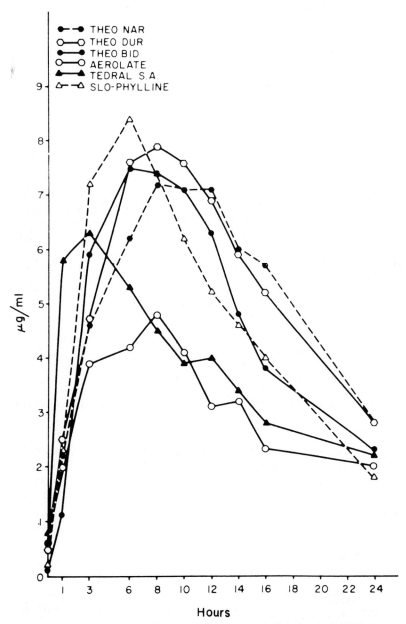

Figure 19–2. Comparisons of the mean plasma theophylline level at different times after 8 mg/Kg dosing with several sustained-release theophylline preparations. (From Sangler D, Kalof DD, Bloom FL, Wittig HJ: Theophylline bioavailability following oral administration of six sustained-release preparations. *Annals of Allergy* 1978;40(1):8, by permission.)

day. Another concern is the variable effect that food induces upon different sustained-release theophylline products. Dissolution of several formulations is dependent on the pH of the small intestine.[39] When pH increases with meal intake, potentially toxic amounts of theophylline can be absorbed from Theo-24.[40] Food consumption also appears to enhance absorption of theophylline from Uniphyl,[39] while interfering with absorption from Theo-Dur Sprinkle.[40] Slo-bid Gyrocaps, Theo-Dur, Theobid, and Somophyllin-CRT are not associated with variable absorption in the presence of food and, in most individuals with slower metabolism, provide for relatively stable blood levels.[38]

To maintain a serum theophylline level within the therapeutic usage of 10 to 20 μg/ml, serum concentration fluctuations must be kept less than 100%. As outlined above, fluctuations of serum theophylline are related to three factors: (1) product formulation, which determines the rate and amount of drug absorbed (Fig. 19–2), (2) patient metabolism of the drug, and (3) physician prescription of the interval between doses. A useful formula[38] to predict the percent of serum theophylline fluctuation is:

$$\% \text{ Fluctuation} = \frac{\text{Peak} - \text{trough}}{\text{trough}} \times 100$$

Patients with rapid metabolism may only avoid excessive fluctuations of serum theophylline with more frequent dosage intervals.

Beta Agonists

In 1948, Ahlquist first proposed the presence of both alpha and beta adrenergic receptors.[42] Since that time, further work has separated the beta receptors into beta-1 and beta-2 subclasses.[43] Beta-1 receptors are located in the heart, while beta-2 receptors are found on bronchial and vascular smooth muscle. More recently, drugs have been developed that are selective for beta-2 stimulation and bronchodilation while avoiding the cardiac irritability associated with beta-1 stimulation.[44, 45] Beta-2 agonists currently available in this country for use as selective bronchodilator agents include isoetharine, metaproterenol, bitolterol, albuterol and terbutaline. All are available in metered-dose inhalers. Isoetharine and metaproterenol are provided in solution form for nebulization and many beta-2 agonists are also available in tablets for oral administration. Beta agonists act by stimulating adenyl cyclase and increasing intracellular concentrations of cyclic AMP. Cyclic AMP, in turn, is thought to mediate many different actions including bronchial smooth muscle relaxation and improved ciliary motility.

Although some beta-2 agonists are marketed for systemic administration, the inhaled route is preferable for the majority of ambulatory patients with COPD.[46, 47] Inhalation enables direct delivery of drug to the site of action with smaller doses required than with oral or parenteral formulations. This results

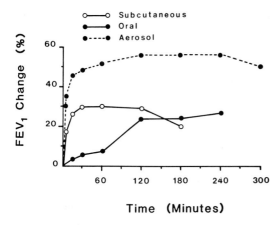

Figure 19–3. Changes in FEV₁ following three different routes of administration of terbutaline. (Modified from Dulfano MJ, Glass P: The bronchodilator effects of terbutaline: Route of administration and patterns of response. *Annals of Allergy* 1976; 37(5):357, by permission.)

in bronchodilation that is greater and more rapid in onset while simultaneously causing less side effects (Fig. 19–3). In addition, beta-2 agonists lose some of their beta-2 specificity when administered systemically. When COPD patients use chronic inhaled beta-2 agonist therapy, the physician and patient must understand that regular dosing (every six to eight hours depending upon the preparation chosen) achieves more continuous bronchodilation and reduces chronic symptoms more effectively than prn use after dyspnea has occurred (Table 19–2).

Certain precautions are needed when using metered-dose inhalers to insure delivery of the beta agonist to the peripheral conducting airways, where beta receptors are found. Although there is controversy regarding the optimal technique of aerosol administration, patients should be instructed to dispense the aerosol at the beginning of a slow, deep inhalation while holding the canister 2 to 3 cm from the mouth.[48] This serves to reduce impaction of the aerosol in the oropharynx. After inhalation, a 10-second period of breath-holding should occur, which aids gravitational forces in distributing aerosol to the peripheral airways and impacting upon the airway walls.[49] Even with proper technique, only 10% to 15% of the administered compound is actually delivered to the lower respiratory tract. In those patients (such as the elderly) with poor inhalation-dispensing coordination, interposing a reservoir between the metered-dose inhaler and the patient may be helpful. The reservoir acts as a drug collection chamber to reduce the requirements for hand-breathing coordination.[50]

Side effects from the beta agonists are often related to inadvertent beta-1 stimulation and include tachycardia and palpitations.[51] Cardiac irritability is a serious complication that limits the use of these compounds in patients at risk for arrhythmias.[52, 53] Hand tremor is the most frequent complaint but fortunately diminishes with continued use. The frequency of developing tachyphylaxis to the bronchodilatory properties of the beta agonists is unclear but probably rare.[44] When reduced responsiveness does occur, withdrawal of the medication for one to two weeks appears to restore bronchodilation on rechallenge.

Table 19–2. Selected Beta-2 Adrenergic Agonists

Agent	Route of Administration	Dose	Onset of Action (min)	Peak of Action (min)	Duration of Action (hr)
Isoetharine	MDI*	2 Inhalations (0.25–0.5 ml)	2–5	5–20	1–4
	Inhaled solution				
Terbutaline	MDI	2 Inhalations	5–30	120	3–4
	Subcutaneous	0–0.25 mg	2–5	30–60	2–4
	Oral	2.5–5 mg	10–30	120–180	4–6
Metaproterenol	MDI	2 Inhalations (0.2–0.3 ml)	2–10	10–60	1–5
	Inhaled solution		3–5	10–60	2–6
	Oral	10–20 mg	10–20	15–60	3–4
Albuterol	MDI	2 Inhalations	2–15	60–90	3–6
	Oral	2–4 mg	10–30	120–180	4–6
Bitolterol	MDI	2–3 Inhalations	3–4	30–180	5–8

*MDI = Metered-dose inhaler.

Corticosteroids

Many studies have attempted to define the role of corticosteroids in the treatment of patients with COPD. Early studies have been criticized for being uncontrolled, reporting on small numbers of patients, or showing reductions in airflow obstruction with steroids in patients who were mislabeled and were truly asthmatic.[54] Two recent studies have examined the use of steroids in treating airflow obstruction in patients with chronic airflow obstruction.[55, 56] In both studies, a subgroup of patients was identified that had a positive bronchodilatory response to corticosteroids.

Albert and colleagues studied 44 patients with acute exacerbations of chronic bronchitis and severe airflow obstruction (mean FEV_1 of 0.61 L) in a prospective, randomized fashion.[55] All patients were hospitalized, and the group given methylprednisolone in addition to bronchodilators showed a greater percent change in FEV_1 than the group treated with bronchodilators alone. Despite the increase in FEV_1, no alteration in morbidity or mortality was demonstrated.

Mendella and associates in a double-blind crossover trial compared 32 mg/day of methylprednisolone to placebo over a two-week period in 46 patients with stable COPD.[56] Eight patients showed a 29% or greater increase in FEV_1 in response to steroid therapy resulting in a significantly greater FEV_1 in the entire steroid-treated group. Baseline characteristics of steroid responders only differed from those of nonresponders by a greater response to inhaled beta agonists. This latter feature raises the question whether steroid-responsive patients had an asthmatic component in addition to emphysema or chronic bronchitis. The distinction between these entities becomes less important when one realizes that chronic airflow obstruction represents a spectrum of airway disorders, and in most clinical situations, more than one abnormality is present. No difference in morbidity was evident between the steroid-responding group and the nonresponding one.

How corticosteroids promote bronchodilation is still not clear. Steroid actions begin with binding to a specific cell receptor that interacts with nuclear DNA and results in RNA synthesis and the formation of new proteins.[57] Since these newly synthesized proteins mediate some steroid actions, there is a time delay of several hours until these effects become evident. Other actions are more immediate and could include the activation of preformed proteins,[58] mobilization of membrane-bound calcium,[59] decreasing beta-adrenergic receptor uncoupling,[60, 61] suppressing the response to bronchoconstrictors,[57] or inhibiting mucous secretion.[62]

A diagnostic trial of oral corticosteroids is recommended in patients with stable COPD who are severely limited despite optimal therapy.[63] Since many patients feel better because of the nonpulmonary effects of steroids, symptomatic improvement may not correlate with physiologic benefit. The effectiveness of steroids should be assessed objectively by serial spirometry. It is necessary to individualize each case and to determine whether the benefit of potentially greater bronchodilatation outweighs the significant side effects of chronic steroid therapy.

Anticholinergic Agents

Anticholinergic compounds used as bronchodilators are quaternary ammonium congeners of atropine (ipratropium bromide and atropine methonitrate) and will soon be released in this country for use in obstructive airways disease. Some evidence suggests that they might have a primary role in the therapy of airflow obstruction in patients with chronic bronchitis and emphysema.[64] These drugs act at a site different than beta adrenergic agents and have demonstrated an additive bronchodilatory response when used in conjunction with beta agonists.[65, 66] In chronic bronchitis, anticholinergic agents have been shown to produce more potent bronchodilatation than that achieved with beta adrenergic compounds.[66] Although atropine has important bronchodilatory properties of its own when inhaled, its use is limited by a low therapeutic index.[64] The quaternary ammonium congeners appear to be as potent inhaled bronchodilators as atropine but, because of their geometric configuration, are not absorbed systemically, and unwanted side effects are avoided.[67] They may become the drug of first choice in patients with airflow obstruction associated with chronic bronchitis,[68] pyschogenic-induced bronchospasm,[69] and beta adrenergic blockade.[70]

Calcium Antagonist

Calcium channel blockers have recently been released in the United States, and their use in the management of pulmonary disorders is currently under investigation. Many events in the pathogenesis of airways obstruction are felt to require the participation of calcium.[71] In vitro studies have demonstrated the role of calcium in releasing chemical mediators causing bronchospasm[72] and smooth muscle contraction,[73] altering electrolyte movement across cells,[74] and affecting mucous production.[75] In vivo studies have demonstrated conflicting results on the ability of calcium channel blockers to inhibit bronchospasm induced by methacholine, histamine, exercise, and various inhaled antigens. Some of the variability in response may be secondary to different potencies of the calcium blocking agents used or to the inability of certain compounds to achieve adequate delivery to the airways.[71] In addition, calcium pools at many different sites may be involved in airways disease (intracellular, extracellular, or membrane-bound), and the ability of individual drugs to affect various pools may have significance. Furthermore, newer agents that have greater potency, or that can be delivered topically, may be successful in achieving adequate airway distribution while avoiding unwanted side effects.[76] What impact these new agents have on the management of airways obstruction is uncertain at the present time.

Initiating Pharmacologic Therapy

Which bronchodilator to use first when initiating therapy must be individualized. Consideration must be given to the benefit of added bronchodilation produced by each class of drugs weighed against potential side effects. Certain side effects may be easily tolerated by one particular patient but be intolerable for another. The most reliable objective parameters used in following the response to bronchodilator therapy are not well defined. Improvement in FEV_1 or forced expiratory flow from 25% to 75% of the exhaled volume ($FEF_{25-75\%}$) of 15% or greater after bronchodilator challenge is considered by many to be indicative of bronchodilator responsiveness. Others consider these measurements too insensitive and suggest changes in airway resistance[77] or improvements in vital capacity and functional residual capacity as better indicators of bronchodilator responsiveness.[78] Complicating the issue of the sensitivity of pulmonary function testing is that a patient's response to one bronchodilator agent may be blunted when using another.[79] Additionally, some beneficial aspects of therapy are not monitored by airflow testing. Improved diaphragmatic performance and mucociliary clearance are well-documented effects of theophylline but might not be observed with commonly used spirometric techniques. Therefore, most authorities recommend a trial of bronchodilator therapy in patients with symptomatic chronic airflow obstruction. If bronchodilator responsiveness is demonstrated, continuation of therapy is indicated. In patients without spirometric responsiveness but clinical improvement by history and physical examination, bronchodilator therapy should continue in the absence of serious medication side effects.

General recommendations for the use of bronchodilators in ambulatory patients with COPD are to initate therapy with either a sustained action theophylline preparation or regular doses of an inhaled selective beta-2 agonist. Although the choice of agents is arbitrary, factors that may influence the decision include the presence of conditions or the use of drugs that modify theophylline metabolism, the patient's ability to correctly use a metered-dose inhaler, and the need for rapid or sustained bronchodilator action. In patients refractory to single-agent therapy, combination therapy with agents of both classes can produce more bronchodilatation with fewer side effects than administering large amounts of either drug alone.[80] If significant limitation continues once therapy with beta agonists and theophylline has been maximized, corticosteroid therapy should be considered. When corticosteroids are used, emphasis should be placed upon changes in objective parameters to avoid reliance on subjective improvement secondary to steroid-induced euphoria. Since complications from steroid therapy are serious and dose-related, inhaled corticosteroids should supplement or replace systemic therapy whenever possible. Although this latter plan is desirable, most steroid-responsive patients cannot be controlled with only the inhaled delivery route.[63] Inhaled steroids may nonetheless allow reductions in the dose of systemic steroids. Guidelines for stepwise management using anticholinergic therapy do not yet exist and calcium channel blockers do not have an established role in the management of chronic airways obstruction at the present time.

MANAGING COMPLICATIONS

Antibiotics

Antibiotics are probably prescribed more frequently than needed in ambulatory patients experiencing exacerbations of COPD. Studies have shown that 15% to 34% of all infectious mediated exacerbations are due to viral or mycoplasmal organisms.[81] The results of a sputum Gram stain and culture are of little use since these patients frequently grow pneumococci or *Haemophilus influenzae* when there is no deterioration in clinical course.[82] Nevertheless, most authorities suggest a 10- to 14-day course of broad-spectrum antibiotics when sputum becomes mucopurulent.[83, 84] Ampicillin or tetracycline are reasonable choices. If beta-lactamase–resistant *Haemophilus influenzae* is a strong consideration, trimethoprim and sulfamethoxazole or cefaclor is recommended.

Vaccines

Patients with significant pulmonary disease are often advised to receive a one-time-only pneumococcal[85] and yearly influenza vaccinations.[86] Since the utility of pneumococcal vaccination in all patients with COPD has recently been questioned,[87] administration of pneumococcal vaccine should be made on an individual basis.

Oxygen

Chronic hypoxemia leads to severe disturbances in end organ function. Altered physiologic processes resulting from tissue hypoxia most noticeably affect the pulmonary vasculature and heart, kidneys, brain, and systemic circulation. The pulmonary vasculature responds to chronic hypoxia by increasing pulmonary vascular resistance while simultaneously increasing cardiac output and decreasing systemic vascular resistance. An increase in renal blood flow can be demonstrated with mild reductions of arterial oxygen, while chronic hypoxemia impairs salt and water excretion and thus can contribute to the presence of peripheral edema.[88] Impaired neuropsychological function manifested by irritability, confusion, seizures, syncope, loss of fine motor coordination, memory loss, and impaired intellectual performance on standardized testing can result from chronic reductions in arterial oxygen concentration.[89] Cardiac arrhythmias are more common in hypoxemic individuals, and persistent elevations in pulmonary vascular resistance can lead to right ventricular hypertrophy[90] and eventual right ventricular failure.[91] Erythropoietin production stimulated by chronic hypoxemia enhances erythrocytosis and leads to secondary polycythemia, which can cause complications secondary to elevated blood viscosity.

Many studies have suggested that oxygen therapy could reverse many of the serious complications of chronic hypoxemia. Long-term oxygen therapy improves mentation[89] and decreases hematocrit,[92] pulmonary artery resistance,[93] and mortality in those patients with severe hypoxemia or cor pulmonale.[94] Moreover, chronic outpatient oxygen therapy is safe, and no untoward decrement in lung function has been demonstrated.[95] However, most of the early studies were plagued by having small numbers of patients or by lack of proper control populations.[96]

Two large prospective studies, one in Britain[97] and the other a multicenter trial in the United States,[98] have demonstrated that oxygen therapy can decrease morbidity and mortality in patients with airflow obstruction and chronic hypoxemia. These studies (summarized in Chapter 8) conclude that continuous oxygen therapy improves survival over nocturnal therapy and that either therapy is better than no oxygen supplementation at all.

Based upon the results of the American trial, COPD patients should be considered candidates for long-term oxygen therapy if they have a $Pa_{O_2} \leq 55$ torr at rest or ≤ 59 torr with clinical evidence of the secondary signs of tissue hypoxia, such as peripheral edema due to cor pulmonale, "p" pulmonale on ECG, erythrocytosis, or impaired mentation (Table 19–3). The measurements of arterial oxygen should be obtained when the patient is in a stable state and after receiving optimal medical management to treat airways disease. Further indications for oxygen must be made on an individual basis and include those patients with normal resting arterial oxygen who desaturate during sleep or exercise.

COPD is probably the most common cause of sleep hypoxemia in the absence of obstructive apnea.[99] While most patients desaturate minimally

Table 19–3. **Indications for Chronic Home Oxygen Therapy**

$Pa_{O_2} \leq 55$ mmHg when patient is stable on optimal therapy.

$Pa_{O_2} \leq 59$ mmHg with associated:
- cor pulmonale
- secondary polycythemia
- central nervous system dysfunction.

Selected patients with Pa_{O_2} during exercise ≤ 55 mmHg.

Selected patients with Pa_{O_2} during sleep ≤ 55 mmHg
with documented:
- cor pulmonale
- cardiac arrhythmia during sleep
- secondary polycythemia
- disordered sleep pattern.

Table 19–4. Forms of Oxygen for Outpatient Therapy*

Form of Oxygen	Reservoir Duration, if Used at 1 L/min	Associated Portable System	Portable Supply and Duration if Used at 1 L/min	Portable Supply, Weight (lbs)	Cost/Month, if Used 24 hr/day 1 L/min	Cost/Month, if Used 24 hr/day 3 L/min	Advantages	Disadvantages
Compressed gas	4.8 days per large "H" cylinder.	Small tanks with wheels or shoulder strap: "E" cylinder "D" cylinder "C" cylinder Mada cylinder	11 hr 7 hr 4 hr 2 hr	17 10 8 5	$300	$900	Widely available. Least expensive for use at home if used at low flow rates or for brief periods.	Heavy and large; hard to move. Portable system rather bulky. Frequent tank deliveries may be needed.
Liquid oxygen	13–14 days per 70–75 lbs of liquid oxygen canister.	Canisters with shoulder strap or wheels: Small canister Large canister	7 hr 13 hr	6.5–7.5 10–12	$400	$850	Portable system easiest to carry and longest lasting. Most convenient and least expensive for extended or high flow.	Most expensive, except for patients on high flow rates (> 3 L/min) and those who spend long periods on portable use. Oxygen slowly evaporates (2%/day) even if system is turned off. Some patients have trouble refilling some models of portable canisters.
Oxygen concentrator	No limit: machine extracts O_2 from air.	Small compressed gas tanks (see above).	Small compressed gas tanks (see above).		$250 for any amount of usage plus cost of electricity and portable tanks.		Most economical for patients who use oxygen 24 hrs/day and stay home. Not dependent on deliveries of oxygen from supplier. Attractive cabinet-like appearance of machine.	Dependent on electricity, so back up system needed. Alternate system needed for portable use. Can deliver up to 4 L/min of > 90% oxygen. Cost of electricity ($25/month) not covered by insurance.

*From Make B: Medical management of emphysema. Clinics in Chest Medicine 1983;4:465, by permission.

during non–rapid eye movement (NREM) sleep secondary to hypoventilation, further severe reduction in arterial oxygen can occur during REM sleep in certain patients. Many hypotheses have been suggested to explain the reductions in arterial oxygen that can occur during REM sleep. These include ventilation-perfusion imbalance,[100] reduction in the contribution of the accessory inspiratory muscles to ventilation,[101] and blunted ventilatory responses to hypoxemia[102] and hypercapnia.[99] Block has suggested that nocturnal desaturation may be a major contributor to secondary pulmonary hypertension in some COPD patients.[103] Clinical predictors of nocturnal desaturation are not yet available. Sleep hypoxemia should be suspected in COPD patients with evidence of pulmonary hypertension or syndromes suggestive of reduced oxygen saturation despite an arterial $P_{O_2} > 60$ torr while awake. Sleep disturbances associated with COPD are reviewed in Chapter 16.

Some COPD patients demonstrate significant hypoxemia only with exercise. Owens has demonstrated that this is more likely to occur in COPD patients whose single-breath diffusing capacity is below 55% of the predicted value.[104] Many studies have demonstrated that oxygen supplementation can improve exercise performance in patients with COPD.[105–109] This beneficial effect on exercise endurance was considered secondary to improved right ventricular performance,[110] decrease in airways resistance,[111] or reduction in minute ventilation.[112] Recent data suggest that respiratory muscle endurance is prolonged and ventilatory muscle fatigue is delayed while exercising with supplemental oxygen.[112–114] At present, oxygen therapy should be considered for those patients who demonstrate oxygen desaturation during exercise. Before oxygen therapy with exercise is implemented in the home, patients should demonstrate improvement in exercise performance and tissue oxygenation with supplemental oxygen in a controlled setting.

Long-term oxygen therapy in the outpatient setting is delivered by nasal cannula. Flow rates of 1 to 4 L/min are usually adequate to maintain a Pa_{O_2} of 60 torr. The supply of oxygen can be delivered in the home setting by compressed gas, liquid oxygen, or oxygen concentrator. The advantages and disadvantages of these three systems are listed in Table 19–4. (See also Chapter 8.)

New oxygen-conserving cannulas that have reservoirs and demand valves that permit oxygen utilization only on inspiration are now being marketed.[116] These devices reduce the amount of oxygen used and expand the useful period for portable oxygen systems.

Mechanical Ventilation

Mechanical ventilation at home may be a viable option in selected patients with COPD and ventilatory failure.[116, 117] Rising hospital costs to care for patients who cannot be successfully weaned from the ventilator following emergency intubation for respiratory acidosis and hypercapnia coupled with improved home ventilatory technology and the success of several rehabilitation programs has created this option for care. Smaller ventilators can easily be accommodated in the home and adapted for automobiles and wheelchairs. Rehabilitation programs have demonstrated that patients and their families can be instructed to adequately perform ventilator and tracheostomy care.[116] Furthermore, ventilated patients can increase exercise endurance and perform daily activities despite their impairment. Patients chosen for home ventilator care should be medically stable and well motivated and have a strong emotional support system.[118] Ventilator teaching and exercise programs are begun in the hospital while assessment of their artificial respiration needs are completed. The time spent on the mechanical ventilator ranges from 24 hours to nocturnal ventilation only and must be individualized. Home ventilation for COPD patients is more difficult than in cases of respiratory failure due to neuromusculoskeletal disorders.

Since the respiratory muscles are placed at a mechanical disadvantage by hyperinflation and are required to work harder in the presence of airflow obstruction, ventilatory muscle failure commonly occurs in severe COPD. If fatigue contributes to the disabling symptoms of these patients, the use of mechanical ventilation may free the respiratory muscles of the burden of breathing by resting them. External negative pressure ventilation has recently been used electively in patients with severe COPD and fatigued respiratory muscles. Braun has reported a favorable outcome with an increase in resting muscle strength, improved exercise capacity, a reduction in the number of hospital admissions and in the length of stays, and reduced Pa_{CO_2} in patients treated with intermittent external ventilation.[119] Other researchers have demonstrated no improvement among externally ventilated patients over those treated with a standard rehabilitation program.[120, 121] All these studies suffer from small patient numbers. Although negative-pressure ventilation could favorably alter the quality of life of a large number of patients, it should be considered as only an investigational tool at the present time.

PULMONARY REHABILITATION

The goal of pulmonary rehabilitation is to restore patients to the highest functional ability by involving them in a comprehensive multidisciplinary program. Pulmonary rehabilitation is therefore appropriate for any individual who has difficulty maintaining his or her lifestyle because of lung disease. Since COPD is a chronic disorder, often with limited reversibility of impairment, teaching patients methods to improve functioning while reducing symptoms has become an accepted form of therapy. See Chapter 13 for a discussion of pulmonary rehabilitation.

The major goal of patient education is to increase compliance with the prescribed therapeutic regime. Education about lung disease also provides patients with realistic expectations about treatment outcomes, enables them to avoid factors that precipitate symptoms, and helps them to recognize signs of evolving complications. The initial educational process can occur in a hospital group setting with further reinforcement given in outpatient visits or by health professionals who periodically evaluate the patient at home. Visiting nurses or respiratory therapists not only provide the patient with proper instruction on breathing techniques, a medication administration, and chest physiotherapy but are also indispensable in monitoring patient compliance and the medical status of individuals with severe COPD in the home. They can evaluate the patient's and family's ability to appropiately use the respiratory equipment and ascertain whether existing systems or location of equipment allows for maximal functioning of the patient. Home health professionals should then recommend modifications to the prescribing physicians in order to improve the patient's functioning at home. Exercise training in patients limited by COPD is valuable and can be divided into two types: ventilatory muscle training and the training of specific muscle groups by a particular exercise. Although ventilatory muscle training has been shown to increase whole body exercise endurance in patients with COPD,[122–124] the converse is not true.[125] Breathing against an inspiratory resistor[122, 123] and isocapnic hyperventilation[124] are effective ways of increasing ventilatory muscle endurance. Inspiratory resistance training has been shown to improve leg cycle performance more than a standard physiotherapy protocol.[122] However, certain precautions should be taken in prescribing this therapy. Patients who demonstrate an improvement in exercise endurance also demonstrated electromyographic evidence of inspiratory muscle fatigue during the training maneuver.[122] Therefore, patients should be supervised in their use of resistive training to avoid precipitating ventilatory failure.

Increased exercise endurance for leg ergometry, treadmill exercise, and a 12-minute walk have all been demonstrated after relatively brief training periods. Walking a defined distance or for a defined period of time is particularly suitable for the outpatient setting, but the patient should be given instructions for self-monitoring with the aid of visits to a health professional. Although a patient may improve exercise tolerance after leg or arm cycling, ventilatory muscle endurance may not be improved.[125]

Some patients show relief from dyspnea with pursed-lip breathing. It has been proposed that this improves gas exchange by altering the equal pressure point and delaying dynamic compression of the peripheral airways.[126]

Chest percussion and postural drainage may be important in hospitalized individuals with acute pneumonia or significant bronchitis, but they have little use for a patient with predominant emphysema and scant secretions.[127] The usefulness of chronic chest physiotherapy in stable outpatients has not been well studied, but patients with excessive secretions often report significant symptomatic improvement with such therapy. Other physical therapy modalities such as the need for pacing, planning of activities, and energy conservation have an even greater role in the outpatient setting. Strategies such as sitting while doing dishes or cooking may allow particular patients to be more productive at home while avoiding disabling dyspnea.

A visiting nurse can be a valuable asset to any outpatient rehabilitation program. The nurse is a trained observer who can record vital signs or a change in secretion or airflow obstruction, recognize developing complications, and insure proper medication administration and necessary equipment care. They also can suggest changes in the environment that may allow a patient to function on a higher level. Eliminating excessive stair climbing or lowering the height of frequently used objects allows patients to experience less dyspnea while performing needed tasks. In their own home, patients may feel more in control and willing to discuss bothersome issues previously inhibited by the doctor-patient relation or hospital environment, so a visiting nurse may more readily discover unrecognized psychosocial or sexual disorders that the patient was not previously comfortable in discussing.

Particular attention should also be paid to psychosocial counseling and vocational training. Patients with chronic debilitating illnesses can suffer from a loss of self-esteem because of their inability to perform their job or role as spouse or parent. By addressing these negative feelings with both patients and their families, major improvements in the quality of life can be obtained.

SUMMARY

The management of COPD requires judicious use of pharmacologic agents, treating complications when present, and devoting attention to the

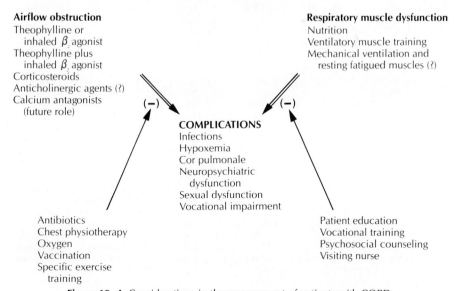

CHRONIC OBSTRUCTIVE PULMONARY DISEASE

Airflow obstruction
Theophylline or
  inhaled β_2 agonist
Theophylline plus
  inhaled β_2 agonist
Corticosteroids
Anticholinergic agents (?)
Calcium antagonists
  (future role)

(−)

Respiratory muscle dysfunction
Nutrition
Ventilatory muscle training
Mechanical ventilation and
  resting fatigued muscles (?)

(−)

COMPLICATIONS
Infections
Hypoxemia
Cor pulmonale
Neuropsychiatric
  dysfunction
Sexual dysfunction
Vocational impairment

Antibiotics
Chest physiotherapy
Oxygen
Vaccination
Specific exercise
  training

Patient education
Vocational training
Psychosocial counseling
Visiting nurse

Figure 19–4. Considerations in the management of patients with COPD.

patient's psychological well-being (Fig. 19–4). New drugs (anticholinergic agents) and technologic innovations (portable volume ventilators and external negative-pressure ventilation) may improve the ability of these patients to cope with their illness. An outpatient comprehensive care program allows individuals with severe COPD to lead more active and productive lives in their homes.

References

1. Bergstrand H: Phosphodiesterase inhibition and theophylline. *Eur J Respir Dis* 1980(suppl);109:37–44.

2. Rall TW: The Xanthines, in Gilman AG, Goodman LS, Gilman A (eds): *The Pharmacological Basis of Therapeutics*, ed 6. New York, MacMillan, 1980, pp 592–607.

3. Horrobin DF, Manku MS, Franks DJ, et al: Methylxanthine phosphodiesterase inhibitors behave as prostaglandin antagonists in a perfused rat mesenteric artery preparation. *Prostaglandins* 1977;13:33–40.

4. Bresson GRJ, Malaisse-Lagal F, Malaisse WJ: The stimulus secretion coupling of glucose-induced insulin release. VII. A proposed site of action for adenosine 3'5'-cyclic monophosphate. *J Clin Invest* 1972;51:232–241.

5. Anderson KE, Persson CG: Extrapulmonary effects of theophylline. *Eur J Respir Dis* 1980;61(suppl 109):17–28

6. Cushley MJ, Tattersfield AE, Holgate ST: Adenosine-induced bronchoconstriction in asthma. *Am Rev Resp Dis* 1984; 129:380–384.

7. Lunell E, Suedmyr N, Andersson KE, et al: Effects of enprofylline, a xanthine lacking adenosine receptor antagonism, in patients with chronic obstructive lung disease. *Eur J Clin Pharmacol* 1982; 22:395–402.

8. Rees HA, MacDonald HR, Bothwick RG, et al: The circulatory effects of aminophylline in man. *Clin Sci* 1969;36:359–369.

9. Aubier M, DeTroyer A, Sampson M, et al: Aminophylline improves diaphragmatic contractility. *N Engl J Med* 1981; 305:249–252.

10. Murciano D, Aubier M, Lecocguic Y, et al: Effects of theophylline on diaphragmatic strength and fatigue in patients with chronic obstructive pulmonary disease. *N Engl J Med* 1984;311:349–353.

11. Clarke SW: The effect of theophylline on mucociliary transport, in Jonkman JGH, Jenne JW, Simons FER, et al. (eds): *Sustained Release Theophylline in the Treatment of CRAO*. Amsterdam, Excerpta Medica, 1984, pp 22–25.

12. Lakshminarayan S, Sahn SA, Weil JV: Effect of aminophylline on ventilatory responses in normal man. *Am Rev Resp Dis* 1978;117:33–38.

13. Gal P, Jusko WL, Yurchak AM, et al: Theophylline disposition in obesity. *Clin Pharmacol Ther* 1978;23:438–444.

14. Piafsy KM, Sitar DS, Rangno RE, et al: Theophylline disposition in patients with hepatic cirrhosis. *N Engl J Med* 1977; 296:1495–1497.

15. Reis G, Pingleton SK, Melethil S, et al: The effect of erythromycin base on theophylline kinetics. *Clin Pharmacol Ther* 1981;29:601–605.

16. Jackson JE, Powell JR, Wandell M, et al: Cimetidine decreases theophylline clearance. *Am Rev Resp Dis* 1981;123:615–617.

17. Reitberg DP, Bernhard H, Schentag JJ: Alteration of theophylline clearance and half-life by cimetidine in normal volunteers. *Ann Intern Med* 1981;95:582–585.

18. Manfredi RL, Vessel ES: Inhibition of theophylline metabolism by long-term allopurinol administration. *Clin Pharmacol Ther* 1981;29:224–229.

19. Renton KW, Gray JD, Hall RI: Decreased elimination of theophylline after influenza vaccination. *Can Med Assoc J* 1980;123:288–290.

20. Bukowsky M, Munt PW, Wigle RD, et al: Theophylline clearance: Lack of effect of influenza vaccination and ascorbic acid. *Am Rev Resp Dis* 1984;129:672–675.

21. Manguis JF, Carruthers SG, Spence JD, et al: Phenytoin—theophylline interaction. *N Engl J Med* 1982;307:1189–1190.

22. Landay RA, Gonzalez MA, Taylor JE: Effect of phenobarbital on theophylline disposition. *J Allergy Clin Immunol* 1978;62:27–29.

23. Tornatore KM, Kanarkowski R, McCarthy

TL, et al: Effect of chronic oral contraceptive steroids on theophylline disposition. *Eur J Clin Pharmacol* 1982;23:129–134.

24. Monks TJ, Caldwell J, Smith RL: Influenza of methylxanthine-containing foods on theophylline metabolism and kinetics. *Clin Pharmacol Ther* 1979;26:513–524.

25. Grygiel JJ, Birkett DJ: Cigarette smoking and theophylline clearance and metabolism. *Clin Pharmacol Ther* 1981;30:491–496.

26. Lohman SM, Miech RP: Theophylline metabolism by the rat liver microsomal system. *J Pharmacol Exp Res* 1976;196:213–225.

27. Mangione A, Imhoff TE, Lee RV, et al: Pharmacokinetics of theophylline in hepatic disease. *Chest* 1978;73:616–622.

28. Staib AH, Schuppan D, Lissnerr ZW, et al: Pharmocokinetics and metabolism of theophylline in patients with liver diseases. *Int J Clin Pharmacol Ther Toxicol* 1980;18:500–502.

29. Vozeh S, Powell JR, Riegelman S, et al: Changes in theophylline clearance during acute illness. *JAMA* 1978;240:1882–1884.

30. Clozel J-P Saunier C, Royer-Morot MJ, et al: Respiratory acidemia and theophylline pharmacokinetics in the awake dog. *Chest* 1981;80:631–633.

31. Westerfield BT, Caider AJ, Light RW: The relationship between arterial blood gases and serum theophylline clearance in critically ill patients. *Am Rev Resp Dis* 1981;124:17–20.

32. Bukowsky JM, Nakatsu K, Munt P: Theophylline reassessed. *Ann Intern Med* 1984; 101:63–73.

33. Zwillich CW, Sutton FD, Neff TA, et al: Theophylline-induced seizures in adults: Correlation with serum concentrations. *Ann Intern Med* 1975;82:784–787.

34. Dutt AK, De Soyza ND, Av WY, et al: The effect of aminophylline on cardiac rhythm in advanced chronic obstructive pulmonary disease: Correlation with serum theophylline levels. *Eur J Respir Dis* 1983;64:264–270.

35. Banner ASJ, Sunderrajan EV, Agarwal MK, et al: Arrthymogenic effects of orally administered bronchodilators. *Arch Intern Med* 1979;139:434–437.

36. McFadden ER: Introduction: Methylxanthine therapy and reversible airway obstruction. *Am J Med* 1985;79(suppl 6A):1–4.

37. Weinberger M, Hendeles L: Slow-release theophylline: Rationale and basis for product selection. *N Engl J Med* 1983; 308:760–764.

38. Hendeles L, Massanari M, Weinberger M: Update on the pharmacodynamics and pharmacokinetics of theophylline. *Chest* 1985;88(suppl 2):103–111.

39. Karim A: Theophylline absorption, controlled release formulations and food. Presented at the 3rd Annual Conference on Current Concepts in Biopharmaceutics and Clinical Trials, University of Maryland, Baltimore, October 4, 1984.

40. Hendeles L, Weinberger M, Milavetz G, et al: Food-induced dumping from a "once-a-day" theophylline product as a cause of theophylline toxicity. *Chest* 1985;85:758–765.

41. Pederson S, Miller-Petersen J: Erratic absorption of a slow release theophylline sprinkle product caused by food. *Pediatrics* 1984;74:534–538.

42. Ahlquist RP: A study of the adrenotropic receptors. *Am J Physiol* 1948;153:586–600.

43. Lands AM, Arnold A, McAuliff JP, et al: Differentiation of receptor systems activated by sympathomimetic amines. *Nature* 1967;214:597–598.

44. Paterson JW, Woolcock AJ, Shenfield GM: Bronchodilator drugs. *Am Rev Resp Dis* 1979;120:1149–1179.

45. Jenne JW: The clinical pharmacology of bronchodilators. Basics of Respiratory Disease 1977; (vol 6) 1:18–23.

46. Dulfano MJ, Glass P: The bronchodilator effects of terbutaline: Route of administration and patterns of response. *Ann Allergy* 1976;37:357.

47. Larsson S, Svedmyr N: Bronchodilating effect and side effects of beta-2-adrenoceptor stimulants by different modes of administration (tablets, metered aerosol, and combinations thereof). *Am Rev Resp Dis* 1977;116:861–869.

48. Dolovich M, Ruffin RE, Roberts R, et al: Optimal delivery of aerosols from metered dose inhalers. *Chest* 1981;80 (suppl): 911–915.

49. Palmes ED: Measurement of pulmonary air spaces using aerosols. *Arch Intern Med* 1973;131:76–79.

50. Newman SP: Aerosol deposition considerations in inhalation therapy. *Chest* 1985;88(suppl 2):151–160.

51. Make B: Medical management of emphysema. *Clin Chest Med* 1983;4(3):465–482.

52. Webb-Johnson DC, Andrews JL Jr: Bronchodilator therapy. *N Engl J Med* 1977;297:476–482.

53. Banner AS, Sunderrajan EV, Agarwal MK, et al: Arrhythmogenic effects of orally administered bronchodilators. *Arch Intern Med* 1979;139:434–437.
54. Sahn S: Corticosteroids in chronic bronchitis and pulmonary emphysema. *Chest* 1978;73:389–396.
55. Albert RK, Martin TR, Lewis SW: Controlled clinical trial of methylprednisolone in patients with chronic bronchitis and acute respiratory insufficiency. *Ann Intern Med* 1980;92:753–758.
56. Mendella LA, Manfreda J, Warren CPW, et al: Steroid response in stable chronic obstructive pulmonary disease. *Ann Intern Med* 1982;96:17–21.
57. Morris HG: Mechanisms of glucocorticoid action in pulmonary disease. *Chest* 1985;88(suppl 2):133–141.
58. Johnson LK, Longnecker JP, Bakter JD, et al: Glucocorticoid action: A mechanism involving nuclear and non-nuclear pathways. *Br J Dermatol* 1982;107(suppl 23):6–23.
59. Grosman N, Jensen SM: Influence of glucocorticoids on histamine release and ^{45}Ca uptake by isolated rat mast cells. *Agents Actions* 1984;14:21–30.
60. Ellul-Micallef R, Fenech FF: Effect of intravenous prednisolone in asthmatics with diminished adrenergic responsiveness. *Lancet* 1975;2:1269–1270.
61. Daries AO, Lefkowitz RJ: Agonist-promoted high affinity state of the B-adrenegic receptor in human neutrophils: Modulation by glucocorticoids. *J Clin Endocrinol Metab* 1981;53:703–708.
62. Marom Z, Shelhamer J, Alling D, et al: The effects of glucocorticoid on mucous glycoprotein secretion from human airways in vitro. *Am Rev Resp Dis* 1984;129:62–65.
63. Anthonisen NR: Glucocorticoids in chronic obstructive lung disease. Clinical Challenge in Cardiopulmonary Medicine 1982;4(2):1–6.
64. Gross NJ, Skorodin MS: Anticholinergic, antimuscarinic bronchodilators. *Am Rev Resp Dis* 1984;129:856–870.
65. Pierce RJ, Allen CJ, Campbell AH: A comparative study of atropine methonitrate, salbutamol and their combination in airways obstruction. *Thorax* 1979;34:45–50.
66. Burderman I, Cohen-Aronovski R, Smorzik J: A comparative study of various combinations of ipratropium bromide and metaproterenol in allergic asthmatic patients. *Chest* 1983;83:208–210.
67. Lichterfeld A: Safety of Atrovent. *Scand J Respir Dis* 1979;103(suppl):143–146.
68. Klock LE, Miller TD, Morris AH, et al: A comparative study of atropine sulfate and isoproterenol hydrochloride in chronic bronchitis. *Am Rev Resp Dis* 1975;112:371–376.
69. McFadden ERJ, Jr, Luparello T, Lyons HA, et al: The mechanisms of action of suggestion in the induction of acute asthma attacks. *Psychosom Med* 1969;31:134–143.
70. DeVries K: The protective effect of inhaled SCM 1000 MDI on bronchoconstriction induced by serotonin, histamine, acetylcholine and propanolol (abstract). *Postgrad Med J* 1975;51(suppl 7):106.
71. Ahmed T, Abraham WM: Role of calcium-channel blockers in obstructive airways disease. *Chest* 1985;88(suppl 2):142–151.
72. Middleton E Jr: Antiasthmatic drug therapy and calcium ion: Review of pathogenesis and role of calcium. *J Pharm Sci* 1980;69:243–251.
73. Coburn RF: The airway smooth muscle cell. *Fed Proc* 1977;36:2692–2747.
74. Al Bazza ZF, Jayaram T: Ion transport by canine tracheal mucosa: Effect of elevation of cellular calcium. *Exp Lung Res* 1981;2:121–131.
75. Balfre K: The effects of calcium and calcium ionophore A23187 on mucin secretion and potential difference in the isolated chicken trachea. *J Physiol* 1978;275:80–81.
76. Ahmed T, Russi E, Kim CS, et al: Comparative effects of oral and inhaled verapamil on antigen-induced bronchoconstriction. *Clin Allergy* 1983;13:119–122.
77. Payne CB Jr, Chester EM, Hsi BP: Airway responsiveness in chronic obstructive pulmonary disease. *Am J Med* 1967;42:554–566.
78. Ramsdell JW, Tisi GW: Determination of bronchodilation in the clinical pulmonary function laboratory. *Chest* 1979;76:622–628.
79. Dull WL, Alexander MR, Kasik JR: Isoproterenol challenge during placebo and oral theophylline therapy in chronic obstructive pulmonary disease. *Am Rev Resp Dis* 1981;123:340–342.
80. Wolfe JD, Tashkin DP, Calvarese B, et al: Bronchodilator effects of terbutaline and aminophylline alone and in combination in asthmatic patients. *N Engl J Med* 1978;298:363–367.

81. Smith CB, Golden CA, Kanner RF, et al: Association of viral and mycoplasma pneumoniae infections with acute respiratory illness in patients with chronic pulmonary diseases. *Am Rev Resp Dis* 1980;121:225.

82. Tager I, Sperzer FE: Role of infection in chronic bronchitis. *N Engl J Med* 1975;292:563–571.

83. Snider GL: Control of bronchospasm in patients with chronic obstructive pulmonary diseases. *Chest* 1978;73(suppl 6):927–935.

84. Anthonisen NR, Manfreda J, Warren CPW, et al: Early antibiotic therapy of exacerbations of COPD (Abstract). *Am Rev Resp Dis* 1986;133(4, part 2):A127.

85. American College of Physicians. Pneumococcal vaccine recommendations. *Ann Intern Med* 1982;96:206–207.

86. Centers for Disease Control: Influenza vaccines 1983–84, Recommendations of the Immunization Practices Advisory Committee. 1983;99:497–499.

87. Williams JH, Moser KM: Pneumococcal vaccine and patients with chronic lung disease. *Ann Intern Med* 1986;104:106–109.

88. Committee Report: Recommendations for continuous oxygen therapy in chronic obstructive lung disease. *Chest* 1973; 64(4):505–507.

89. Krop HD, Block AJ, Cohen E: Neuropsychologic effects of continuous oxygen therapy in chronic obstructive lung disease. *Chest* 1973;64:317–322.

90. Heath DA, Williams DR: *Man at High Altitude*. New York, Churchill Livingstone, 1977.

91. Fishman AP: *Pulmonary Diseases and Disorders*. New York and Toronto, McGraw-Hill, 1980, p 463.

92. Levine BE, Bigelow B, Hamstra RD, et al: The role of long-term continuous oxygen administration in patients with chronic airway obstruction with hypoxemia. *Ann Intern Med* 1967;66:639–650.

93. Abraham AS, Cole RB, Bishop JM: Reversal of pulmonary hypertension by prolonged oxygen administration to patients with chronic bronchitis. *Circ Res* 1968;23:147–157.

94. Neff TA, Petty TL: Long-term continuous oxygen therapy in chronic airway obstruction. Mortality in relationship to cor pulmonale, hypoxia and hypercapnia. *Ann Intern Med* 1970;72:621–626.

95. Petty TL, Standford RE, Neff TA: Continuous oxygen therapy in chronic airway obstruction. Observations in possible oxygen toxicity and survival. *Ann Intern Med* 1971;75:361–367.

96. Anthonisen NR: Hypoxemia and O_2 therapy. *Am Rev Resp Dis* 1982;126:729–733.

97. Fenley DC, Douglas NJ, Lamb D: Nocturnal hypoxemia and long term domiciliary oxygen on blue and bloated bronchitics. *Chest* 1980;77:305–307.

98. Continuous or nocturnal oxygen therapy in hypoxemic chronic obstructive lung disease. *Ann Intern Med* 1980;93:391–398.

99. Anthonisen NR: Long-term oxygen therapy. *Ann Intern Med* 1983;99:519–527.

100. Fletcher EC, Gray BA, Levin DC: Nonapneic mechanisms of arterial oxygen desaturation during rapid-eye-movement sleep. *J Appl Physiol* 1983;54:632–639.

101. Tusiewicz K, Moldofsky H, Bryan AC, et al: Mechanics of the rib cage and diaphragm during sleep. *J Appl Physiol* 1977;43:600–602.

102. Bradley CA, Fleetham JA, Anthonisen NR: Ventilatory control on patients with hypoxemia due to obstructive lung disease. *Am Rev Resp Dis* 1979;120:21–30.

103. Block AJ, Boysen PG, Wynne JW: The origins of cor pulmonale; a hypothesis. *Chest* 1979;75:109–110.

104. Owens GR, Rogers RM, Pennock BE, et al: The diffusing capacity as a predictor of arterial oxygen desaturation during exercise in patients with chronic obstructive pulmonary disease. *N Engl J Med* 1984; 310:1218.

105. Cotes JE, Gilson JC: Effect of oxygen on exercise ability in chronic respiratory insufficiency. *Lancet* 1956;1:872–876.

106. Raimondi AC, Edwards RHT, Denison DM, et al: Exercise tolerance breathing a low density gas mixture, 35% oxygen and air in patients with chronic obstructive bronchitis. *Clin Sci* 1970;39:675–685.

107. Bradley BL, Garner AE, Billur D, et al: Oxygen-assisted exercise in chronic obstructive lung disease. *Am Rev Resp Dis* 1978;118:239–243.

108. Scano G, Van Meerhaeghe A, Willeput R, et al: Effect of oxygen on breathing during exercise in patients with chronic obstructive lung disease. *Eur J Respir Dis* 1982;63:23–30.

109. Vyas MN, Banester EW, Morton JW, et al: Response to exercise in patients with

chronic airway obstruction. *Am Rev Resp Dis* 1971;103:401–412.

110. Olvey SK, Reduto LA, Stevens PM, et al: First pass radionuclide assessment of right and left ventricular ejection fraction in chronic pulmonary disease. *Chest* 1980; 78(1):4–9.

111. Libby DM, Briscoe WA, King TKC: Relief of hypoxia-related bronchoconstriction by breathing 30% oxygen. *Am Rev Resp Dis* 1981;123:171–175.

112. Bye PTP, Esau SA, Levy RD, et al: Ventilatory muscle function during exercise in air and oxygen in patients with chronic airflow limitation. *Am Rev Resp Dis* 1985;132:236–240.

113. Criner GJ, Rassulo J, Celli BR: Ventilatory muscle recruitment and exercise endurance in normoxia and hyperoxia in severe chronic obstructive pulmonary disease (COPD). *Chest* 1985;88:38S.

114. Bye PTP, Esau SA, Walley KR, et al: Ventilatory muscles during exercise in air and oxygen in normal men. *J Appl Physiol* 1984;56:464–471.

115. Tiep BL, Nicotra BM, Carter R, et al: Low concentration oxygen therapy via a demand oxygen delivery system. *Chest* 1985;87(5):636–643.

116. Make B, Gilmartin M, Brody JS, et al: Rehabilitation of ventilator-dependent subjects with lung diseases. *Chest* 1984; 86:358–365.

117. Fischer DA, Prentic WS: Feasibility of home care for certain respiratory-dependent restrictive or obstructive lung disease patients. *Chest* 1982;82:739–743.

118. O'Donohue WJ, Giovannoni R, Goldberg AJ, et al: Guidelines for the care of ventilator-assisted individuals at home and alternate community sites. *Chest* 1986; 90 (Suppl 1):1–37.

119. Rochester DL, Braun NMT, Laune S: Diaphragmatic energy expenditure in chronic respiratory failure. The effect of assisted ventilation with body respirators. *Am J Med* 1977;63:223–230.

120. Lee H, Criner G, Rassulo J, et al: A controlled study of rehabilitation versus rehabilitation and respiratory muscle resting with negative external ventilation in patients with severe COPD (Abstract). *Am Rev Resp Dis* 1986;133(4, part 2):A168.

121. Pluto LA, Fahey PJ, Sorenson L, et al: Effect of 8 weeks of intermittent negative pressure ventilation on exercise parameters in patients with severe chronic obstructive lung disease. *Am Rev Resp Dis* 1985;131:A64.

122. Pardy RL, Rivington RN, Despas PJ, et al: The effects of inspiratory muscle training on exercise performance in chronic airflow limitation. *Am Rev Resp Dis* 1981;123:426–433.

123. Sonne LJ, Davis JA: Increased exercise performance in patients with severe COPD following inspiratory resistive training. *Chest* 1982;81(4):436–439.

124. Belman MJ, Mittman C: Ventilatory muscle training improves exercise capacity in chronic obstructive pulmonary disease patients. *Am Rev Resp Dis* 1980;121:273–280.

125. Belman MJ, Kendregan BA: Physical training fails to improve ventilatory muscle endurance in patients with chronic obstructive pulmonary disease. *Chest* 1982;81:440–443.

126. Mueller RL, Petty TL, Filley GF: Ventilation and arterial blood gas changes including pursed lip breathing. *J Appl Physiol* 1970;28:784–789.

127. Murray JF: The ketchup-bottle method. *N Engl J Med* 1979;300:1155.

20

THE ROLE FOR EARLY IDENTIFICATION OF COPD*

THOMAS L. PETTY

It is well established that chronic obstructive pulmonary disease (COPD) is a smoking-related disease state that clusters in families and is more common in men than women.[1] Now, with men and women smoking in almost equal numbers, the incidence of COPD is rising in women and may equal the male frequency in the future. The course of COPD probably covers 20 to 30 years before the symptom complex becomes manifest as a prelude to premature morbidity and mortality. Today, smoking cessation, pharmacologic therapy, and inoculations against influenza and pneumococcus are given to many patients once symptomatic and advanced COPD is present. Whether or not these therapies alter the course and prognosis of advanced COPD is not known.

The presumption is that these therapies are beneficial, and the author's own experience keeps him enthusiastic about the systemic management of advanced COPD. Pulmonary rehabilitation and oxygen are offered to selected patients with advanced disease. Oxygen clearly alters the late natural course

*Adapted from Flenley DC, Petty TL (eds): *The Early Pathogenesis and Identification of COPD*. New York, Churchill Livingstone, 1986.

of COPD (see Chapter 8), and it has been suggested that pulmonary rehabilitation may have a favorable effect on survival.[2] Chapter 13 briefly presents the details of a pulmonary rehabilitation program.

EARLY PATHOGENESIS

A growing body of evidence indicates that inflammatory damage of small airways and surrounding alveoli occurs in relatively early stages of COPD. Respiratory bronchiolitis,[3] small airways inflammation and fibrosis,[4, 5] and loss of surrounding alveolar attachments[6–8] have been identified in smokers in early stages of COPD. Probably, inflammatory changes of the large airways are also present. Inflammation of the large airways results in mucus hypersecretion and presents clinically as chronic cough and expectoration. Damage to small airways and surrounding alveolar attachments finally results in airflow limitation.[4, 5] It is believed that these two processes, emphysema and airways inflammation, parallel one another as a result of common factors (mostly smoking) that cause inflammation. It may be an oversimplification, but emphysema generally results in airflow obstruction (limitation) and airways inflammation in mucus hypersecretion and cough with expectoration. In any case, prognosis is clearly related to the degree of airflow obstruction and age.[9] Mucus hypersecretion does not relate to prognosis.

Mechanisms of Damage to Alveoli and Small Airways

The mechanisms of inflammation, damage, and destruction have also been elucidated for the most part. It is highly probable that proteolytic damage from leukocyte and possibly macrophage elastases or both causes the pathologic changes involved. The reduction of antiproteinases on a hereditary basis leads to very early damage and destruction, often distributed diffusely throughout the lungs as in panlobular emphysema.[10] This hereditary abnormality, however, accounts for only 3% to 5% of patients with COPD. Individuals with normal amounts of proteinase also apparently develop COPD via proteolytic mechanisms. This probably occurs from oxidative damage to the normally present antiproteinases.[11] Why some patients develop proteolytic damage via these oxidative mechanisms and others do not remains a mystery. One hypothesis is that antioxidant defense mechanisms may defend the majority of smokers against oxidant damage of the antiproteinase screen of the lungs. Whatever the exact biochemical mechanism may be, it is certainly related to smoking and clusters in families. The pathologic result is manifest by impaired air flow, dyspnea, cough, and expectoration.

A 20-year prospective study has now shown that smoking cessation in early stages of airflow obstruction slows the rate of decline of lung function.[8]

Even smoking cessation late in the natural course of COPD has a substantial survival benefit. This fact plus the possiblity of pharmacologic therapy directed at bronchial hyperreactivity, which would hopefully alter the early (or at least the earlier-than-heretofore) course of COPD, has stimulated an interest in early identification. In their book *The Lung in Transition Between Health and Disease*, Macklem and Permutt comment:

> It is likely that in every case of significant chronic airflow limitation, there was a time in the past history of the patient when airflow limitation was minimal and that the development of chronic airflow limitation from that earlier time is an insidious process.

They also say:

> In considering the simplicity of determination of FEV_1 and its potential use in detecting individuals who are headed toward serious trouble at a time when *intervention* might have prevented a disastrous outcome, it is interesting to explore the reasons why the spirometer has not achieved a position comparable to the clinical thermometer, the sphygmomanometer, the ophthalmoscope, the chest x-ray and the EKG.

Finally, they commment:

> Perhaps even greater responsibility for the near absence of the use of pulmonary function in the *prevention* of chronic airflow limitation must be borne by the expert in pulmonary medicine, especially in relation to the non-specialist.*

Thus, physicians should ask themselves why not measure FEV_1 in all patients at risk, e.g., smokers, those in dusty industries, and those with a family history of COPD. Prospective studies have clearly established the accuracy of the FEV_1 in estimating the risk of premature morbidity and mortality from COPD.[9, 12]

Other tests to identify small airways dysfunction or disease have been extensively evaluated. These include the nitrogen washout test to measure the closing volume or closing capacity of the lungs,[13] maximum expiratory flow volume test using gases of different densities,[14] and frequency dependency tests of compliance[15] and resistance.[16] Although these tests distinguish smokers from nonsmokers and also correlate with inflammatory changes of small airways, they may be no more sensitive or specific than simple flow-time curves in identifying clinically significant disease.[5] In any case, more elaborate tests of so-called small airways disease are not suitable for most clinics or physicians' offices. A simple, dry, direct recording device for the measurement of FEV_1, FVC, and $FEV_1\%$ of FVC is the most practical method of assessing the risk of developing COPD. To repeat and re-emphasize, it has been established that spirometry is a better predictor than actual symptoms in assessing the prognosis of patients with COPD.[9]

---

*Macklem PT, Permutt S: *The Lung in Transition Between Health and Disease*. New York, Marcel Dekker, Inc, 1979, by permission.

If airflow abnormalities are found, smoking cessation should be emphatically prescribed. It appears that knowledge of a pulmonary function abnormality can be used to motivate people to stop smoking.[17] Today, the public is aware of the universal risk of heart attack and cancers (not just lung cancer) from smoking. Thus, patients may be encouraged to invest in their own health after understanding normal lung function and realizing that years of smoking have not (yet) caused serious lung damage!

Improved methods of smoking cessation are currently under study. The availability of nicotine chewing gum, used as part of a comprehensive smoking cessation program, offers the physician a prescription item for the nicotine-addicted patient.[18] When properly used, nicotine gum can assist certain patients during the early withdrawal period from tobacco by replacing low levels of nicotine through oral absorption of the alkaloid.

In addition to smoking cessation, the annual use of the influenza virus vaccine and the once-in-a-lifetime inoculation of polyvalent pneumococcal vaccine is recommended and offers substantial protection against two common infections. *Haemophilus influenzae* B vaccine may also have value. Beyond these preventive measures, what else can be offered patients when they have early stages of COPD? The use of broad-spectrum antibiotics for purulent bronchitis appears wise, even though the role of infection in the progressive deterioration of lung function has to be established.

The role of bronchodilators in improving airflow in COPD has been the subject of numerous studies. One of the most impressive recent studies showed that a substantial number of patients participating in a multicenter clinical trial of IPPB therapy using bronchodilators compared with patients receiving the same bronchodilator by a pump-driven nebulizer had a substantial improvement in airflow by the administration of beta-agonist aerosols.[19] Those with the highest FEV_1 levels had the greatest improvement in airflow. In some instances, airflow improvement was marked in spite of severe airflow limitation.

That COPD cannot be distinguished from asthma by bronchodilator response alone is an emerging concept.[19, 20] In addition, the hypothesis that bronchial hyperreactivity affects the early course and prognosis of COPD is being evaluated in an NIH-sponsored multicenter trial in North America. If the systematic use of inhaled bronchodilators in this stage of disease results in a reduced rate of decline of airflow measurements, new therapeutic strategies will be created for the emerging stages of COPD.

According to current concepts, the *fact of airflow obstruction* must be identified by simple spirometric measurements of FEV_1 and FVC. If airflow abnormalities are present, bronchodilators should probably be used by both the inhaled and oral routes. The availability of potent, long-acting, and specific beta-2 agonists and long-acting theophyllines offers a convenient strategy in bronchodilator therapy. If the course of COPD is altered by long-term bronchodilator therapy in conjunction with smoking cessation, the outcome of millions of patients with various stages of COPD could be vastly improved.

COPD represents a major health challenge for all industrialized nations and wherever smoking is common. Society expends large sums for intensive care units treating acute respiratory failure and perhaps even larger sums on domiciliary oxygen and pulmonary rehabilitation. Now is the time to spend precious and scarce health care resources on health itself. The alternative is to spend it on disease.

References

1. Higgins M: Epidemiology of COPD—state of the art. Chest 1985;(Suppl):3S–8S.
2. Petty TL: Pulmonary rehabilitation, in Petty TL (ed): Chronic Obstructive Pulmonary Disease. New York, Marcel Dekker, 1985, pp 339–354.
3. Niewoehner DE, Kleinerman J: Pathologic changes in the peripheral airways of young cigarette smokers. N Engl J Med 1974; 291:755–758.
4. Cosio MG, Ghezzo H, Hogg JC, et al.: The relations between structured change in small airways and pulmonary function test. N Engl J Med 1978;298:1277–1281.
5. Petty TL, Silvers GW, Stanford RE: The morphology and morphometry of small airways disease. (Relevance to chronic obstructive pulmonary disease). Tran Am Clin Climat Soc 1982;94:130–140.
6. Saetta M, Ghezzo H, Kim WD, et al.: Loss of alveolar attachments in smokers. Am Rev Respir Dis 1985;132:894–900.
7. Petty TL, Silvers GW, Stanford RE: Radial traction and small airways disease in excised human lungs. Am Rev Respir Dis 1986; 133:132–135.
8. Cosio MG, Hale KA, Niewoehner DE: Morphologic and morphometric effects of prolonged cigarette smoking on the small airways. Am Rev Respir Dis 1980;122: 265–271.
9. Peto R, Speizer FE, Cochrane AL, et al: The relevance in adults of airflow obstruction but not of mucus hypersecretion to mortality from chronic lung disease. Am Rev Respir Dis 1983;128:491–500.
10. Kueppers F, Block LF: Alpha antitrypsin and its deficiency. Am Rev Respir Dis 1974;110:176–194.
11. Janoff A, Carp H: Inactivation of alpha-1-antitrypsin by cigarette smoke. Am Rev Respir Dis 1977;116:65–72.
12. Petty TL, Good JT, White DP: Long-term followup of a random population observed for the prevalence and outcome of COPD, in Petty TL (ed): Chronic Obstructive Pulmonary Disease. New York, Marcel Dekker, 1985, pp 93–103.
13. Buist AS, Ross BB: Predicted values for closing volume using a modified single breath nitrogen test. Am Rev Respir Dis 1973;107:444–452.
14. Hutcheson M, Griffin P, Levison H, et al: Volume of isoflow (a new test in the detection of mild abnormalities in lung mechanics). Am Rev Respir Dis 1974;120: 458–465.
15. Woolcock AJ, Vincent NJ, Macklem PT: Frequency dependence of compliance as a test for obstruction in small airways. J Clin Invest 1969;48:1097–1106.
16. Kjelgard JM, Hyde RW, Speers DM, et al: Frequency dependence of total respiratory resistance in early airway disease. Am Rev Respir Dis 1976;114:501–508.
17. Hepper NG, Drage CW, Davies SF, et al: Chronic obstructive pulmonary disease: A community-oriented program including professional education and screening by a voluntary health agency. Am Rev Respir Dis 1978;121:97–103.
18. Hughes JR, Miller SA: Nicotine gums to help stop smoking. JAMA 1984;252: 2855–2858.
19. Anthonisen NR, Wright EC, and the IPPB Trial Group: Bronchodilator response in COPD. Am Rev Respir Dis 1986; 133:814–819.
20. Eliasson U, De Groff AC: Criteria for reversibility and obstruction in bronchodilator trials. Am Rev Respir Dis 1985; 132:858–864.

21

COURSE AND PROGNOSIS IN COPD

BENJAMIN BURROWS

The term "chronic obstructive pulmonary (or lung) disease" was originally introduced to avoid the semantic confusion that existed 25 years ago in regard to diseases characterized by chronic airflow obstruction. While such patients were generally classified under the broad heading of chronic bronchitis in the United Kingdom, emphysema was the category used more often in the United States. In both countries, however, these cases were considered distinct from asthma, even from the persistent form of that disease sometimes seen in older adults.

Unfortunately, COPD has come to be used in a broader context and may now include virtually all patients with persistent obstructive ventilatory impairment, even when such impairment is accompanied by stigmata suggesting an asthmatic disorder or when there is marked improvement in response to bronchodilator and/or corticosteroid therapy. These latter cases, subsequently referred to as chronic asthmatic bronchitis, were deliberately excluded from early studies of COPD, a fact that must be remembered in interpreting available data on the long-term course of the disease. As will be discussed, patients with chronic asthmatic bronchitis may have a less predictable and more favorable course than those whose disease results primarily from emphysematous destruction of the lung.

In the 1960s, there was considerable concern with distinguishing different forms of COPD, even after excluding all recognizable forms of asthma.[1, 2] Based on their clinical presentations, patients were sometimes characterized

268

as "pink puffers" or "blue bloaters." Alternatively, they were arbitrarily classified, respectively, as type A or B. Since features of type A disease were often found when there were grossly emphysematous lungs and since features of type B disease were thought to be associated with disease that lay in or adjacent to the bronchial or bronchiolar walls, the terms "emphysematous" versus "bronchial" were substituted for types A and B. In addition, typical pink puffers often had an emphysematous type of disease, while the most characteristic blue bloaters often had findings more compatible with the bronchial type of illness. These distinctions may have played a useful role in pointing out the spectrum of nonasthmatic airways disease that used to exist on the two sides of the Atlantic, but they may have little applicability to current chest practice.

The most characteristic cases of the bronchial type B disease seem to be disappearing; they may have been dependent on uncontrolled infection and even on a degree of underlying bronchiectasis that was common earlier in the century. Findings in a recent series of cases indicate that emphysema itself is almost always present in nonasthmatic forms of airways obstruction and that intrinsic disease of the small airways, while possibly critical in the pathogenesis of the disease, is less well correlated with disease severity than emphysema in later stages of illness.[3] Variations in the severity of blood gas abnormalities and cor pulmonale appear to be better explained by inherent differences in ventilatory drive or by unexplained differences in ventilatory pattern than by the nature of the underlying anatomic alteration. Thus, emphysema is the appropriate term for the vast majority of these cases and is certainly more descriptive than the overworked acronym COPD.

While the distinction between bronchial and emphysematous forms of chronic airflow obstruction may have decreasing clinical relevance, an increasing number of elderly subjects seem to be presenting with a persistent variant of asthma. There have been few long-term studies of such patients, and criteria for distinguishing them from those with emphysema are imperfect. However, if there are any findings suggesting an asthmatic bronchitic disorder or if the typical features of emphysema are absent, it is probably better to overdiagnose an asthmatic type of disease. This discourages therapeutic nihilism, emphasizes appropriate therapeutic approaches, and does not imply a more dire prognosis than may actually be indicated.

THE COURSE AND PROGNOSIS OF EMPHYSEMA

There is still some debate concerning the preclinical history of this disease. Most authorities appear to accept the concept that it begins quite early in adult life in "susceptible smokers" and is characterized by a slowly progressive deterioration in function that persists for many years prior to the development of clinically significant illness. However, periods of quite rapid decline in function have sometimes been observed, and in some patients, the disease may progress from near-normal lung function to disabling airways obstruction in a relatively short time. Once clinically significant airways obstruction has developed, however, either the rate of progression must become relatively slow or the patient will soon die of his or her disease. Thus, all studies of rates of decline in function in clinically ill individuals must include a survivor effect.

Several other points require emphasis in regard to interpreting the rates of fall in lung function over time. Many patients first seek medical help during an acute or subacute exacerbation of their disease. Even if this is not the case, most emphysematous patients have some degree of reversible airways obstruction when they first see a physician. Thus, they are likely to show some improvement when first placed on a therapeutic regimen. The apparent course of the disease over a short time span depends largely on whether one uses the pre- or post-treatment test as a baseline. If one uses the pretreatment value, there may appear to be no decline or even an improvement in function

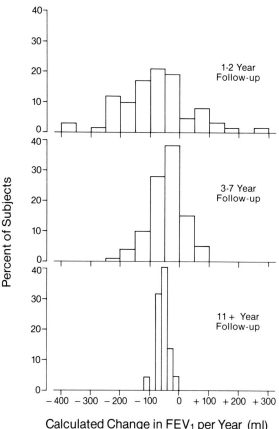

Figure 21–1. The decreasing variability in calculated rates of decline in FEV_1 with increasing length of follow-up in COPD patients. (From Burrows B: An overview of obstructive lung diseases. *Medical Clinics of North America* 1981; 65:455–471, by permission.)

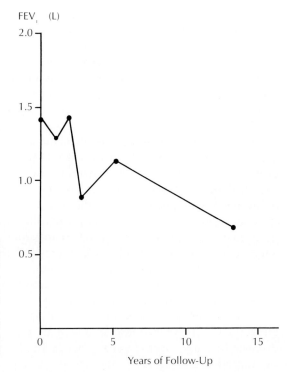

FEV$_1$ (L)

Figure 21–2. The course of one individual with COPD exemplifies the fluctuations in lung function that frequently occur. The calculated overall decline is − 54 ml/yr, very close to the mean decline in a large series of cases. (From Burrows B: Prognostic factors in chronic obstructive pulmonary disease. *Practical Cardiology* 1980; 6:61–69, by permission.)

Years of Follow-Up

for the first few years of follow-up. In contrast, most patients show some deterioration of function following their initial response to therapy.

Even if one begins follow-up with the post-treatment level of function, the intrinsic variability in lung function measurements causes calculated rates of change to be unreliable until follow-up is quite prolonged. The problem is evident in Figure 21–1, which shows the great dispersion of apparent rates of decline in patients followed for only a few years but a progressively more uniform rate of change as follow-up becomes more prolonged. The reason for this is apparent in Figure 21–2, which shows the successive annual FEV$_1$ measurements in a patient whose overall rate of change is close to the mean for a relatively large series of cases (− 54 ml/year). Calculations of rates of change based only on the first few years of follow-up would be meaningless.

The apparent rate of change in lung function over time also depends on the specific measure used to assess such change. Since both the FEV$_1$ and the VC tend to decrease with increasing severity of the illness, their ratio may remain relatively stable. In fact, any value that depends on the size of the FVC may be misleading. Instantaneous flows at some fraction of the FVC (e.g., the $\dot{V}_{max\ 50\%}$ or $\dot{V}_{max\ 75\%}$) or even the flow over the middle half of the forced expiration (FEF$_{25-75\%}$) may all appear to stabilize only because they are being measured closer to total lung capacity as the disease progresses. While these values (especially the FEV$_1$/VC ratio) may be the most reliable guides to the presence of an airways obstructive problem, they are not reliable indicators of its severity or change in severity. The FEV_1 itself is far preferable for evaluating progression of the illness.

Among survivors, reported annual rates of decline in FEV_1 have generally been in the range of 50 to 60 ml/year.[4] As already noted, however, a survivor effect must be present in such data, and the actual mean decline may be closer to 75 ml/year, the rate observed in milder cases of the disease.

From a clinical standpoint, however, it is more important to emphasize the extreme variability in rates of change than to be concerned with its mean value. Remarkable stability of the disease has been noted in a few patients even after 10 to 20 years of follow-up while other show an inexplicably rapid decline despite optimum therapy.[5] If a patient or family insists on a prediction of the rate of progression of the illness, it is fair to say that, with any luck, the change in function will be no greater than that which occurs with aging in normal individuals. With proper management, the patient may actually improve their quality of life despite any worsening of lung function. As discussed elsewhere in this book, the latter is certainly the case for patients who are able to improve their general physical conditioning and in those whose symptoms are related to hypoxemia.

Most other pulmonary function test also show progressive abnormality, though they are even more erratic than the FEV_1. In general, exertional dyspnea increases over the years, but as implied above, this can be modified by appropriate therapeutic approaches. Cough and sputum may improve, especially when the patient discontinues smoking.

The influence of smoking cessation on the overall course of the illness requires special emphasis. Clearly, smoking cessation before the onset of symptoms can dramatically delay the development of disabling disease. Even later in the illness, progression of ventilatory impairment is slowed by smoking cessation. All of the clinical series reported to date have dealt with patients who were receiving some type of medical supervision, and a large proportion of the subjects had discontinued smoking even before their first definitive evaluation. The average rate of progression of the disease would certainly have been more rapid if this were not the case.[6]

Blood gas abnormalities may be at least as critical as ventilatory impairment in assessing the course of the disease. Unfortunately, there are few data documenting progression of hypoxemia and hypercapnia in individual cases. Based on cross-sectional studies, carbon dioxide retention generally is found relatively late in the disease, when the FEV_1 is well below 1 L. Significant hypercapnia with a lesser degree of ventilatory impairment suggests some disorder of ventilatory control, which may be amenable to therapy.

Chronic hypercapnia without rapidly progressive clinical deterioration appears to be well tolerated by some patients, and if the concomitant hypoxemia is controlled, there may be remarkable stability of the $Paco_2$. There is a group of patients, however, who maintain normal or even slightly low $Paco_2$ levels until very late in their disease. They may then show a rapid decline in their general clinical condition with weight loss, weakness, and a steady increase in their arterial carbon dioxide. In this setting, the progressive carbon dioxide retention is an ominous sign.

Arterial hypoxemia is also extremely variable and is even less closely related to the level of ventilatory impairment than the $PaCO_2$. Serial studies documenting the development of hypoxemia are not available, and with the widespread use of oxygen therapy, such studies will probably never be carried out.

It is also doubtful that the natural evolution of pulmonary hypertension and cor pulmonale, which are closely related to hypoxemia, will ever be fully elucidated. Cross-sectional observations suggest that, in the early stages of emphysema, the pulmonary artery pressure is generally near normal at rest, but the compromised pulmonary vascular bed leads to pulmonary hypertension on exertion even in relatively mild disease. With progression of the illness, two different patterns of cardiovascular abnormalities may be seen. In the absence of severe hypoxemia, there may be a low cardiac output that allows the resting pulmonary artery pressure to remain relatively low despite a high pulmonary vascular resistance. There is a clinical impression that this pattern may be associated with the cold extremities, weakness, and easy fatiguability of some emphysematous patients. When there is more severe hypoxemia, cardiac output tends to be better maintained, resulting in severe pulmonary hypertension and, finally, classic cor pulmonale. This type of problem may respond dramatically to supplemental oxygen therapy.

A number of studies begun more than 25 years ago have documented the mortality of patients with emphysema.[4, 5] Among elderly subjects, survival is relatively short, but it is difficult to be sure how much of this is related to complicating illnesses and how much to the emphysema itself. In younger subjects (<65 years of age), survival is closely related to the initial level of ventilatory impairment and particularly to the postbronchodilator FEV_1. In early studies, median survival was only two to three years in the most impaired subjects ($FEV_1 < 30\%$ of predicted) and was close to five years in those with an FEV_1 between 30% and 42% of predicted.[4] In patients with milder degrees of obstruction, mortality was only slightly increased over normal for the first five to seven years of follow-up, and the 50% survival point was close to 10 years.

Many other factors also adversely influenced survival, including clinical or ECG evidence of cor pulmonale, hypercapnia, and in the most impaired patients, a very low pulmonary diffusing capacity. A marked increase in pulmonary vascular resistance was also associated with a very poor prognosis.[6]

These data may have been antiquated by the widespread use of supplemental oxygen therapy for hypoxemic patients. Clearly, survival is markedly prolonged by such therapy in those patients who originally had the poorest survival.[7] Furthermore, survival of nonhypoxemic patients appears to be much more favorable than that found in earlier studies of unselected patients. Thus, the mortality rates noted in earlier studies are almost certainly higher than expected in modern practice where hypoxemic subjects are identified and given appropriate therapy.

In any event, overall mortality data are difficult to use in clinical practice for a disease as variable as emphysema. There are patients who survive for very long periods despite markedly impaired function, and it is prudent to avoid providing patients or families with specific life expectancies.

THE COURSE AND PROGNOSIS OF CHRONIC ASTHMATIC BRONCHITIS

As already noted, patients with stigmata of asthma or with marked reversibility of their disease were often excluded from earlier series of patients with chronic airflow obstruction, and data concerning their course and prognosis are very limited. However, such patients do not necessarily show a progressive downhill course since they often survive for many years despite marked ventilatory impairment. Since their disease is often responsive to bronchodilator or steroid therapy and their lung function may show considerable fluctuation, it is difficult to calculate simple rates of change in their FEV_1 values over time.[8]

Data collected in the Netherlands over many years suggest that there are different patterns of change in FEV_1 in patients with chronic airflow obstruction and that patients who show marked improvement in function in response to corticosteroid therapy generally have an excellent prognosis.[9] The different patterns are exemplified in Figure 21–3, and their relationship to mortality is indicated in Figure 21–4. Indeed, in these studies, even acute responsiveness to bronchodilators proved a better guide to long-term survival than the initial level of function.

In the author's experience, the major late problems of many of these asthmatic-bronchitic patients are related to the side effects of prolonged corticosteroid therapy. These are the type of patients who develop disabling osteoporosis and in whom cataracts are distressingly common.[8] However, one has the impression that they rarely die of progressive respiratory insufficiency, and frank cor pulmonale does not appear to be a common complication of their illness.

It is always dangerous to generalize from one's personal observations, especially when these are not supported by firm data in a large series of cases. However, the author has observed the following scenario frequently enough to suspect that it is a relatively common pattern of disease. The patient is often an elderly female with a history of smoking a relatively small number of cigarettes. Although there may be no past history of overt asthma, the patient often recalls relatively minor symptoms suggesting a reactive airways problem prior to the more recent development of severe dyspnea and wheeze. A family history of asthma is not uncommon. Although the symptoms are now persistent, they fluctuate considerably in severity. In the author's expe-

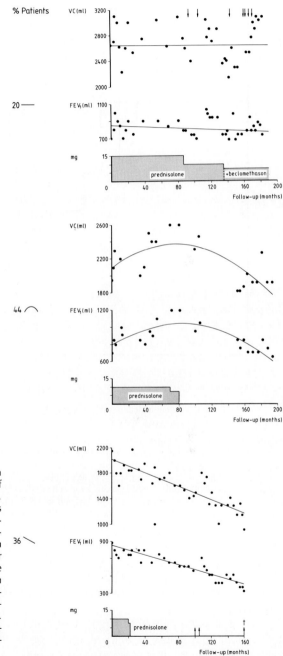

Figure 21–3. Three subgroups with a different pattern of the course of FEV$_1$ and VC. Of every subgroup, one patient is shown. Small arrows indicate clinical observation because of pulmonary infection. (Reproduced with permission from Postma DS, Steenhuis EJ, van der Weele LT, Sluiter HJ: Severe chronic airflow obstruction: Can corticosteroids slow down progression? *European Journal of Respiratory Diseases* 1985;67:56–64. Copyright © 1985 Munksgaard International Publishers Ltd., Copenhagen, Denmark.)

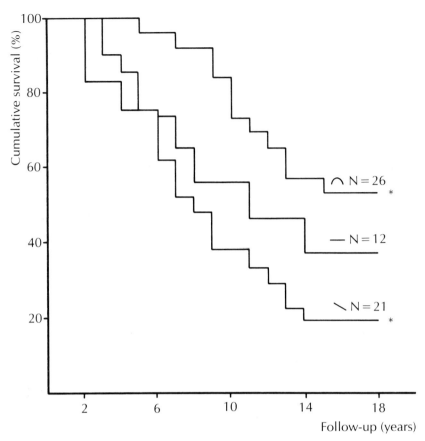

*P < 0.05 compared with survival
in—, by log-rank test

Figure 21–4. Effect of subgroups with different FEV_1 and VC patterns on survival: convex (⌒), no change (—), and linear decrease (⌍). Subjects with the worst survival rate, who had a relatively steady decline in function as shown in Figure 21–3, were noted despite the fact they had the highest initial mean FEV_1 level. Only 50% of the subjects with a convex course of FEV_1 were smokers compared with 75% of those with a linear decrease and 91% of those showing no systematic change in FEV_1. (Reproduced with permission from Postma DS, Steenhuis EJ, van der Weele LT, Sluiter HJ: Severe chronic airflow obstruction: Can corticosteroids slow down progression? *European Journal of Respiratory Diseases* 1985; 67:56–64. Copyright © 1985 Munksgaard International Publishers Ltd., Copenhagen, Denmark.)

rience, eosinophilia of blood and sputum is frequently present in these patients.

There is often little improvement with simple bronchodilator therapy, but the patient may show a marked remission with oral steroids. Often, the symptomatic improvement appears to exceed the objective changes in lung function measurements, which continue to show moderate airways obstruction. Initially, it may be possible to discontinue oral steroid therapy, either substituting inhaled corticosteroids or maintaining the patient on bronchodilators alone. Over time, repeated courses of oral steroids become necessary to deal with exacerbations, and eventually, maintenance oral therapy (preferably on an every-other-day basis) becomes necessary. Unfortunately, some patients seem to require daily medication to remain functional, and in some cases, quite high doses may be needed. As the years progress, the patient may appear to become less responsive to bursts of steroids given for exacerbations, and the chronic impairment becomes more severe. A curious phenomenon develops in some cases. As patients become less responsive to steroid bursts, they also become less dependent on maintenance steroids to prevent acute symptoms. At this point, it may be possible to discontinue oral steroids despite persisting airflow obstruction. In the very elderly subject, the chronic airways problem may be reasonably well tolerated in the absence of acute exacerbations. As this stage of the illness, the asthmatic component, which was so prominent earlier, may be much less evident, and the patient's symptoms would be difficult to distinguish from more persistent forms of airflow obstruction. If serious complications of steroid therapy do not develop, some of these elderly patients are remarkably functional for the level of their FEV_1.

The basic mechanisms involved in the type of illness just described are totally obscure. While there may be a past history suggesting an allergic predisposition, it is usually impossible to implicate a specific allergen as a cause of the respiratory disease, and even allergy skin tests are often negative. There is a distinct impression that immunologic problems may play an early role in the disease but that these "burn out" with age, leaving the patient with severe small airways damage but with little remaining tendency to bronchospasm.[8]

There are a great many variations of the syndrome just described. What appears to tie these cases together is the very late onset (often when patients are in their sixties or seventies) of an asthma-like disorder that is only partially reversible with therapy and in which steroid dependence is likely to develop rapidly. Death from disease itself appears relatively uncommon and few of these patients develop severe hypoxemia, chronic hypercapnia or cor pulmonale. They tend to die with their disease rather than from it. However, adequate long-term follow-up of an unselected series of patients with this syndrome has not yet been reported.

References

The first two papers deal with the different forms of COPD described in the early 1960s and their anatomic correlates.

1. Mitchell RS, Ryan SF, Petty TL, et al: The significance of morphologic chronic hyperplastic bronchitis. *Am Rev Respir Dis* 1966;92:720–729.

2. Burrows B, Fletcher CM, Heard BE, et al: The emphysematous and bronchial types of chronic airways obstruction. *Lancet* 1966; 1:830–835.

The following study is from a relatively recent series of cases and suggests that emphysematous destruction is the important lesion in most cases of nonasthmatic airways obstructive disease.

3. Nagai A, West WW, Thurlbeck WM: National Institutes of Health intermittent posi-

tive-pressure breathing trial: Pathology studies II. Correlation between morphologic
findings, clinical findings, and evidence of
expiratory air-flow obstruction. *Am Rev
Respir Dis* 1985;132:946–953.

*The next two papers report on the predictors
of survival in a series of patients with chronic
airflow obstruction. The first deliberately excluded subjects with features of asthma and
found that the initial FEV₁ level was most
predictive of longevity. The second, originating
in the Netherlands, examined a wider range of
airways disorders and found that response to
therapy was the best predictor of survival regardless of the level of function.*

4. Traver GA, Cline MG, Burrows B: Predictors of mortality in chronic obstructive pulmonary disease. *Am Rev Respir Dis*
   1979;119:895–902.
5. Postma DS, Burema J, Gimeno F, et al.:
   Prognosis in severe chronic obstructive pulmonary disease. *Am Rev Respir Dis*
   1979;119:357–367.

*The following paper presents the author's view-
point in regard to the overall problem of
chronic airways obstruction.*

6. Burrows B: An overview of obstructive lung
   diseases. *Med Clin North Am* 1981;65:
   455–471.

*The effectiveness of continuous oxygen therapy
in prolonging survival in hypoxemic patients is
evident from the following widely cited reference.*

7. Nocturnal Oxygen Therapy Trial Group:
   Continuous or nocturnal oxygen therapy in
   hypoxemic chronic obstructive lung disease. *Ann Intern Med* 1980; 93:391–398.

*The first article below summarizes some of the
recent data suggesting that immunologic factors
may play a role in the pathogenesis of chronic
asthmatic bronchitis. The second reference is
less readily available but represents the most
complete description of the patterns of airways
disease identified in patients in the Netherlands.*

8. Burrows B: Possible pathogenetic mechanisms in chronic airflow obstruction. *Chest*
   1984;85(suppl):13S–15S.
9. Postma DS, Steenhuis EJ, van der Weele
   LT, et al: Severe chronic airflow obstruction: Can corticosteroids slow down progression? *Eur J Respir Dis* 1985;67:56–64.

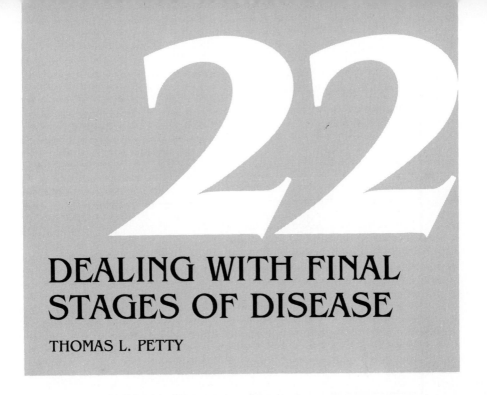

DEALING WITH FINAL STAGES OF DISEASE

THOMAS L. PETTY

Practical and Ethical Issues

Chronic obstructive pulmonary disease (COPD) is characterized by premature morbidity and mortality. Many chapters in this book have shown that modern treatments, such as pharmacologic therapy for specific complications including chest infections and emerging respiratory failure, can be effective. When necessary and appropriate, intubation with mechanical ventilation can buy time until reversible features of the disease are resolved. It is also certain that, in selected patients, long-term oxygen therapy in the home can improve survival. Part-time oxygen is better than none, and continuous oxygen therapy offers additional survival benefits (Chapter 8). A patient's quality of life and brain function are better with continuous ambulatory oxygen.

The ability to ambulate and participate in normal activities of daily living is probably a major reason for the improved survival in selected patients who receive continuous oxygen therapy.

Rehabilitative techniques (Chapter 13) are valuable in improving activities of daily living and the quality of life and probably in extending life as well. Any discussion of the management of COPD would be incomplete without considering the final phases of illness. Accordingly, this chapter is devoted to that purpose.

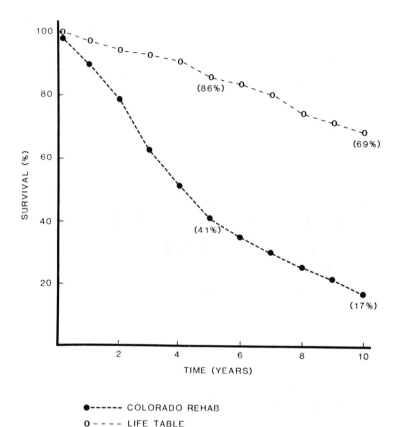

Figure 22–1. Survival of patients with severe COPD who participated in the University of Colorado Pulmonary Rehabilitation Program (solid dots) compared with the actuarial survival curve of white men, aged 61 years, in 1968. The 10-year survival curve reveals a 17% versus a 69% predicted survival in the general population. (From Sahn SA, Nett LM, Petty TL: Ten-year follow-up of a comprehensive rehabilitation program for severe COPD. *Chest* 1980;77 (suppl):311–314, by permission.)

CAUSE OF DEATH IN PATIENTS WITH COPD

Data from my own rehabilitation program have clearly shown that patients with advanced COPD finally die of their basic underlying lung disorder. Figure 22–1 shows the survival of patients originally entered into a pulmonary rehabilitation program.[1] Their demographic and physiologic background factors are listed in Table 22–1 and compared to survival predictions from actuarial tables. Table 22–2 lists the causes of death of the patients within the study's 10-year observation period. Patients identified as suicides might be better listed as respiratory deaths, since it was the respiratory problem that

Table 22–1. **Background Factors in a Consecutive Series of Patients Entering the University of Colorado Pulmonary Rehabilitation Program and Study—1966 to 1968**

		Range	SD
Number	182	–	–
% Men	87	–	–
Age	61	–	–
FVC	2.58 L	1.22–5.17	0.79
FEV$_1$	0.94 L/sec	0.26–2.21	0.38
MVV	36 L/min	6.4–80.9	15.1

may have caused the depression and despair that led to suicide. This act of terminating life is common in any chronic disease state and is less often chosen when patients have a good social support system.

HOME CARE

The overwhelming majority of patients with advanced COPD can live comfortably and happily at home, sometimes for prolonged periods of time. Thus, a brief discussion of home care methods follows. The concept of home care is appropriate for those who cannot or should not come to the hospital for either acute care or their maintenance management. However, these patients still need a dedicated and committed physician supervisor, family support or equivalent meaningful friendships, and a home health provider, such as a nursing or respiratory therapy service. Emphasis on coping with the dyspnea associated with the necessary daily activities and other aspects of prescribed medical care are fundamental in the home care setting.

The medical care used at home has been described in other chapters, i.e., pulmonary rehabilitation (Chapter 13) and home inhalation and respiratory therapy (Chapter 8). Patients must become independent or be assisted in their regular use of nebulized bronchodilators. Antibiotics for intercurrent

Table 22–2. **Causes of Death During the 10-Year Colorado Rehabilitation Program (N = 143)**

Pulmonary		Nonpulmonary	
Progressive COPD	58	Myocardial infarction	8
Progressive COPD with right heart failure	35	Suicide	5
Pneumonia	12	Other cardiovascular problems	3
Pulmonary embolus	1	GI bleeding	3
Lung cancer	1	Other known causes	9
Other pulmonary disorders	3	Unknown causes	5
Total	110	Total	33

infections, courses of corticosteroids when necessary, and home oxygen require a prescription and the supervision of a managing physician and other health care providers. A few patients live at home with the assistance of mechanical ventilators to promote rest of the respiratory muscles and to support them during the hours of sleep. Ventilators are sometimes used continuously in highly selected individuals. In these cases, skilled assistance for care of the airway and use of the mechanical ventilator is required. When negative-pressure, body wrap, or cuirass-type ventilators are more practical, short- or long-term ventilatory assistance may be possible without the requirement of a permanent airway.

Beyond the brief discussion of these technologic details, however, are more serious considerations about dealing with the final stages of disease. These include nutrition, maintenance of personal hygiene and socialization, and preparing for the transition to death.

Nutrition

It is extremely important for patients with advancing disease to be given at least maintenance calories. Although concern over the choice of calories occupies many scientific articles, it is basically true that patients with advanced COPD should and can eat essentially anything that suits them. This includes liberal use of carbohydrates as an energy source and a limited amount of salt or salt substitute for seasoning. Far too many people are denied carbohydrates for fear of increased carbon dioxide production and are prescribed a bland diet because of inappropriate restrictions in seasoning. It should be constantly borne in mind that chronic compensated carbon dioxide retention is, in fact, adaptive to the severe work of breathing caused by advanced emphysema. Reason dictates that carbon dioxide retention is good in these instances. One study from our center showed the favorable prognosis of patients living at home on oxygen when a high level of chronic, compensated carbon dioxide retention could be achieved.[2] Since this process is adaptive by virtue of appropriate reclamation or generation of bicarbonate to maintain an acceptable pH, one could easily argue that a high carbohydrate diet could be useful in encouraging this level of carbon dioxide retention. Dyspnea usually abates when a chronic compensated carbon dioxide retention of 75 mmHg or more occurs, and the mechanism for this symptomatic relief is likely the release of brain opioides (endorphins) to blunt respiratory drives.

Only in states of uncontrolled and uncompensated cor pulmonale with edema should salt restriction be enforced. Prudence is always wise, but imposing a bland diet for someone without edema just doesn't make sense. Unnecessary sodium can be avoided by simply avoiding the obviously highly salinated condiments and snacks and by using "light-salt" products, which contain half the sodium of ordinary table salt. Keeping a diet appetizing and encouraging frequent feedings probably helps to prevent the nutritional deprivational state often encountered in patients with advanced COPD. The moderate use of alcoholic beverages, such as a glass of beer, wine, or even a cocktail, is also acceptable unless alcohol abuse is a problem. Excessive consumption of alcohol, of course, should be avoided for its health consequences, as in all disease states.

Personal Hygiene

Even patients with very limited activity should plan to arise early in the morning or preferably at sunrise in order to keep sleep patterns appropriate for the time of day. Bathing, hair grooming, shaving, and other necessary or desired grooming procedures should be performed each day as a regular ritual. Dressing in loose and comfortable clothing as opposed to remaining in bed clothes or bath robes orients the patient's mood to appropriate daily activities. These are necessary steps in socializing for obvious reasons. Grooming and bathing routines are particularly difficult for many individuals, and instructions in energy saving methods should be taught and encouraged. The use of pursed-lip breathing during hair combing and shaving can be helpful. Sitting in front of the sink on a wooden chair for sponge bathing or putting a wooden stool or chair in the shower are effective techniques. Showering or bathing while receiving oxygen is no major problem. Appropriate assistance from family members or home health care visitors can be helpful.

Venturing out of the home for a trip to the barber shop or hair dresser should be encouraged at necessary or desired intervals. The maintenance of proper grooming has a very beneficial effect upon the patient's mood and self-esteem. Shopping for new clothes is equally important. It must be stressed and re-emphasized that many patients seemingly with end-stage disease may live for a number of years and that it would be totally inappropriate to allow them to abandon their usual styles of dress and grooming. Proper grooming, of course, aids in the socialization component of the home care program as well.

Socializing

The main aspect of socialization involves friends and family visiting in the home. When possible, this should be structured on a regular basis but with sufficient spontaneity. In recent years, the development of emphysema groups such as the nationwide Emphysema Anonymous Association with headquarters in Fort Myers, Florida, and the Pep Pioneers of the Little Company of Mary Hospital in Torrance, California, have shown how active patients can be despite advanced stages of disease. The group at Little Company of Mary Hospital has now participated in two ocean cruises with a rehabilitation team serving patients who may require continuous oxygen therapy. These adventures were organized by Mary Burns, the nurse director for the program. Regular meetings for potluck lunches and dinners, educational programs, bingo games, and lectures offer a popular focus for group socialization.

At Little Company of Mary Hospital, the annual spring rally is particularly exciting. The patients with advanced COPD who are able to walk or even those in wheelchairs participate in a contest where they negotiate a marked-off distance in a competitive fashion. I participated in one of these events myself in the spring and was impressed with this strategy that involves all the patients and staff with the project. Patients are asked to estimate the time it will take for them to complete the walk or distance by wheelchair, and they pace themselves so the goal can be reached over a measured distance. It is not the speed of walking that is important, but the ability to complete the task at one's own pace that offers the necessary strategy for success.

Additional socialization through writing letters and making phone calls offers opportunities for social interaction. In fact, phoning or writing the physician at appropriate times not only offers important guidance for the medical regime but also serves as a form of socialization in itself.

For those patients with a religious ethic, the church community can be a significant source of comfort and loving care. Close communication regarding the patient's needs among the patient's clergyman, hospital chaplain, and attending physician can help to provide crucial support for such individuals.

Recreation

There are a varity of opportunities for recreation. Listening to radio and television, of course, is quite popular. The daily reading of newspapers and weekly and monthly magazines is easily accomplished. Having hobbies within the home, such as caring for plants and even small animals, can be pleasant. A cat, small dog, or goldfish can offer relaxing recreation and an important measure of companionship. Light gardening, driving in the countryside, golfing, and fishing have been accomplished by many of my patients either with or without continuous oxygen and in spite of very severe degrees of disabling airflow obstruction.

Preparing the Emphysema Patient for Death

Patients with progressive and irreversible obstructive lung disease who face death often prefer to remain at home in the comfort and security of their family. Counseling about dying at home becomes extremely important in this instance. Patients have fears of suffocation and struggling to breathe. That this almost never occurs in COPD should be stressed. Death itself is described as a long, peaceful sleep. Family members also need counseling regarding the mechanism of death, instructions in determining when death, in fact, has occurred, and counseling to avoid a last-minute panic that might send the patient to the emergency room of a hospital for unnecessary intubation and mechanical ventilation, which would only prolong the terminal state.

This form of care has been quite successful in our rehabilitation program. Of the 135 patients in the study (see Fig. 22–1 and Table 22–2), 36 died at home and nine required final care in a nursing facility because of the family's inability to cope with the problems. In addition, 12 patients were brought to the hospital for a final one- or two-day illness where mechanical ventilation was purposely not instituted, and the patient was simply kept comfortable with fluids until death finally occurred.

RESUSCITATION DECISIONS

The withholding or withdrawing of life-support systems raises fundamental ethical questions. These are discussed in some detail with particular reference to the management of the final stages of patients suffering from COPD.

Modern medical care presumes a sustaining of life.[6] Knowledge of how to resuscitate patients with sudden cessation of circulation and respiration is taught to everyone on the medical team. Emergency medical technicians and the lay public alike rightfully assume that all reasonable resuscitative efforts should commence immediately when otherwise healthy people collapse. Few would quarrel with these practices in most situations.

But it occurs to me that nobody ever dies anymore. Patients have cardiac arrests, respiratory arrests, shock, terminal seizures, or asystole, but they don't just die. Nature's final process, guaranteed at birth to every human being, is often interfered with by inappropriate actions or gestures that may cause more harm than good, particularly for some patients with advanced COPD. Thus, it is appropriate to discuss some of the principles involved in making resuscitation decisions and the aftermath, which is often mechanical ventilation and circulatory support in critical care units. I base the comments below on more than 20 years of experience as head of the Respiratory Care Unit of the University of Colorado Health Sciences Center where I have faced the ethical and moral decisions dealt with in this section on numerous occasions.

Patients' Expectations of the Health Care System

Today's public is well aware of the marvelous life-support systems available in our nation's hospitals. Many have had family or friends who have been saved from critical illness. Newspaper articles and television shows continue to dramatize this important aspect of modern medical care. Against the excitement of success, however, is the growing specter of endless suffering with no expectation of reasonable outcome and loss of human and personal dignity. The fundamental right to self-determination and the right to privacy guaranteed by common law and the United States Constitution are being liberally discussed by both medical and lay groups.

The right to refuse medical care has been clearly established. In addition the President's commission for the study of ethical problems in medicine has stated loud and clear that, from an ethical point of view, there is no substantial difference between withholding and withdrawing life support in patients who are hopelessly ill.[3, 4] Courts have held that decision making belongs in the hands of patients and their physicians, and at this writing, there have been no legal or civil judgments against physicians for withholding or withdrawing life support. How these decisions are made, however, is not purely a legal or ethical matter. It becomes a matter of personal conscience and morality, which may have different individual implications than ethics and legalities. Some of the considerations that help decide whether to resuscitate a patient or to withdraw life-support care follow.

Ethical Principles

The Principle of Benevolence

There is a long history in the medical and nursing profession dealing with beneficence to the patient. This begins with the oath of Hippocrates ("I will come for the benefit of the sick") and includes the Florence Nightingale pledge ("and devote myself to the welfare of those committed to my care"). These guiding principles, so simply stated, must not only be forever remembered but practiced daily by the entire health care team.

The Principle of Autonomy

The autonomy of the individual is guaranteed by fundamental legal principles. These include the United States Constitution, which guarantees the right to privacy, and common law, which determines the right to bodily self-determination. The principle of autonomy includes the fundamental right to confidentiality. Thus, all decisions regarding resuscitation or withdrawing life-support systems must consider these established legal and moral obligations.

The Principle of Informed Consent

Informed consent is a fundamental matter that deals with a clear understanding and, indeed, a contract between patient and physician concerning the patient's wishes and desires about his or her care during any medical circumstance, be it a single procedure or long-term care. In the opinion of many experts, the do-not-resuscitate decision and/or order becomes part of the doctrine of informed consent. The patient consents to be treated or not, and the patient can demand that life-support systems be withdrawn. How this informed consent is documented is another matter. Written informed consent is largely mechanical and ceremonial, but it also carries some weight. Oral informed consent is a far deeper human process, implying a level of trust and understanding that often goes beyond the written word. Yet, when informed consent regarding life-and-death medical decisions is achieved and fully understood by all parties, this fact should be recorded somewhere, particularly on the official medical record, for possible later reference. The principle of informed consent, of course, embodies the fundamental of truth-telling.

Surrogate Decision Making

The Principle of Substituted Judgment

The process of substituted judgment embodies the principle that a patient, who no longer can articulate, write, or otherwise communicate his wishes, can leave written or verbal instructions for someone else to convey these wishes and make the necessary decisions.

Today, 35 states have living-will legislation with the rights of the individual and directives to physicians written in somewhat different language. There is a great need for a uniform rights act throughout the United States. All 50 states embrace the principle of durable power of attorney, which permits surrogate decision making even if the person who gives this legal power is mentally incompetent. It is interesting that the District of Columbia still does not recognize durable power of attorney. Although living wills are perhaps better known to the public, durable power of attorney is more powerful and allows for flexibility. Yet, it goes without saying that living wills and durable power of attorney are subject to constant review, revision, and revocation. Both provide for surrogate decision making in the event of a mentally incompetent or unconscious patient. The goal, of course, is to carry out the final wishes of the patient in the most dignified and humane way possible. In the absence of a provision for substituted judgment, the next best approach is to invoke the principle of the patient's best interests.

The Principle of the Patient's Best Interests

Much of this principle, or rather a method of arriving at a decision, is embodied in the paragraphs above. It includes the principles of beneficence and individual autonomy as well as substituted judgment. The problem here is that opinions differ at times as to what the patient's best interests are. This occurs when families come into conflict or there is a difference of opinion between the care giver and one or more family members. If there is a disagreement, negotiation and final reconciliation are required. These may be aided materially by an ethics committee. Ethics committees do not make decisions but rather serve as a board of review where all parties can express their opinions and feelings. Often an open airing of the dispute results in reconciliation. In the final analysis, all parties must agree that the patient is the only one who really knows how he or she feels about what life means. The burdens of illness and therapy and the patient's hopes and expectations for the future must dictate the final decision, no matter whether the patient is in a competent state or the surrogate decision maker has the final responsibility.

The Principle of Reason

Human beings are endowed with various levels of reason and judgment. The issues of beneficence, autonomy, confidentiality, informed consent, best interests, and substituted judgment must be aired, reviewed, and re-reviewed. At this point, it becomes obvious that what is considered reasonable to one may be thought folly by someone else. Here again, the process of reconciliation must apply.

Medical Decisions Concerning Resuscitation

The Decision Not to Resuscitate

Sudden death, whether at a hospital or not, almost always calls for a rush of emergency medical teams to re-establish respiration and circulation. Though few would question that useful lives have been saved, there is also the nagging feeling that many should have been allowed to die without resuscitative efforts. It is inherently wrong to deny human beings one of nature's most fundamental events, life's transition into death at the appropriate time. Some time ago, I wrote an editorial designed to help guide decision making in the event of sudden cardiopulmonary arrest.[5] This statement is appropriate for any disease state where the effort to try to maintain life is not appropriate, as in many patients with very advanced COPD. This has been widely quoted, but I have taken the liberty of reproducing this commentary:

> Faced with a patient with sudden cessation of respiration and cardiac function, how does one decide whether intubation, mechanical ventilatory support and reestablishment of cardiac function with closed chest massage and/or pharmacologic agents should be instituted? The systematic review of four basic questions provides major assistance in this important decision. These questions are as follows:
>
> a. Do I know the patient's underlying disease process and its course and prognosis?
> b. Do I know the patient's quality of life in the context of his disease

process? (I now must add and reemphasize, do I know the patient's wishes for the future?)

c. Do I have anything more to offer the patient by resuscitative efforts designed to gain more time?

d. Do I wish to gain more time through resuscitative efforts to resolve these other questions? (Now I must add, wish on behalf of my patients).

The physician and nurse (or therapist) should be able to answer these questions quickly in order to determine if the patient is best served by initiating respiratory and/or cardiac support. If one is unable to answer the first two questions in the affirmative, it is still highly likely that support should be offered until the answers become clearer. One should not fear making a mistake in the direction of vigorous support, for certain patients will be saved to lead meaningful lives once again. If "yes" is the clear answer to the first two questions and the third and fourth are "no" then the physician, nurse or allied health worker should simply stand by and offer whatever comfort and assistance they can to the patient or the family or both. When the patient's life is known to be miserable at best, and when the patient has indicated no wish to have his suffering extended by technological means, in short where there is nothing to be gained by the additional hours, days or weeks one might achieve by supporting respiration and circulation—the intervention such as tracheal intubation, mechanical assistance and cardiopulmonary support should be set aside on behalf of the patient. Classic examples of these situations might include patients with advancing, disabling emphysema with no hopes for recovery from respiratory failure or patients with uncontrolled metastatic carcinoma in whom respiratory failure develops.*

Today, I would add to this list a fifth question:

e. Do I have a verbal or written contract with my patient about how I should handle situations when further medical care to sustain life is not appropriate?

The Decision Not to Ventilate

One could use approximately the same check list in order to make the decision not to ventilate when such intervention would only create pain and sorrow or postpone an otherwise inevitable death.

The Decision to Discontinue Ventilatory Support

As stated above, there is no fundamental, moral, or ethical difference between withholding or withdrawing life support. The decision to stop ventilatory or circulatory support in cases of certain hopelessness are governed by the same principle as that not to initiate support. This same principle applies to withdrawing supplemental oxygen, food, electrolytes, fluids, and pharmacologic agents.

---

*Reprinted with permission from Petty TL: Don't just do something—stand there! *Archives of Internal Medicine* 1979;139:920–921. Copyright 1979, American Medical Association.

The Decision to Continue Ventilatory Support in Patients Destined to Become Ventilator-Bound

These are perhaps the most difficult situations because they usually involve patients with advanced COPD who are awake and alert and whose life clearly can be sustained with mechanical ventilatory support but who are destined to be tethered to their life-support system for prolonged periods of time. But there are patients who can enjoy life in such situations, and their rights must be recognized. It must also be recognized by patient and family that living in the hospital, or more commonly today in the home, supported by a mechanical ventilator for months or years creates its own burdens. There can be no clear-cut rules to guide everyone in this difficult medical decision because the considerations are almost endless and the complexities profound; but the rights of the individual to self-determination must be the overriding consideration. More and more people will have life sustained—hopefully, happily and productively—with mechanical ventilatory support in extended care facilities or, preferably, in the home.

Economic Issues

Even though continued life support carries severe economic burdens, it has been clearly stated by experts and at conferences that economics and burdens on health care resources cannot carry any weight in resuscitation or the decision to continue life support in the hospital or home. The economic considerations become trivial in the face of ethical and moral principles defined above.

CASE EXAMPLES

Some aspects of the ethical and moral principles involved in resuscitation and continued life support are cited in the two case examples below.

Patient No. 1

FC was a 72-year-old retired businessman who had enjoyed life until disabling emphysema first limited his activities at age 62. He retired from his successful business at age 65 and entered a pulmonary rehabilitation program. His exercise tolerance improved only slightly with breathing training and conditioning. Because of severe sustained hypoxemia and congestive right heart failure from cor pulmonale, he was given continuous ambulatory oxygen. This caused a dramatic improvement in his ability to participate in activities of daily living and his mood and quality of life. He traveled extensively with his wife and visited his children and grandchildren. However, as the years passed, be became progressively dyspneic on exertion and finally at rest. Ultimately, he was housebound because of unrelenting dyspnea in spite of continuous oxygen and other pharmacologic therapy. He and his personal physician had an excellent relationship, and the wife, patient, and physician often discussed the future and the fact that resuscitation would not be appropriate should death occur at home and the patient should not enter a hospital during final stages of disease.

The patient became progressively forgetful as chronic carbon dioxide retention emerged. His dyspnea nearly disappeared when the Pa_{CO_2} gradually became elevated above 80 mmHg with appropriate bicarbonate compensation. Following a very mild upper respiratory illness, the patient became semistuporous. The physician made a house call and determined that death was probably imminent but not certain. The physician and the patient's wife agreed that transfer to the hospital and intubation with mechanical ventilation was not the wish of the patient because of the verbal contact made on numerous occasions via meaningful discussions when the patient was totally lucid. The patient was maintained at home with oxygen. He remained comatose for approximately 24 hours with the wife in attendance. After approximately 36 hours of "deep sleep," the patient awakened gradually one morning and asked for some breakfast. He then rapidly emerged from a stuporous state and felt relaxed and at ease. He had nothing but pleasant recollections of his emergence into the carbon dioxide narcosis. It was springtime and he took an interest in sitting out in the sunshine on the patio and even puttering a little bit with the flowers. After several visits from his children and grandchildren in the fall of the same year, the wife realized one morning that her husband had died in bed during the night.

COMMENT

This is an example of ideal preparation for death and a clear directive against intervention. This man died at age 73 in peace and the quiet of his own home. The interesting rally from a comatose state is not unusual in advanced emphysema. The late Alvan Barach even termed this "sleep therapy." The gradual buildup of carbon dioxide, a potent smooth muscle relaxant, may well provide some bronchodilation, and it probably engenders an outpouring of brain endorphins that blunt respiratory drives and mitigate dyspnea. No matter what the mechanism may be, I have seen numerous patients, such as this private patient of mine described above, emerge through "the short sleep" into a period of détente with death. At times, the period of détente may be six to 24 months of meaningful life. The détente, of course, is followed by what I describe to my patients as "the long sleep."

Patient No. 2

JC was a 63-year-old man I had treated for 15 years. He had advanced emphysema caused by hereditary alpha$_1$-antitrypsin deficiency. When he was seen in 1968, his FEV$_1$ was 0.8 L and his FVC was 2.1 L. By 1977, the patient required continuous oxygen, but he continued to work as a stockbroker until 1978, when he retired. After retirement, he remained active in social circles and continued to work on a limited basis as an investment counselor. His exercise tolerance gradually deteriorated in spite of oxygen therapy, full doses of bronchodilators, and corticosteroids. Early in 1983, I had a frank and detailed discussion with the patient about the certain progress of his disease and the fact of death, which I estimated to be six to 12 months hence. The patient was adamant that he did not want any heroic or resuscitative efforts, and he signed a living will, a portion of which read:

> If at any time I should have an incurable injury, disease, or illness regarded
> as a terminal condition by my physician and if my physician has
> determined that the application of life-sustaining procedures would serve
> only to artificially prolong the dying process and that my death will occur

whether or not life-sustaining procedures are utilized, I direct that such procedures be withheld or withdrawn and that I be permitted to die with only the administration of medication or the performance of any medical procedure deemed necessary to provide me with comfort care. In the absence of my ability to give directions regarding the use of such life-sustaining procedures, it is my intention that this declaration shall be honored by my family and physician as the final expression of my legal right to refuse medical and surgical treatment and I accept the consequence from such refusal.

This living will was witnessed by his wife, and a copy of it was kept in the medical record. I continued to care for the patient via house calls and by telephone. Shortly before Christmas, the patient could not be awakened. Since it had been predetermined that the transition to death would be difficult for the wife to handle at home, I admitted him to a private hospital. He was placed in a private room and given intravenous fluids because of his dehydration and thirst, which he occasionally complained of when awake. Usually, he remained semistuporous and comatose. Blood gases were not obtained to assess the degree of respiratory failure. Nasal oxygen was continued empirically. The patient slept for 24 hours and then awakened remarkably refreshed just before Christmas. He enthusiastically greeted his family, which included his sister and brother-in-law, who had traveled from another state to see him. He rallied further, began to take food, and ambulated limited distances in the hall. I joined him in a small New Year's celebration with his family in attendance. We enjoyed a glass of champagne together. He was discharged home the next day. He wrote family and friends and even discussed business ventures with his son during the two weeks that followed. However, one day, while sitting in a chair, he suddenly became glassy-eyed and simply stopped breathing. Later, shallow breathing returned but he was not responsive. His wife again called for a private ambulance to take the patient to the same private hospital where, by my prearrangement, death could occur quietly. However, the private ambulance was intercepted by the city's emergency ambulance team, who overheard the radio dispatcher of the private ambulance service. Emergency personnel rushed into the patient's house and, over his wife's prostestations, began resuscitative efforts and intubated the patient. His wife was told that they had no choice but to resuscitate a patient who appeared to be dying and to take the patient to the nearest hospital, which was **not** the hospital where I had arranged for the patient's admission. In the emergency room, the patient was placed on a mechanical ventilator, but he had a sudden ventricular arrhythmia and died in spite of the inappropriate heroic efforts that were being imposed upon him and his family.

COMMENT

The ethical issues here were quite profound, and even legal issues came into play. It is clear that the rights of the patient and family were violated by inappropriate intrusion. The patient's autonomy and right to privacy were violated. In the judgment of many, those who interfered had exposed themselves to legal action and could have been charged with criminal or civil assault.

GUIDING PRINCIPLES FOR THE INDIVIDUAL CARE GIVER

How the above ethical considerations impact upon each doctor, nurse, or other health worker becomes a matter of personal conscience. Those working at the bedside must be comfortable with the decision not to resuscitate, the withholding of mechanical ventilation, or the withdrawing of it. It is far easier to recite the ethical principles previously discussed than it is to deal with them on a personal and emotional basis. Decision makers need help with their feelings about life and death, and open relationships with other members of the health care team are extremely helpful. The hospital ethics committee can be an effective sounding board for the airing of all feelings and views. In the end, a consensus must be reached about the best interests of the patients. It is best and, in fact, possible for these decisions to be made only between patients and their physicians on an individual basis. Decisions cannot be made by committees, and it should not be their responsibility. It is the responsibility of the physician and other health care givers to have the capacity and courage to serve patients in their final hours in a kind and dignified manner. This is the hallmark of the complete person who can and does choose to serve his or her dying friend.

References

1. Petty TL: Pulmonary rehabilitation, in Petty TL (ed): *Chronic Obstructive Pulmonary Disease*. New York, Marcel Dekker, 1985.
2. Neff TA, Petty TL: Tolerance and survival in severe chronic hypercapnea. *Arch Intern Med* 1972;129:591–596.
3. President's Commission for the Study of Ethical Problems in Medicine and Biomedical and Behavioral Research: *Defining Death*. Washington, DC, Government Printing Office, 1981.
4. President's Commission for the Study of Ethical Problems in Medicine and Biomedical and Behavioral Research: *Making Health Care Decisions*, Vol 1. Washington, DC, Government Printing Office, 1982.
5. Petty TL: Don't just do something—stand there! *Arch Intern Med* 1979;139:920–921.
6. Nett LM, Petty TL: Reconciling ethical principles and new technology: A commentary on critical care medicine and mechanical ventilation. *Resp Care* 1985; 30:610–620.

23

ISSUES DESERVING FURTHER INVESTIGATION

THOMAS L. PETTY
JOHN E. HODGKIN

The foregoing chapters have presented an immense amount of information about the nature and treatment of chronic obstructive pulmonary disease (COPD). Although a tremendous revolution in our understanding about the course and prognosis of this disease and effective treatments has been established, many issues deserve further inquiry.

It is now known that simple measurements by spirometry identify the clinically significant stages of COPD. Why don't we recognize this fact and establish spirometry as a fundamental tool for all physicians' offices? Why don't we begin to make simple measurements of volume and flow in all symptomatic patients, all smokers, and all those with pulmonary abnormalities on chest roentgenograms? Spirometric testing is particularly important in all patients who have a family history of COPD. It is now known that the prognosis of COPD relates closely to the age at which the FEV_1 deviates significantly from normal. Even more important is the response to bronchodilators. The postbronchodilator FEV_1 is probably the best indicator of prognosis.[1] And it appears that failure to treat patients with bronchial hyperreactivity is, in fact, detrimental. This statement comes from longitudinal studies that show patients with bronchial hyperreactivity have a more rapid loss of lung function.[2] The assumptions here are that bronchospastic airways develop fixed airways obstruction and that this phenomenon could have been prevented with the use of bronchodilating aerosols or systemic pharmacologic agents.

At this writing, the national Heart, Lung, and Blood Institute is initiating a controlled clinical trial in early stages of airflow obstruction. Persons over the age of 35 but not yet 60 will be randomly assigned into either an ordinary care or a special care group. Ordinary care will include smoking cessation and reduction of work hazards along with whatever other measures the patient's personal physician wishes to employ. These measures will likely include the use of antibiotics for episodes of purulent bronchitis, expectorants, and hopefully influenza virus vaccine each fall. Special care patients will receive the elements of ordinary care including attempts at smoking cessation and the avoidance of occupational and environmental irritants. In addition, they will be randomized to receive an inhaled bronchodilator or a placebo. All patients will be followed longitudinally, looking at global outcomes including the rate of change of ventilatory function over time. Methacholine challenges to indicate patients with nonspecific bronchial hyperreactivity will be performed so that the clinical researchers can learn whether or not nonspecific bronchial hyperreactivity is an effective marker of those patients at risk of premature loss of ventilatory function. The corollary of this study will be to discover whether or not the regular use of bronchodilators compared to placebo alters bronchial hyperreactivity and ameliorates the accelerated loss of ventilatory function over time.

There are many therapeutic issues that need further evaluation. Probably the most important of these is what effect corticosteroids have on the course and prognosis of advancing COPD. Well-conducted, long-term prospective evaluations have strongly suggested that corticosteroids can stabilize at least the late phase of COPD.[3] Although no prospective placebo-controlled longitudinal clinical trials have been conducted, experienced physicians recognize that modest doses of corticosteroids, such as 10 to 20 mg of prednisone each morning, may improve pulmonary function, reduce the symptom complex, and develop a period of stability in the lives of these patients, which probably would not have occurred otherwise. Although the definitive study to answer the question about corticosteroids in regard to course and prognosis would be difficult to design and conduct, such studies could answer this very important question.

More data needs to be collected to help clarify which patients with a reactive airway disease component could benefit from allergy testing and desensitization therapy. Allergists use these techniques commonly while pulmonologists are much less likely to refer patients for this intervention.

Major questions remain in the area of oxygen therapy. Probably the most compelling need is a study to compare the effectiveness of continuous oxygen from stationary sources with oxygen that permits ambulation and increased activities of daily living. It is highly likely that the improved survival rate reported in the Nocturnal Oxygen Therapy Trial was due to both the increased duration of oxygen and the effect of exercise.[4] Patients receiving continuous oxygen in this study actually took it approximately 20 hours per day as indicated by estimates of compliance. Those on nocturnal oxygen received it an average of 12 hours a day, including the hours of sleep. The ambulatory patients could be much more active including getting outside of the home. It is reasonable to believe that the increased activity allowed by oxygen from ambulatory sources was responsible for at least part of the benefit. This benefit could come through improved strength of the respiratory muscles; better appetite, diet, and sleep; and psychosocial factors. Whether or not such a study will ever be conducted remains to be seen, but it would be of great interest to those in the field as well as to third-party payers.

A second issue focuses on the possibility that nocturnal events with severe hypoxemia, i.e., sleep-disordered breathing, result in early reactive pulmonary hypertension. Studies could be designed to determine if oxygen corrects this by providing better sleep quality or by preventing nocturnal hypoxemia.[5, 6] Another issue is the long-term value of transtracheal oxygen. Is it simply better because of cosmetics and conservation of oxygen or are there other reasons for preference in selected patients?[7] Conversely, are there long-term complications?

Although many experts recommend the use of pneumococcal vaccine once in a lifetime, even this form of extremely safe, preventive therapy remains controversial.[8, 9] Perhaps additional data will be gathered to learn more about the protective effect of the new pneumococcal vaccine containing 23 antigens in patients with advanced COPD.

Other therapies require further evaluation. Although the metered-dose inhaler is a highly convenient and extremely effective way of delivering aerosol bronchodilators, there are those who still prefer the use of the same medication by solution and a pump-driven nebulizer. Certainly, larger quantities of medication can potentially be delivered with a pump-driven nebulizer. Whether they can reach more bronchodilating receptors is not known, and further controlled clinical trials are needed to determine this.

The potential contributions of anticholinergic agents needs further investigation. Preliminary studies strongly suggest that the parasympathetic nervous system is more active in COPD than previously believed.[10] Anticholinergics are the oldest medications used to treat bronchospasm in asthma. It appears that atropine derivatives may have an important role to play in the various stages of COPD. Atropine is available in solution and dissolvable tablets for nebulization at the present time. The role of ipratropium (Atrovent) in the pharmacological armamentarium will need to be established through clinical trials and the experience of physicians who prescribe these agents.

The best way to employ antibiotics in COPD requires further study. Common practice is to use broad-spectrum antimicrobials at the first sign of purulent bronchitis. This is when the normally white or gray sputum becomes yellow-green and increases in volume. Most experienced physicians are aware of the fact that the liberal use of antibiotics on an empiric basis shortens the course of episodes of purulent bronchitis. The widespread use of trimethoprim and sulfamethoxazole, ampicillin and derivatives, tetracyclines, erythromycin, and even occasionally chloramphenicol probably does a lot more good than harm. Common organisms invading the airways of patients with advanced COPD are *Haemophilus* bacilli, the pneumococcus, anaerobes, and occasionally *Mycoplasma* and *Legionella*. Thus, the agents listed above are appropriate on empiric grounds. Certainly, no one would use chloramphenicol as a first line of defense against microbial invaders, but in fact, chloramphenicol is one of the drugs of choice for *Haemophilus influenzae* that is beta-lactamase–positive. It is also highly effective against anaerobes. Being a small molecule, it penetrates the lung extremely well. In addition, since it is not widely used, there are very few organisms that are resistant to it. Accordingly, it remains an ace in the hole for recalcitrant, purulent bronchitis.

The widespread use of expectorants and mucokinetics in some countries is not paralleled in the United States. It may be that we do not have the best mucokinetics available. A derivative of bromhexine (Bisolvon), ambroxol seems to be advantageous in mucus clearance, at least in some patients.[11] We need to understand the basic mechanisms of mucus transport in order to find methods and drugs to help promote mucociliary clearance.[12] The basic nature of human respiratory mucous glycoproteins must also be better understood.[13]

Other pharmacologic agents are of interest. The drug almitrine, which is both a respiratory stimulant and an agent that improves the matching of airflow and blood flow at the tissue level, has received a certain notoriety.[14] Obviously, pharmacologic agents that improve oxygen transfer across the lung would be valuable.

A concerted effort must be made both to encourage people not to start smoking and to help others with smoking cessation. Although knowledge that a personal commitment, behavioral modification, and replacement therapy in using a nicotine substitute offer a valuable strategy, there may be other methods useful in smoking cessation.[15, 16] The most effective method must be found.

The whole area of nutrition in COPD requires intense re-evaluation. All experts in the field recognize the malignant triad of dry weight loss, progressive dyspnea, and resting tachycardia. Can this be overcome by nutritional manipulations? Would using more lipids and less carbohydrates be advantageous in COPD patients with carbon dioxide retention? Or, by contrast, would increased carbohydrate feeding promote slow compensated carbon dioxide retention? This could foster a "re-acclimatization" to a higher P_{CO_2}, which might allow carbon dioxide homeostasis to occur at a lower minute ventilation. This could reduce the work of breathing and the accompanying dyspnea in patients with the most advanced degrees of airflow obstruction. Much research in nutrition is needed to answer these questions.

More work on respiratory muscle training is required before it can be considered as an integral part of comprehensive care. Although the value of pulmonary rehabilitation programs on an outpatient basis is no longer in doubt, how to best provide such services to an aging and expanding population is a challenge.

More pragmatic approaches to the assessment and awarding of Social

Security disability benefits on the basis of impairments assessed in physicians' offices are necessary. Simple spirometry does not often provide reliable information regarding a patient's functional ability on a specific job. But the spirometer remains the best estimate of the impairment of lung mechanics.

We must finally learn much more about the basic nature of COPD. Does it begin in childhood as a result of chest infections or other factors?[17] What is the basis for the familial clustering that goes beyond the alpha-antiproteinase phenotype?[18]

We must look at the immense and growing problem of COPD from a holistic point of view. After all, this disease is caused by smoking, clusters in families, and worsens with age. A concentrated effort to prevent smoking in the first place would change the whole outlook for all stages of COPD. A nonsmoking generation would have a far lower prevalence of disease, and thus, many of the therapies described in this book would be unnecessary. Better understandings of the basic biology of lung injury through elastase and oxidative mechanisms and pharmacologic agents to correct or forestall this damage could end emphysema by the end of this century. It seems almost too much to hope for, but it is possible.

References

1. Burrows B: Course and prognosis in advanced disease, in Petty TL (ed): *Chronic Obstructive Pulmonary Disease* ed 2. New York, Marcel Dekker, 1985.
2. Kanner RE, Renzetti AD, Stanish WM, et al: Predictors of survival in subjects with chronic airflow limitation. *Am J Med* 1983;74:249–255.
3. Postma DS, Steenhuis EJ, van der Weele L Th, et al: Severe chronic airflow obstruction: Can corticosteroids slow down progression? *Eur J Respir Dis* 1985;67:55–64.
4. Nocturnal Oxygen Therapy Trial Group: Continuous or nocturnal oxygen therapy in hypoxemic chronic obstructive lung disease. *Ann Intern Med* 1980;93:391–398.
5. Boysen PG, Block AJ, Wynne JW, et al: Nocturnal pulmonary hypertension in patients with chronic obstructive pulmonary disease. *Chest* 1979;76:536–542.
6. Block AJ, Boysen PG, Wynne JW: The origins of cor pulmonale; a hypothesis. *Chest* 1979;75:109–110.
7. Christopher KL, Spofford BT, Brannin PK, et al: Transtracheal oxygen therapy for refractory hypoxemia. *JAMA* 1986;256:494–497.
8. LaForce FM, Eickhoff TC: Pneumococcal vaccine: The evidence mounts. *Ann Intern Med* 1986;104:110–112.
9. Williams JH, Moser KM: Pneumococcal vaccine and patients with chronic lung disease. *Ann Intern Med* 1986;104:106–109.

10. Gross NJ, Skorodin MS: Role of the parasympathetic system in airway obstruction due to emphysema. *N Engl J Med* 1984;311:421–425.
11. Bertolic L, Rizzato G, Baufi F, et al: Action of ambroxol in mucociliary clearance, in Cosmi EV, Scarpelli EM (eds): *Pulmonary Surfactant Symposium.* New York, Elsevier, 1984.
12. Warwick WJ: Mechanisms of mucus transport. *Eur J Respir Dis* 1983;64(suppl 27):162–167.
13. Shelhamer JH, Marom Z, Logan C, et al: Human respiratory mucous glycoproteins. *Exp Lung Res* 1984;7:149–162.
14. Howard P: Almitrine bimesylate (Vectarion). *Bull Eur Physiopathol Respir* 1984;20:99–103.
15. Jarvis MJ, Raw M, Russell MAH, et al: Randomized controlled clinical trial of nicotine chewing gum. *Br Med J* 1982;285:537–540.
16. Higenbottam T, Chamberlain A: Giving up smoking. *Thorax* 1984;39:641–646.
17. Phelan PD: Does adult chronic obstructive lung disease really begin in childhood? *Br J Dis Chest* 1984;78:1–9.
18. Keuppers F, Miller RD, Gordan H, et al: Familial prevalence of chronic obstructive pulmonary disease in a matched pair. *Am J Med* 1977;63:336–342.

Glossary
PULMONARY FUNCTION ABBREVIATIONS

AM	Alveolar macrophage
AT	Anaerobic threshold
BHR	Bronchial hyperresponsiveness
CC	Closing capacity
CV	Closing volume
DL_{CO}	Diffusing capacity for carbon monoxide
ERV	Expiratory reserve volume
fb	Breathing frequency
FEF	Forced expiratory flow
fs	Sigh frequency
FEV_1	Forced expiratory volume in 1 second
FRC	Functional residual capacity
FVC	Forced vital capacity
HCF	High molecular weight chemotactic factor
IC	Inspiratory capacity
IRV	Inspiratory reserve volume
LCF	Low molecular weight chemotactic factor
$MEF_{50\% VC}$	Mid-expiratory flow at 50% vital capacity
$MIF_{50\% VC}$	Mid-inspiratory flow at 50% vital capacity
MPO	Myeloperoxidase
MVV	Maximal voluntary ventilation
Pa_{CO_2}	Arterial partial pressure of carbon dioxide
Pa_{O_2}	Arterial partial pressure of oxygen
P_{CO_2}	Partial pressure of carbon dioxide

P_{O_2}	Partial pressure of oxygen
PEF	Peak expiratory flow
PVC	Predicted forced vital capacity
$\dot{Q}$	Perfusion
R_{AW}	Airway resistance
RV	Residual volume
SaO_2	Arterial oxygen saturation
SV	Sigh volume
TLC	Total lung capacity
V	Lung volume
$\dot{V}$	Ventilation
$\dot{V}_A$	Alveolar ventilation
VC	Vital capacity
$\dot{V}_{CO_2}$	Carbon dioxide production
V_D	Volume of dead space
$\dot{V}_{O_2}$	Oxygen consumption
$\dot{V}_{O_2}max$	Maximal oxygen uptake
$\dot{V}_{O_2}(SL)$	Peak oxygen consumption symptom-linked
$\dot{V}/\dot{Q}$	Ventilation-perfusion ratio
V_T	Tidal volume

Index